Whole Person Self-Healing: A Science and Art

Authored by

Phillip Shinnick

&

Laurence Porter

Whole Person Self Healing Institute, Inc. New York
New York, USA

Bentham Science Publishers Ltd.
Executive Suite Y - 2
PO Box 7917, Saif Zone
Sharjah, U.A.E.
Email: subscriptions@benthamscience.org

CONTENTS

FOREWORD i

PREFACE iv

ACKNOWLEDGEMENTS vi
CONFLICT OF INTEREST vi

ABOUT THE ARTWORK vii

CHAPTER 1 INTRODUCTION AND OVERVIEW 3
PRIMARY AUTHOR'S BACKGROUND, BOOK OVERVIEW AND CO-AUTHOR'S INTRODUCTION 3
A FEW WORDS ON LAURENCE PORTER 8
A FEW WORDS FROM LAURENCE PORTER 9
ACKNOWLEDGEMENTS 11

CHAPTER 2 HISTORICAL DEVELOPMENT OF PULSED ELECTROMAGNETIC FIELDS, PEMF (COULOMB, GAUSSIAN AND PHOTONIC) WITH IMPLICATIONS FOR DIAGNOSIS, TREATMENT, AND HEALING IN MEDICINE 12
SAFE AND EFFECTIVE ELECTROTHERAPY 21
SUBTLE MEASUREMENT OF COULOMBIC, GAUSSIAN, AND PHOTONIC FIELDS 23
THE HEART HAS MEMORIES AND RETAINS MORE THAN ORGANS 24
PULSE GENERATORS 26
Photonic Energy 27
THE HEART'S PULSE GIVES INFORMATION FOR HEALTH AND NOXIOUS CONDITIONS 28
Cavity of Earth: Schuman Resonance 33
NOTES 34
REFERENCES 34

CHAPTER 3 PARALLEL PROPERTIES OF ONENESS IN THE MOST STABLE INORGANIC AND ORGANIC STATES 39
INTRODUCTION 39
PHYSIOLOGIC STATE OF ENLIGHTENMENT 41
ATTENTION TO THE PRESENT: LEARNING AND EMOTION 46
MASTER VERSUS TECHNICIAN 49
SYSTEM OF UNITY: SHARED AND PARALLEL PROPERTIES 49
REFERENCES 50

CHAPTER 4 A MEDITATION ON MEDITATION FOR BEGINNERS: A CREATIVE ODYSSEY FROM YEARS OF PRACTICE 52
A PERSONAL INTRODUCTION TO MEDITATION 52
A BASIC PHILOSOPHICAL APPROACH 56
BEGINNING WITH THE ESSENTIALS: THE BREATH FOR BEGINNERS . . . APHORISMS ON MEDITATION 57
NUMBERS . . . FOR GOOD AND FOR BAD 64
ANOTHER ASPECT OF NATURE: COLOR & VIBRATION 67
MEDITATION, ILLNESS AND DISEASE 73
Impulses Come from Deep Seated Habitual Happenstance Propensities and Not What We Think We are Rationalizing 74
THE SELF IS OUR TEACHER . . . AND NO PARTICULAR FORM OF MEDITATION IS THE WAY TO GO 83
TRAUMA, OPPOSITES, EMOTION, FEELINGS 86
FOOD AND OUR EATING HABITS 90

TOWARD A MORE TRANSCENDENT SEXUAL UNION 91
NON ATTACHMENT TO LIFE AND TO DEATH 93
REFERENCES 93

CHAPTER 5 THE SCIENTIFIC MEASUREMENT OF "QI": TECHNIQUES FOR QIGONG BEGINNERS AND FOR QIGONG ADDICTION THERAPY 95
INTRODUCTION 95
DEFINITION OF QIGONG AND METHODICAL RESTRICTIONS 97
MAJOR METHODS OF MEASUREMENT EQ (EMITTED QI) AND RESULTS 98
Physical Signal Detectors 98
Utilizing a Far-Infrared Detector (8-14 mμ) 98
AGA Thermo Gram 99
GE Micro- Pressure Detector (Placed from 0.5m to 2m) 99
8 mm Microwave Radiation Meter 99
Infrasonic Sound Detector (Denmark B-K Corp's Infrasonic Sound Detector 1,3,5,6,10 or 40 cm Distance) 100
Chemical Dynamic Methods Using Qigong with Yi or Intention and Directionality 100
Detector Using Biological Materials 101
Liver Cancer Cell and Lung Cancer Cell Cultures, DNA Synthesis and DPPC Liposomes 101
Detectors Using Living Sensors 102
Effect of EQ on Cancer Growth 102
Effect of Qigong on Anti-Cancer and Anti-Tumor Effect of EQ on the Immunologic Functions of Tumor Bearing Mice (TBM) 102
The Effects of EQ on Human Bodies 103
MAJOR TECHNIQUES OF QIGONG PRACTICE ACCORDING TO HE BIN HUI2 103
Adjustment of Body Posture 104
I. External Maneuver 105
a. Posture Maneuver 105
1) Standing Posture 105
2) Sitting Posture 107
3) Lying Posture 109
a) Supine Position 109
4) Other Postures 110
5) Movement Maneuver 110
ADDICTION THERAPY 117
REFERENCES 117

CHAPTER 6 ORGAN PULSED ELECTROMAGNETIC FIELDS (PEMF): CRITICAL EVALUATION OF TRADITIONAL CHINESE MERIDIAN THEORY AND O-RING CONTRIBUTION TO MEDICINE 120
INTRODUCTION TO THE O-RING TEST 120
APPLICATION TO ORT TO CARDIOVASCULAR SYNDROME 134
FOOD AND DRUG COMPATIBILITY TO PATHOGENIC MICROORGANISM 137
INFORMATION PROPAGATION WITH LASER 137
CHANGES IN BIOCHEMISTRY DUE TO PAIN 138
BIOCHEMICAL PRECURSORS TO CANCER AND CIRCULATION DISTURBANCES 138
LONGEVITY 139
PEMF EFFECTS ON HUMANS BIOCHEMISTRY 139
COMPARISONS OF ORIENTAL PATHWAYS TO CLINICAL TESTING WITH O-RING 140
Summary 148
ACKNOWLEDGEMENTS 152
REFERENCES 152

CHAPTER 7 SELF HEALING IN CHRONIC HEART DISEASE: A CLINICAL STUDY USING HEART MEDICATION 156
INTRODUCTION 156
BEFORE, DURING AND AFTER THE "QUIET" 159
DESIGN AND METHOD 160
MEDICATION 162

MEDITATION: VOLUNTARY 162
BREATH CONTROL 162
QIGONG 164
INVOLUNTARY USE OF THE WILL OR VOLITION 164
RESULTS AND DISCUSSION 165
CONCLUSION AND SUMMARY 166
APPENDIX A 167
Treatment Strategies 167
APPENDIX B 172
Summation of Variables 172
REFERENCES 173

CHAPTER 8 WHOLE PERSON FAMILY HEALING: HOW A DAUGHTER HEALS HER MOTHER 175
THE OATH OF HIPPOCRATES 175
INTRODUCTION 176
TWO SIDES OF THE SAME COIN 177
WHOLENESS 178
HEALING MEDICINE IS AN ART 180
PROGRESS REPORT 189
CONCLUSION 190
REFERENCES 191

CHAPTER 9 MULTI CULTURAL SELF HEALING FOR A SPINAL INJURY 192
INTRODUCTION, REPORTS, TECHNIQUES, HISTORY, AND STRATEGY 194
Heart Agitation, Arrhythmia, and Relief Procedures 197
Self Help Treatment 200
Involuntary Meditation: 201
Voluntary Meditation 202
Background of Voluntary Meditation: Yoga, Kung Fu and Native Americans Animal Forms 204
Animal Healing Arts 205
The Law of Action/Reaction in Emotional and Physical Pain 209
Physical and Emotional Reactivity: 209
Therapist Progress Notes 210
Summary 212
Mung Bean and Rice to Aid Digestion by Yogi Bhajan, Ph.D. 214
Photonic Image 214
Computerized Axiomatic Thermography 214
REFERENCES 217

CHAPTER 10 WHOLE PERSON CONSIDERATIONS FOR SELF HEALING IN ATHLETICS 218
CREATING A NEW SPORTS CULTURE 218
A MORE NATURAL APPROACH TO ATHLETICS AND COMPETITION 220
COACHES, MASTERS AND ATHLETIC SELF-HELP 223
OLYMPIC PREPARATION, COMPETITION, MEDITATION AND INJURIES 224
TRAINING FOR STRENGTH, ENDURANCE, SPEED, FLEXIBILITY AND COMPETITION 231
PRACTICING FOR FUTURE DISEASES 232
GENERAL CONCLUSION 232
SHINNICK AND FREED BACKGROUND 232
GLOSSARY 234
REFERENCES 240

SUBJECT INDEX 241

FOREWORD

So called evidence based medicine is not scientific. It cannot be accepted as evidence in a criminal court because studies are done on heterogeneous groups of people, but the results of the studies are then applied to patients who are not representative of those groups. Case studies produce more valid evidence. The history of medicine is replete with instances of doctors who have a greater consideration for the size of their practice and income than they have for their own medical progress or for the welfare of their patients. The currently rigid and narrow views being expressed by mainstream science are not ideal. Long-term audits reveal that many of our highly touted technologies can be ineffective -- or even downright dangerous. Let us encourage people to think more freely. Let us not condemn new ideas that do not agree with our limited tunnel vision.

During the last ten years, Dr. Phillip Shinnick and I belonged to a nexus of scientists, physicians, inventors, healers and researchers from all around the world. We met periodically in various locations because we felt we must do something about the many things that had gone wrong in the worlds of science and medicine. It was urgent that we find ways to get back on track and advance healing. These enlightening gatherings have been most beneficial. Our time spent together gave birth to new ideas, different approaches to improving the human condition, the quality of our medicine and our science. We have found new ways to alleviate pain, suffering and disease.

Rustum Roy, Ph.D., an Emeritus Professor and founder of the Material Science Department at Penn State University in College Park, was the impetus. The late Professor Roy was one of the greatest thinkers I ever met. He, Dr. Shinnick and I were very close. During the last few months of his life, Dr. Roy urged us to meet with him to discuss the future of medicine and science.

We both grew up in India. Dr. Roy was born to a Brahmin family that converted to Christianity, although they maintained great social status in the Hindu population. Deep insight into both religions gave Dr. Roy a profound understanding of the differences between Western and Eastern approaches to life. Dr. Roy was brought to the US at an early age. By his 20s, he was a full professor at PSU. The first person to replicate rare earth minerals, he and other scientists made fire come out of water. Dr. Roy founded Alcoholics Anonymous. Celebrated all over the world, he received many Academy of Science awards. In 2002, he was given the Order of the Rising Sun, 3rd Class, Gold Rays, with Neck Ribbon in Japan.

Dr. Shinnick cared for Dr. Roy during the last six months of his life. I observed that only Dr. Shinnick was able to help alleviate Dr. Roy's suffering. Although Dr. Roy was being treated with pain medications, Dr. Shinnick did acupuncture on him and gave him a meditation tape. He listened to it twice a day, and that helped usher Dr. Roy to the other side in peace. The tape had been created during the time of Dr. Shinnick's friendships with He Bin Hui, the Abbot of the Ninth Heaven Taoist Temple in China and with Kevin Chen, Ph.D., M.P.H.

Dr. Roy had urged Dr. Shinnick to bring to light the work of Dr. Yoshiaki Omura, M.D, Sc.D., electrical engineer, editor of an international journal and President of the International College of Acupuncture & Electro Therapeutics. Dr. Shinnick worked as his research assistant for eight years. He became Dr. Omura's secretary and an editor of his research journal. Dr. Omura had developed the Omura O-ring Test, a non-invasive diagnostic technique, and he needed an interpreter to bring out his work. Since Dr. Shinnick was already so familiar with Dr. Omura's work, he was the ideal person for the job.

When testing the traditional Chinese medicine main meridian system with the Omura O-ring for the first time, it was revealed that -- under toxic conditions -- pathways of Qi energy differentiate into new pathways based upon an organ's pathology. Some pathways, like those of the diaphragm and the heart, undergo phases changes after stimulation. When tested with the Omura O-ring, hormesis, a biological phenomenon discovered by Ed Teller, shows that a small amount of bio-positive radiation is effective when higher doses would be lethal. Dr. Shinnick and Dr. Omura have been able to determine the compatibility of a drug to any individual and its proper dosage by using the O-ring. Throughout this book, Dr. Shinnick will offer constructive criticism, but he will also show us significant ways to surmount the shortcomings of both Occidental and Oriental medicine.

Dr. Roy also set up meetings between Dr. Shinnick and Guy Obolensky, a child genius, inventor, engineer and physicist. Obolensky developed a healing instrument, which showered negative ions onto a subject who is placed in a Faraday cage. Dr. Shinnick, from working for ten years with Obolensky, has published insightful, relevant articles on electromagnetism, coulombic, gaussian and photonic energy and various, related, significant case studies.

A couple of months before he died, Dr. Roy arranged for me to meet Dr. Shinnick. He and I have similar interests. My background is in cardiology, and he spent eight years at the Heart Disease Research Foundation. He has published material on the memory of the heart influencing body and mind physiology. We agreed on how important it is to publish case studies, and we discussed ways to approach new understandings of medicine, heart disease and science. Dr. Roy and I founded The Journal of the Science of Healing Outcome, which I now edit. I later appointed Dr. Shinnick as associate editor.

In this book, Dr. Shinnick presents experimental physiological research showing that viscera -- from outside stimulation -- conditions digestion. Yet this noxious stimulation will fade eventually. Long afterward, the heart realizes approximation of these original noxious stimuli after being neglected by the digestive tract. He suggests that the purkinje fiber and vascular fluids may be involved in retaining harmful memories that might cause regression into past injuries, injustices or emotional trauma. He not only describes unconscious conditions that cause our pain and suffering, he also presents us with ways we can help ourselves overcome them through deconditioning and by synchronizing the mind/body/spirit Whole Person.

To gain a deeper understanding, this view of medicine needed more research. In Dr. Shinnick's juxtapositions of inorganic and organic, the most stable Bose-Einstein states show aspects of Oneness that transcend the normal laws of physics and gravity. His research points toward a new medicine, one that is not driven by profit. This new medicine would help everyone to gain a deeper, more connected, new understanding of self-healing. Dr. Roy, Dr. Shinnick and I agreed that it is necessary to translate traditional, ancient techniques of healing and the use of natural medicines into a modern, cultural consciousness.

This book is a product of our years of scientific meetings. It shares some of the data, meticulously gathered for more than 30 years, from the clinical work of the best minds the world has known in physics, chemistry, biochemistry, physiology, philosophy and history.

Human beings are capable of self-healing with no outside help when thoughts and emotions are positive, filled with universal compassion. If the mind or the consciousness is negative or hateful, we suffer. Disease can occur. Thoughts and emotions change energy probabilities into physical matter. Man must change the concept of "I" into "We" in order to change his state of illness into one of wellness because we are all interconnected. Dr. Shinnick complained to Dr. Roy about the presentation given by Hans Peter Durr at one of our gatherings. He said that Durr, co-editor of our journal, was all over the place. Dr. Roy replied to Dr. Shinnick, "That is where we are at this point in history. We are doing our best to bring it all together, to make the connections." And that is just the point. It is what you will find in this book -- making the connections on the path to self healing.

Monappa Hegde
Padma Bhushan awardee
The Journal of the Science of Healing Outcome
Cardiology, London University
Manipal University,
India

PREFACE

The industrial revolution marked an important change in the evolution of humankind. It uses machines and dead sources of energy to mass produce food and material goods, this process tends to increase disorder. It creates greater fragmentation because it uses human beings to exploit nature and other human beings. We can now see that the U.S. health care systems, by following the mass production model under Capitalism, treat patients like commodities or cattle. Health care private capitalism is a system designed to fill the pockets of shareholders through dividends, and stock values; executives of insurance companies are rewarded for denying health benefits (particularly for more traditional or alternative medicine). The medical profession no longer offers benefits that treat the Whole Person due to time limits demanded by the insurers. Instead, it primarily recommends taking high risk drugs and surgery. Drug companies subsidize physicians each year 6.5 billion, with physicians holding a billion in stocks. Scientific research funds just an interior reductionist approach on the molecular level not the Whole Person (response to the diagnosis, behavior, and circumstances causing disease). Companies that create new technological instruments promote expensive, high tech diagnostic tests that have questionable benefits. While the healthcare system profits from pain and suffering, these practices continue to move us away from nature sources of disease and toward instrumental, mechanistic thinking ignoring the totality of the situation..

We are neither machines nor commodities from which to make a profit. We are living organisms. According to negative entropy, all living things preserve their internal order by exchanging energy with their surroundings. How could we return to a more natural state without going backward in time? We can practice cultural healing techniques that were used successfully in the past to raise human consciousness in the present day. How can we naturally restore our health and our environment? How might we integrate the deep knowledge of past masters with the modern age of science? Dr. Shinnick, Dr. Roy, Dr. Freed, Dr. Omura, Guy Obolensky, Dr. Sancier and Dr. Chen have dedicated their lives to answering these questions. Though their work is scientific, their research has always centered on helping people learn to heal themselves. The work they have done helps us to understand life enhancing energies, how to connect to them and how to benefit from the natural forces that maintain life.

Mankind created Medicine, Science, Meditation and Art to satisfy its great desire to understand life and give it meaning. The healing medicine this book proposes is derived from the integration of science, art and meditation. Like us, these systems are open, flowing, and they impact deeply upon each other. Scientists might learn about the benefits of meditation by studying brain waves. Artists can use science to explore new directions in their work. Science, Medicine, Art and Meditation function as an interactive whole, but each system activates a different center in us. Art touches our heart, our emotional center. Science challenges our rationality and intellect, while meditation grounds us in the center located below our navel. The flow between these systems heals us.

Our body is at the center of Life. It is Life. We are responsible for our lives, but we often dissociate ourselves from the source of our aliveness. Then our lives are run by myriad thoughts and a limited ego. This creates suffering and violence toward ourselves, other human beings and the whole of life. By being present to the health of our bodies, our minds and our behavior, we can learn to balance our systems and synchronize them. By taking responsibility, we heal ourselves. Then all human beings and the whole of life will benefit from the good energy our healing generates.

Phillip Shinnick
Whole Person Self Healing Institute, Inc.
New York,
USA

ACKNOWLEDGEMENTS

Thank you to the following people for the valuable contribution of their ideas and helpful feedback that informed and inspired us as we created this book: Quincey Shinnick, R.P.N., Stephen Spahn, Jamie Taicher, Naomi Taicher, Baptiste Nicolas, Novak Djokovic, Chloe Porter, Kevin Chen, Ph.D., M.P.H., Patrick La Riccia, M.D., M.A., B. J. Cling, Ph.D., J.D., Guy Obolensky, Monappa Hegde, M.D., Ph.D. John Pinto, Donna de Varona, Dave Meggyesy, Marlon Raichel, Elias Dakwar, M.D., Effie Chow, Ph.D., R.N., Franklin Porter, Ph.D., Roger Guettinger, Ph.D., S.J., Lakshumi Bai Ramachandran, John Eschmeyer, Ph.D., Roger Jahnke, OMD, Adriano Borgna, M.D. L.Ac., Richard Malter, Kim A. Jobst, MA, DM, MRCP, MFHom, DipAc. Bill Tiller, Ph.D., Yoshiaki Omura, M.D., D.Sc., Bill Dittman, M.D., Nelson Shinnick, M.A., Christopher Mandigo, M.D., Joe Maize, Ph.D., Roberta Flack, Carol Carlson, Larry Tan, Doug Naidus, the late Celia Blumenthal, M.D., Morton Stavis, J.D., Ken Sancier, Ph.D., Hans Peter Durr Ph.D., Simon Freed, Ph.D., Sri Chinmoy, Rustum Roy, Ph.D., Richard Bachrach, D.O., Brother Michael Losco, M.S., and Abbott He Bin Hui of the Ninth Heaven Taoist Temple.

The original studies for this book were supported by the Research Institute of Global Physiology, Behavior and Treatment, Inc., a nonprofit established in 1993. In 2014, the name was changed to Whole Person Self-Healing Institute, Inc. The initial funding came from the estate of Simon Freed, Ph.D. and from contributions by various individuals. We received institutional support from The Heart Disease Research Foundation, The International College of Acupuncture & Electro Therapeutics, New York Medical College, the Center for Dance and Sports Medicine and the Rusk Institute.

A very special thank you to Herman Costa and Shannon Smock for helping us edit the manuscript.

CONFLICT OF INTEREST

The authors confirm that they have no conflict of interest to declare for this publication.

About the Artwork

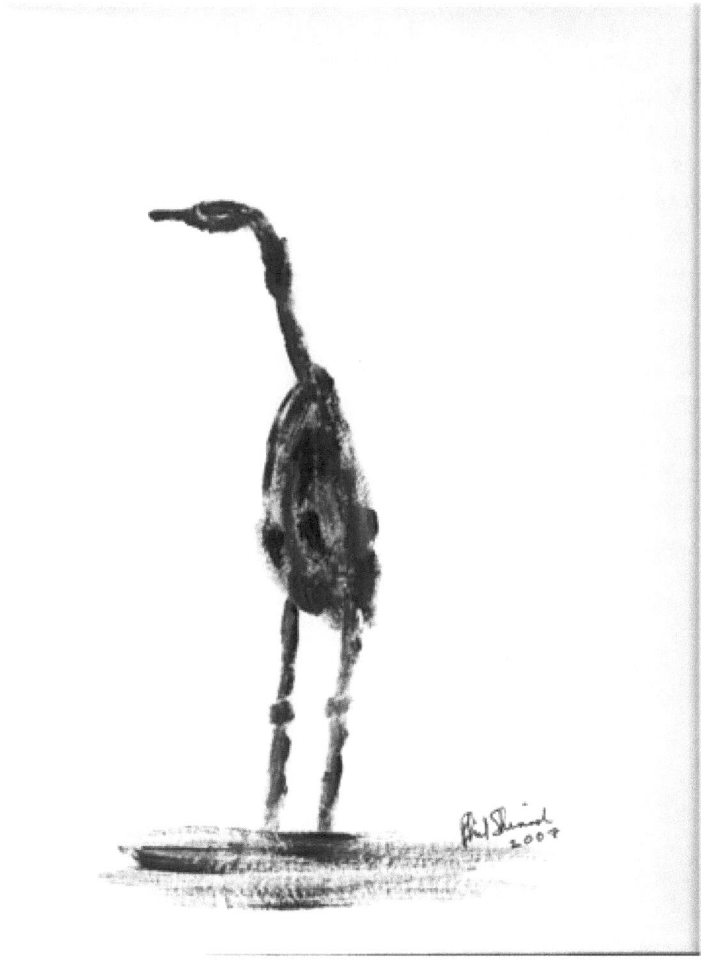

Fig. (1). Crane in the River. PKS. 2008. (This figure is reproduced by special permission of the artist, Phillip Shinnick).

Meditating alone by a river without moving, after some time, creates bird curiosity, in this case a crane, looking back.

All that man does is a kind of art, and this implies skill in doing things, as well as perception of how things fit or do not fit. This is indeed self-evident for the visual or musical artist as well as for the artisan. It is true also for the scientist and the mathematician, but less evident....It is clear, then, that reasoning is to be regarded as an art. And thus, in a deep sense, the artist, the scientist, and the mathematician, are concerned with art in its most general significance, that is, with fitting". -- David Bohm

Cezanne: *The landscape becomes reflective, human and thinks itself through me. I make it an object, let it project itself and endure within my painting. I become the subjective consciousness of the landscape and my painting its objective consciousness (Fig.* ***1****).*

In this book art and science cannot be separated. They are integral to "fitting" into a greater whole. Art and science link the visible and the invisible, form and no form, the whole and the parts, meditative and waking states, creation and decreation. The paintings in this book are manifestations of what has been seen when looking at inner space. The photographs are also moments of vision, but of outer space. They reflect the singularity of a moment that is never twice the same. Human beings are singular. As a species, we all have similarities, yet each individual has unique qualities, which is important in medicine because this singularity can make all the difference when treating an individual. Doctors, scientists and artists explore subtle energies that exist in our current reality. We all experience the processes of nature. The challenge is to neither separate nature from its flow nor to fall into a fragmented or mechanical view of nature. Art and science are both at the core of the human adventure. When used for the benefit of humanity, science and art contribute to our healing of ourselves. They can help us to find our place and to fit better into the world.

Whole Person Self-Healing: A Science and Art

Author: Phillip Shinnick & Laurence Porter

ISBN (eBook): 978-1-68108-259-2

ISBN (Print): 978-1-68108-260-8

First published in 2017.

2

CHAPTER 1

Introduction and Overview

Abstract: This book is a multi-disciplinary attempt to unite the branches of science in physics and biology of organic and inorganic energies focusing on the evolution of pulsed Coulombic, Gaussian and Photonic fields (PEMF). PEMF is explored in relationship to cultivating negative entropy and methods of diagnosis and treatment for pain and suffering. To be sure, clinical case studies are presented in heart disease, spinal injuries, family healing techniques, Qigong for addiction therapy, athletic injuries and meditation techniques in involuntary and voluntary methods.

Keywords: Bose-Einstein stable state, Diagnostic tests, Electrotherapy, Fragmented global physiology, Gung Fu, Healthcare system, Heart disease, Helium, History, Inorganic, Low temperature, Meditation, Nonequilibrium, Organic, Palpation, PET Scan, Physicians, Pulsed electromagnetic fields (PEMF), Qigong, Sociology, Spinal injury, Synchronization, Tai Chi, Thermodynamics, Traditional Chinese Medicine.

PRIMARY AUTHOR'S BACKGROUND, BOOK OVERVIEW AND CO-AUTHOR'S INTRODUCTION

This book reflects upon my lifelong attempt to comprehend the unification of the science of man by uncovering impediments which hide that understanding from us. The purpose of this book is to help human beings who are suffering to acquire the knowledge to better understand the root of their suffering and to give them the tools they need to free themselves from that suffering.

In 1979, I taught in the History and Sociology Departments at Rutgers University. Earlier, I had created a Sports Studies program, which focused on the physiological and cultural context of modern sports. It featured a critical analysis of performance enhancing drugs and of restorative drugs that were prescribed for injuries. Dale Johnson, the Chair, asked me to teach the Sociology of the Health Care System in the US. The job was suitable for me with my background in Systems Analysis as an officer in Air Force Systems Command. During a long career in athletics, I was twice on Olympic teams in track and field. After

Phillip Shinnick & Laurence Porter

competing around the world on many national teams, I naturally gravitated away from the quick fix of restorative drugs or surgery. Intuitively, I always preferred the slower, healthier process of rehabilitation and rest based upon a consideration of my own healthy future.

It became clear from the data that the high costs of health care were due more to the use of technological diagnostic tests than they were to physician's salaries. At the same time the actual treatment of patients by physicians was decreasing due to time constraints inflicted by insurance providers. Now physicians do not treat, nor do they carefully examine patients, by means of traditional palpation or by taking an extensive patient history. Expensive diagnostic tests originated from an advanced understanding of coulombic, gaussian and photonic energy fields. Consequently, we need to go back in history and see the evolution of these developments in physics, biology and clinical understandings.

A main topic of this book is the physics of pulsed electromagnetic fields (PEMF) and its application to biology. Life itself is non-equilibrium. There are flaws in medicine from the lack of uniting scientific understandings in inorganic and organic energy. We are looking at the juxtaposition of positive entropy -- always moving toward loss of energy through time -- with negative entropy, which is central to the reversal of disease and the survival of life. External negative entropy for human organisms consists of an exchange of energy between the organism and the food, water, air, and sun it consumes. To maintain a stable emotional balance, internal negative entropy is enhanced by techniques like meditation, heart-cranium synchronization, yoga, Qigong, dance and martial arts. An integrated person recognizes the terrain of mind, body and spirit. The goal of this book is to reach as many people as possible with that basic information.

Safely using modern electro therapeutics for self-healing according to frequency and intensity of coulombic fields on cell structure and healing will be discussed.

Dr. Simon Freed, Ph.D., studied in Paris at the beginning of the last century. He attended lectures and seminars with Madame Curie and studied mathematics at the Sorbonne. During the Cold War, he was the first scientist to study physiology with Gant and Bykov at the Interacademy Exchange in Moscow. Dr. Freed was in residence in Leiden at the Kamerlingh-Onnes low temperature lab, and he traveled to Japan and China where he studied meditation. Dr. Freed and I co-authored many works during a 10-year period. This book reveals some of the global scientific vision we shared.

Dr. Freed and I measured the global physiological characteristics of wholeness and synchronization that occur during meditation. From our measurements, we deduced the general properties found in the deepest state of meditation. We looked at the parallel analogous inorganic matter when it was subjected to low temperature. For 70 years, science has been examining changes at low temperatures in the state of molecules and the macro-molecule occupying a macro-cell of the lowest energy in Bose-Einstein statistics. Experiments have confirmed and authenticated the theoretical "condensate" quantum liquid possessing super fluidity.

This experiment showed the similarities between inorganic and organic matter when these states are most stable -- the Bose-Einstein states. In inorganic stable states, lowering the temperature creates more stability. Nature seems to be more together without the agitation of heat. In organic nature, the whole organism is in its ideal state to synchronize when the global, physiological parameters of the heart and the brain are at one, and when, biochemically, the blood lactate, consumption of oxygen and the harmonization of brain waves are not distracted by mental or physical agitation.

Many thought the traditional Chinese medicine idea of "Qi" was just an Eastern concept that could not be scientifically proven. In China, scientists have been studying Qigong since the late '70s. Some U.S. scientists have attempted to prove to other scientists that Qi energy exists. The proliferation of studies have shown that Qi can be measured. Newer scientific instruments, able to sense this subtle energy, have been able to measure Qi. Since Qi energy can be measured, it is now accepted as a fact. The results are discussed in this book. "Qi", when externally emitted onto chemical processes by known Masters, shows that changes occur more rapidly than they ordinarily would. In this book, Qi is expressed as a form of negative entropy, which can reverse positive entropy in disease and the aging process. Ken Sancier, Ph.D., was a student of Dr. Freed at Brookhaven National Lab. Later, Dr. Sancier became a research scientist at Stanford University. He founded the Qigong Institute **http://www.qigonginstitute.org**. He helped us incorporate a research institute, now called the Whole Person Self-Healing Institute, Inc. He also helped us raise funds for the Qigong Institute in its inception.

Dr. Sancier recommended that the Institute work with Dr. Kevin Chen, which resulted in a pilot study by me, by Dr. Chen, *et al*. The result of Qigong research, done from 1977 to the present, is available through the Qigong Institute database, which was compiled by Dr. Sancier. It has thousands of references and is available to researchers at the Qigong Institute website. Dr. Chen translated key Chinese studies and published the findings. Formerly an assistant professor at Rutgers Medical School, Dr. Chen is now an associate professor at the University of Maryland Medical School.

The Institute proposed that Dr. Chen conduct a pilot study on the inhibitory effects of external Qi emission on transplanted hepatocarcinoma in mice. Since research in China had already proven that Qigong could be measured and has an effect upon biological materials, Dr. William Tiller, Ph.D., our scientific advisor, suggested that we simply compile a summary of the research. Dr. Chen's first effort, from autumn 2002, will be summarized in subsequent chapters. When Dr. Chen and Master He Bin Hui founded the World Institute of Self Help (WISH), I joined them as a trustee. WISH was established in order to address the problem that not only are many chronic diseases incurable with external modern medicines, but that those very medicines often have damaging long-term side effects. In 2001, the Institute financially supported WISH's First World Symposium on Self-Healing and Consciousness Power. WISH provided self-help training in internal Qigong, particularly for cancer patients.

Tragically, Master He died from complications after a car accident. Although he was a traditional master, he understood the need for research and offered to be a subject for our external Qi experiments.

Due to changing life circumstances, we explore many different kinds of meditation. An already translated, but as yet unpublished, Chinese manuscript on Qigong meditations, written by Master He Bin Hui, is included. The abbott explores all the different positions and mental aspects of Qigong. This book also shares the results of a major study on Qigong in the treatment of addiction.

Dr. Roy and Dr. Effie Chow, Ph.D., RN. have urged me to incorporate my athletic background into the framework of what has been learned about Qi and energy in the last few decades.

Science has developed all sorts of performance-enhancing and restorative drugs, such as anti-inflammatories or anabolic steroids, that have undermined the need to master mind/body unity. With drugs, modern science is exploring ways to create a superman who has no culture and no soul but has a corporate logo stamped on his forehead. A better alternative would be a more integrated science that synchronizes mind and body and is, therefore, of real value to society. This alternative could create a healthier athletic culture through training and performing, and voluntary or involuntary meditation can assist athletes in their endeavors.

President of the Institute, Dr. Patrick La Riccia, MD, of the University of Pennsylvania, published PET scans of the brain taken before and after acupuncture. The results showed that acupuncture changed the structure of brain flow from asymmetry, when there is pain, to symmetry, when there is no pain. We will look at this phenomenon more fully in Chapter 6.

Inexpensive discoveries in diagnosis, such as the Bi-digital O-ring Imaging Test, invented by Dr. Yoshiaki Omura, will be presented in this book. Dr. Freed and I worked closely together with him for 10 years and published our results. Using the Omura O-ring, we critically examined the whole concept of the Qi organ meridian system. Imaging the organ pathway with organ tissue, we found that under pathological conditions, these pathways shift. The acupuncture points -- larger areas than previously known -- invert when stimulated, eliciting internal biological changes, reversing the pain. We also identify the biochemical process involved in each organ pathway as seen in traditional Chinese meridians.

Dr. Freed and I were professors at New York Medical College and research scientists at the Heart Disease Research Foundation. Familiar with the physiology of wholeness, we were eager to change a fragmented or diseased state into a whole or healthier state through self-help practices. When he was 95, Dr. Freed suffered an acute episode of chronic heart disease. We treated his fragmented, diseased state with meditation and Qigong, and we measured the changes in his condition. This became a case study of Chronic Heart Disease in its terminal phases. By supplementing modern drugs and treatment with meditation, Qigong and breathing techniques, we experienced some remarkable results We understood that those results were because of the meditation and Qigong. He still died three months later in peace, but from cancer of the esophagus.

The modern family often has a crisis to manage when dealing with today's medical profession. We present a case study where a daughter had to intervene when a dangerous situation arose due to unnecessary surgery being performed on her elderly mother. We will look at ways in which people can help their family members to heal themselves. The daughter, Laurence Porter, healer and co-author of this book, has worked for 10 years as a research assistant in traditional negative entropy techniques.

What I understand about energy comes mostly from my athletic training and from competing in sports, where the integration of mind, body and spirit is necessary in order to excel. In 2013, I was thrown up in the air on a speeding launch in rough seas. My ability to integrate mind, body and spirit was crucial then because my spine was struck and severely damaged when the boat struck me on my spine.

My spine was fractured and compressed at the tenth thoracic. The vertebrae diagnostic tests showed herniation at the fourth thoracic, spondylolisthesis of the lumbar vertebrae at the fourth lumbar spine and posttraumatic stress disorder due to the violence of the accident. This will be discussed at greater length in Chapter 10. From the beginning, I wrote in a diary every day, charting the course of how things unfolded. I had a few appointments with a neurosurgeon, Dr. Christopher Mandigo, at Columbia. We had a good feeling of mutual understanding for therapy. The traditional approved surgical therapy was to insert a steel rod in the spine. He was open to discussing various ways we might proceed toward healing without surgery which showed no better results than doing nothing, which was a big help to me. For months, Laurence Porter worked on me every day to redirect the damaged energies of my body and my mind.

This resulted in the writing of a case study that examines how a serious spinal injury can be healed without the use of drugs and without resorting to surgery. From practicing Qigong, Yoga and meditation, by receiving physical therapy and hands on palpation treatments, I slowly healed. After studying the fractured spine, global treatments of Zazen, Taoist Qigong, Gung Fu, Yoga and Native American animal healing were considered for treatment. The latter practice added a spiritual dimension to the more traditional science used in the healing of body and mind. The animal form and spirit is part of India's culture with the snake coiled at the bottom of the spine in Kundalini Yoga. In China there are animal forms in Gung Fu and Qigong. The Native North American animal healing spirits shine a new light on healing by bringing forth the animal spirit in severe pain. It is particularly significant for healing the spine with its reptilian history of a snake that opens up the spine.

A FEW WORDS ON LAURENCE PORTER

Fourteen years ago, Laurence Porter became my patient, but she also did healing work on me. When she worked on my back, I realized that she was truly a gifted intuitive healer. I felt the same emanation of external Qi I had experienced in China. Although she was well read in science, I recommended other books that would further benefit her. She quickly grasped my scientific papers and made significant contributions to them. I taught her the principles of acupuncture. Since she was a dancer, and I was an athlete, we understood the human body and spoke a common language. She began treating patients. Her deep feminine intuition appealed to women. In a healing practice, there is greater value when shared masculine and feminine energies reveal a deeper level of insight or understanding. I shared with Laurence the one-on-one teaching I had received from Masters who had bestowed their knowledge on me through initiations during my years of world travel. She has now become an integral part of the wheel of healing.

A FEW WORDS FROM LAURENCE PORTER

What does it mean to be human, to be alive? How can we get involved in our society? How do we bring drastic change while still honoring our authentic selves without getting destroyed in the process? Monks and sadhus isolate themselves from the world in order to meditate. They choose to live in silence and avoid the surrounding affairs of the world. In the Tantric tradition of yoga, a key to liberation is confronting our fears, our demons and our egos while still living in the world.

When our natural state is free, we will no longer be controlled by anything or anyone. In order to liberate ourselves from the oppression and tyranny, we might seek a Master who could selflessly guide us along our path. The Master would act as the true Self until we are able to see our true Self directly. How can we look at ourselves directly, look at reality without confusion and be our own Master? How do we live to the fullest in an everyday life that appears to be competitive and stressful? How do we elevate ourselves above the confusion that is all around and within us? How do we empower ourselves to truly become who we are meant to be? There is no single answer. There are as many paths as there are human beings; the different paths that we take are various manifestations of consciousness. There is even a path of "no path". These are various questions that are being explored in this book. It reminds us that science and medicine are arts. We are all artists and our lives are our creation.

The Buddha meditated until he found the fundamental truths of suffering. Philosophers investigate the mind. Physicists explore matter and study the nature of the universe. Medicine probes the human body to see what brings illness and physical suffering. A gardener deeply connects to nature to grow flowers and plants. Artists leap into the unknown to create new forms. The East and the West have developed vastly different societies based upon disparate ideas about the nature of reality. What do we do with all the knowledge that is constantly being generated and how can we benefit from it in a creative way? What we learn through the thought process cannot tell us the whole story about the human experience. There are other energies beyond the mind. Some of us are able to channel those energies and create new information from them. When that information is unleashed, it, in turn, gets informed and on it goes. What is crucial is not to fossilize information. Since information exists all around us and within us, we must keep all channels open to allow the information to flow. Taking a bird's eye view will help us to see that reality works like Russian dolls. Each level contains further levels and each level contains the whole. The relationship amongst processes is the element of constant creation.

Healing oneself is a science based on observations and a creative act that is slightly different for each of us. Acts of creation might be similar, but they can never be the same. The original paintings reproduced in this book, visions seen during meditation, evoke the originality, fluidity and subtlety of consciousness. Though all Life emerges from the same Oneness, each living organism is absolutely unique.

The body is the vehicle that grounds us in both dimensions, the horizontal dimension of life with its multiplicity and the vertical dimension of Oneness. The body itself has both dimensions. To take responsibility for our lives is to take responsibility for our bodies. To take care of ourselves is often misunderstood as being selfish. On the contrary, it means to honor the spirit of life by inviting the body to join in the joy of being alive. It is to see the different dimensions of life. As we take care of ourselves we nourish our whole being down to its more subtle expression. When we connect the horizontal to the vertical, we reside at their intersection, which is our center. This is true with density in space, when coulombic and gaussian energy intersects.

Dr. Shinnick comes from a lineage of scientists who did not forget that art was the first expression that men used to communicate life's mysteries. As much as science reveals and explains the universe and our role in it, the mystery remains. Artists and scientists use imagination and observation to probe into the abyss. All great insights into the nature of reality are beyond our senses or our thoughts, but upon later reflection, they might be examined through the process of thought in order to more fully understand them.

Dr. Shinnick glides high up in the blue sky of consciousness. From this perspective, he does have the bird's eye view of all that stretches before him. Occasionally, he meets another on his journey. They communicate in their own special language. Dr. Shinnick translates the knowledge that he has received, and he shares an accessible version of it, which will benefit anyone reading this book. Dr. Shinnick has lived a life of commitment -- to his own world class athletic achievements, to social justice for all, to health, to healing medical practices, such as acupuncture and the many forms of meditation; he explores human behavior, which reveals a deeper understanding of human suffering. In exploring this deeper understanding, he has come to realize that, with commitment, the simplest things can help us take better care of ourselves. We automatically receive and transmit energy, and we are all responsible for keeping our energy alive.

The breath is one beautiful example of taking responsibility for one's own energy. We all breathe to live, but when we practice conscious breathing, it brings us to a higher Self. From form to no form, the breath moves all of creation and energy. From formless air inside of a created form (us) and out again to no form, the breath takes us where we need to be. Let us breathe. Let us read this book creatively. Let us understand its meaning, learn its lessons and perform its practices individually and collectively. Let us see that Information is Love. Let each of us become his or her own Master.

As co/author I am honored to acknowledge and continue the work of the creative scientists whose work is brought to light in this book. Since we can't get to the ultimate truth we go through layers and layers of "truths", simply knowing that they fit within a whole that is constantly shifting. As the spirit of healing moves through us, we will find unexpected solutions to the difficult problems we are here on this Earth to solve. The great participants who are part of the lineage represented in this book made the clear choice to benefit humanity by looking at problems creatively and handling them with great compassion.

ACKNOWLEDGEMENTS

The case studies presented here were funded by the Research Institute of Global Physiology, Behavior and Treatment, Inc. a not for profit private foundation supported by individual contributions. (In 2014 the Institute's name was changed to Whole Person Self Healing Institute, Inc. Informed consent forms were signed by all patients who were part of any of these studies).

CHAPTER 2

Historical Development of Pulsed Electromagnetic Fields, PEMF (Coulomb, Gaussian and Photonic) With Implications for Diagnosis, Treatment, and Healing in Medicine

Abstract: This article explores Coulombic, Gaussian, and Photonic fields starting at their historical roots up to their use in modern medicine for diagnosis and treatment. These pulsed electromagnetic field (PEMF) understandings slowly evolved through time. It took almost 400 years to have a clear scientific delineation of the different forms that these phenomena can have, from static generators, batteries (direct current), rotating coils of copper spun around a magnet to create alternating current, and photonic waveforms such as the laser. At first, in the nineteenth century, treatments proliferated but many people were injured from a lack of understanding of the effects that these inventions had on human tissue. Melzack and Wall in the 1960s put forth the control gate theory and the role of serotonin and the neuro transmitters in pain relief. Concomitant to this was research into forms of meditation, both involuntary and voluntary with the use of electrocardiography ECG and electroencephalogram EEG. For neurological disease came the test of the velocity of nerve conduction from the normal standard traveling through a given distance with the electromyography EMG. The use of these diagnostic methods resulted in a less direct patient/doctor relationship. Palpation, as well as the historical patient report, key to situate the patient's condition into an appropriate context receded. Research by Bykov and Gant showed that the heart is susceptible to noxious adverse conditioning to organ stress and adverse stimulation. Acupuncture and electro-therapeutics have been shown to overcome psychosomatic responses such as the phantom limb effect, emotional turmoil, neurological problems, such as reflex sympathetic dystrophy and to calm the heart and viscera. The concept of entropy is refuted for organic life due to the lack of application of inorganic equilibrium scientific experiments to organic non equilibrium conditions espoused by Prigogine. The electrophysiology of the heart with the sinoatrial (SA) node and the atrioventricular (AV) node are the primary pacemaker cell groups in the heart and may be implicated in diseased conditioning of the heart through de-synchronization and body trauma.

Keywords: Alternating current, Atrioventricular (AV) nodes, Auricular therapy, Coulombic, Cranium, Direct current, Electrocardiogram, Electroencephalogram, Electromagnetic spectrum, Electromagnetic therapy, Electromyography, Entropy,

Phillip Shinnick & Laurence Porter

Heart conditioning, Nerve measurement, Omura O-ring test, Pacemaker cells, Photonic fields, Pulsed electromagnetic fields (PEMF), Purkinje fibers, Red blood cells, Sinoatrial (SA) nodes, Static electricity, Symmetry.

This article might be hard for lay persons to read but they should try to go through it to understand negative entropy. Scientists will see that the presentation was scaled down for lay persons and is not a pure scientific presentation yet is important to understand and read for current medical practises. This is a fusion of human natural energy and natures energy (Figs. **1, 2**). Medical therapy has radically changed in diagnosis and treatment over the last 400 years. Today's symptomatic reductionist approach is simply based on experimental (statistical) evaluation of *only* useful *short-term* chemical effects. It is thus divorced from the concept of do no harm in whole person healing given modern scientific experiments that investigate oriental medicine and the three primary classes of Electric, magnetic, and electro-magnetic medicine. Historically, unidirectional electric current (Coulombic field energy) was simply identified as resinous (negative charged) and vitreous (positive charged) without understanding the down side of the positive charged nuclear-particle field energy. Today, we understand that the atom's (planet like) *small negative electron* is known to orbit a *gigantic equally positive* thermonuclear sun. "As above so below". See Glossary page 264.

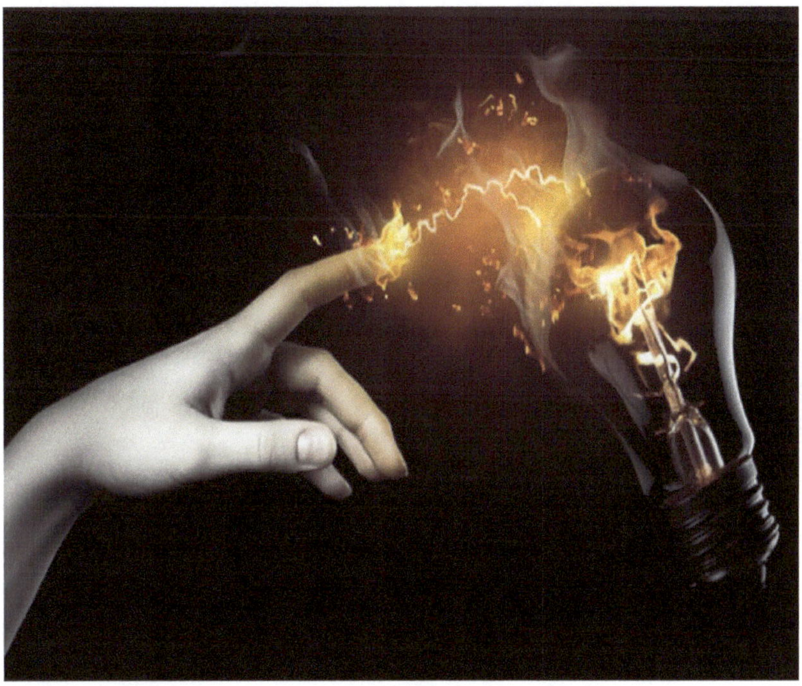

Fig. (1). Spark of life and electromagnetic energy. (With special permission of Hagda).

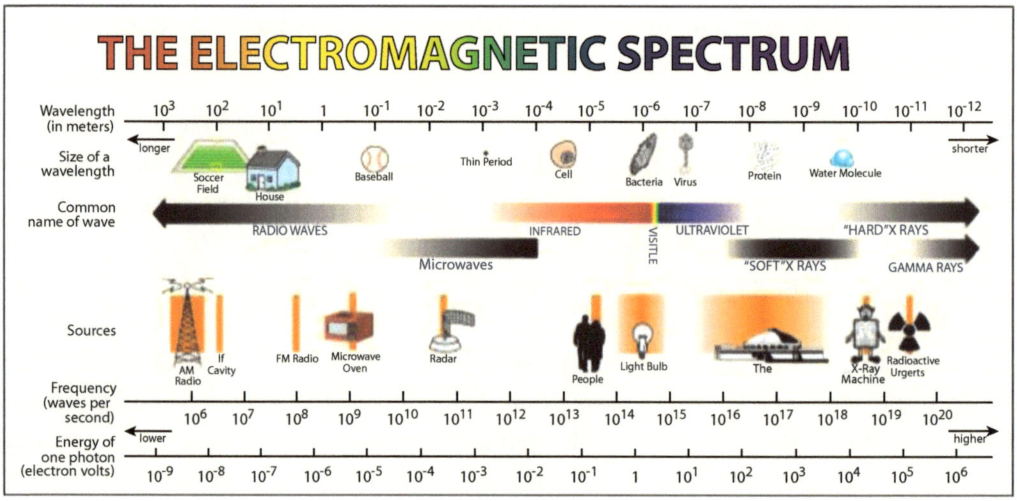

Fig. (2). Nature's Electromagnetic spectrum reflecting wavelength, frequency and energy of one photon. (With special permission of Hegda).

The Chinese system of medicine (Traditional Chinese Medicine, TCM) taught throughout the world is largely unchanged because traditionally established Chinese Medicine does not consider the PEMF electromagnetic/acupuncture connection. What has been learned about electromagnetism since ancient times, which greatly influences Oriental and Occidental medicine today? Moreover, how can modern understanding of the atom and its electromagnetism helps us in healing pain and suffering? What are the advantages and safeguards for PEMF? This chapter will explore the roots of Gaussian, Coulombic and Photonic fields in inorganic sciences (the domain of physics) and organic sciences (the domain of biology). Ancient Greek and Chinese doctors used their intuitive understanding to invent advanced natural procedures that healed without harming patients.

Ancient Greek Doctors put a patient's feet in a bucket of water with an electric eel (torpedo fish), the eels PEMF shocks exceeded 100 volts. This was enough to successfully treated gout and arthritis. The torpedo eel was also wrapped around a patient's head to treat migraine headaches. In 1660, a glass globe when rotated rapidly to increase friction with cloth pressed against it produced electric sparks. It was subsequently discovered that vitreous (glass) and resinous (Sulphur) spheres produced a different kind of electrical spark called (positive) and (negative) respectively. In 1746, the Leyden Jar, a glass jar separating metal foils inside and outside, became the first capacitor to accumulate this vitreous and resinous electricity on the inside foil when the outside foil was connected to the earth and became the first PEMF generator to produce robust sparks. Benjamin Franklin (1752), during his time in France, learned about this pulsed electric generator. When he returned to the USA, he proved that lightning was simply our planet's natural static electricity regulator and subsequently produced a practical PEMF therapeutic machine. It was reported that his patients lined up around the block to simply experience it. He treated sciatica using bonnet needles for his first electro-acupuncture experiment. His belief that an electric current flowed from a positive to a negative terminal is still accepted by public at large even though it was later established that electric current flows from a negative to the positive terminal.

In 1791, Galvani observed that inserting a copper and silver wire into a frog's nerve, made the leg muscle contract. By 1799, Volta created the first reliable Voltaic pile or electrical battery. His pile alternated silver and zinc disks with wet paper between each disk. It produced a continuous electric current and contradicted Galvani assumption by proving that a Voltaic pile would provoke muscle contraction. He also showed, that the initial electric stimulation muscle contraction occurred and that a second contraction occurred when the electricity was removed. This was the first understanding of the on and off current needed to produce a muscle contraction, increase blood circulation, affect nerve stimulation and provide relief from paralysis. While initial reports were encouraging, the electrical understanding was incomplete. By 1800, Coulomb was able to measure the nature of an invariant electric force but not the PEMF effect.

In China, in 1816, electricity was used with needles. In 1960, electro acupuncture was used successfully during surgical operations that received world television attention [1]. Shinnick witnessed this, in 1976, in China when Mao TseTung was alive. After straining his hip and back muscle, playing basketball in the snow in a Commune, he received treatment in a barefoot doctor's clinic (these clinics were run by peasants who treated people using old techniques that they had learned from their ancestors).

In 1831, Michael Faraday invented the first industrially significant electro-magnetic power generator. He discovered that a wire moving at right angles to a magnetic field would produce either a positive or negative electric current, the polarity depending on the direction of motion. In addition, two wire coils wound on a closed iron loop could transform this mechanically generated voltage, whose polarity depended on the coil's relative winding direction, with the relative magnitude dependent on the coil's turn ratio. Faraday's electro-magnetic discoveries allowed James Clark Maxwell to create his legendary quaternion equations. In fact, modern electro-medicine depends on the mathematical understanding advanced by Faraday, Maxwell and Karl Friedrich Gauss (1777-1855), who in 1839, published his general treatment of the mathematically non-commuting inverse-square electric force, having invented (with Weber) instruments for the Absolute Measurement of the linear (mathematically commuting) magnetic field. This connected the earlier (1801) astrophysics discoveries of Gauss to the understanding of "As above, so below" to the force that quantizes a planet's orbit around the Sun like the negatively charged small electron that orbits the atom's enormously massive nuclear engine whose positive electric field is more than 1000 times weaker. The magnetic force is created by electronic spin which has no mass. Whereas the electric force has the mass of the electron. Thus electro magnetism has two qualities. With this similitude, one can understand why living tissue is killed by positively-charged nuclear force and healed by negatively-charged electronic force.

In summation, magnetic-spin field (PEMF) energy is beneficial because its field energy is always non-nuclear. The thermodynamic-equilibrium speed of light is the absolute quotient of electricity and magnetism, given unitary electric field permittivity and magnetic field permeability, based on the absolute CGS Gaussian Metric System. Maxwell's quaternion electric magnetic force ratio for the speed of light required this which could only be proven with a torsion balance not a mass balance because one had mass the other had no mass. They both have force and one has to compare these two forces to determine the speed of light. The only force balance which could work would be a torsion balance to confirm the speed of light which is the force ratio.

The electric force manifest in metric system by the term permittivity. The magnetic force of permeability is not linear so there is only one place where they could be joined and that is unitary or based upon one unit of each. One has mass the other no mass.

Why did Gauss make the electric field permittivity force unitary and the magnetic field permeability unitary (given the unit one)? These don't fit together because they have a different quality yet they both have force. One has mass the other has spin, but spin has no mass. Maxwell recognized that the absolute metric system that made it possible to measure or balance the electric force against magnetic with torsion. Maxwell's twenty quaternion equations were reduced to four vector equations but still called erroneously Maxwell's equation by Oliver Heaviside. Heaviside has to ignore Maxwell's original twenty quaternion equations to only deal with the most elementary aspects of the electric magnetic force.

To experimentally prove that his unitary non-linear electric and linear magnetic force could remain perpetually balanced, like the spinning earth in orbit around the sun required Maxwell to invent and construct his electric/magnetic torsional-force field scale. Unfortunately, at this point in the history of politically acceptable dogma established commerce favored the Marconi and Edison financial empires not true science, so Nikola Tesla's 1900 patented to extract energy from the ambient medium using Maxwell's experimentally established force torsion electro/magnetic force balance that could be pigeonholed until 1908. Now, the true Maxwell's equations and Absolute Measurement would be replaced by the Heaviside's revision so, Practical Measurement could replace Absolute Measurement and old text books would be burned. To close this truth in reality summation, Marconi sued the USA for millions in unpaid royalty for using his radio patents. Less than a year after Tesla's died penniless, the Patent Office declared that Tesla not Marconi had invented Radio, citing Tesla's four tuned-circuit inventions employed by Marconi.

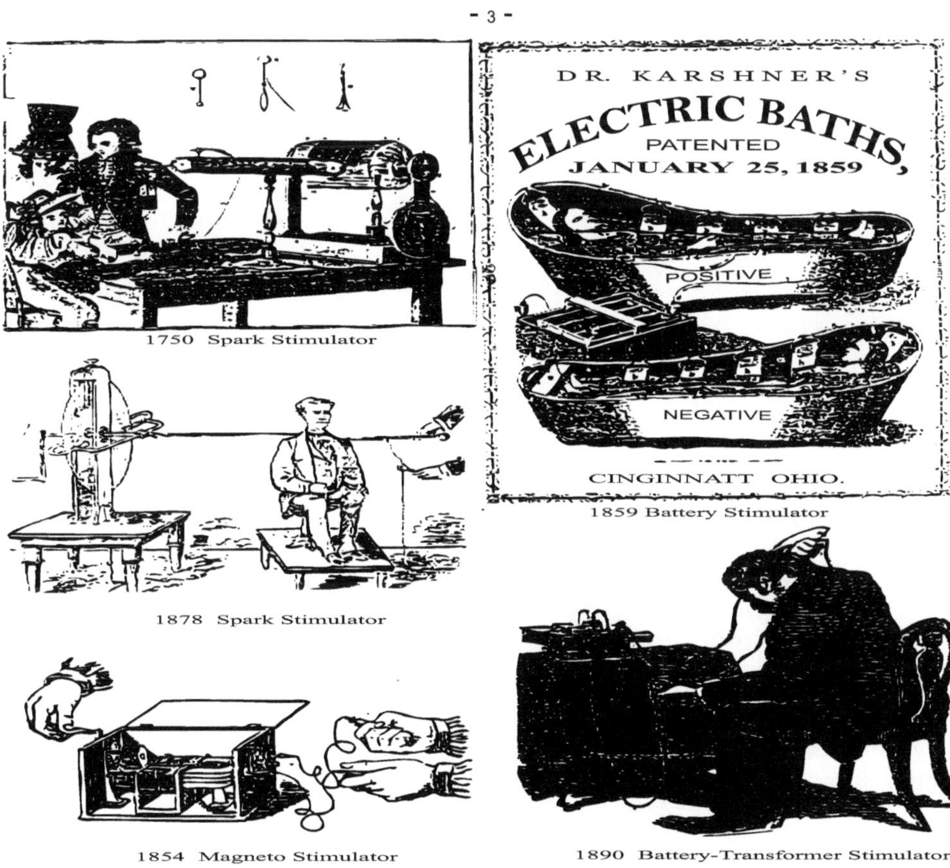

Fig. (3). Electro therapeutics in the 19th century. (With special permission of Hegda).

Later in 1870, many devices were invented with little understanding of their effects on the body and thus harming patients (Fig. **3**). Nevertheless, most physicians used some kind of electrical device in their office (1890-1920) with no real understanding despite the fact that Nikola Tesla perfected and patented the first viable PEMF healing machine, in 1898. Subsequently, Augustus Waller in early 1900's using a capillary electrometer, developed the electrocardiogram which Einthoven improved, to be shown later as instrument graphics that reveal various phases of the heart. De-oxygenated blood comes to the left atrium which flows towards the right ventricle and supplies to the lungs first and then the left atrium discharges oxygenated blood into the left ventricle then expelled into the body.

In the field of medicine, research into the effects of electromagnetic influences on healing and biological changes has also been impeded by the limitations of the simplified Giorgi system and its limiting assumptions. As far back as the beginning of the 20th Century, Nikola Tesla applied for Patents on a Magnifying Transmitter that suppressed dispersive, light-speed-limited, transverse Hertzian waves to create non-dispersing, faster-than-light, longitudinal mode shock waves. If the speed of light was truly invariant, it would have precluded Tesla's longitudinal wave mode. It is inconsistent with present-day use of the nonlinear permittivity of atmospheric water and earth resonance to give biological organisms healing information—a practise that challenges prevailing assumptions about the irreversibility of disease. The general presumption of the invariant speed of light has inhibited acceptance of and advancements on Tesla's Magnifying Transmitter and its earth resonance links to health [22].

Augustus Waller, in early 1900's using a capillary electrometer and developed the electrocardiogram which Einthoven improved on Fig. (**4**). A modern waveform shown on a graph represents various phases of the heart. Firstly, the contraction of heart from the right ventricle to the lungs occurs and then the left atrium discharges blood into the right ventricle and then from the right ventricle to the body after discharging from the right atrium to the ventricle. These phases and its synchronization determine the health of the heart.

In 1907, Bordet was the first to understand nerves damaged or denervation of the nerve that could be measured electrically which is regularly done with electromyography which measures the velocity of the nerve to see its healthy potential. In 1931, Albert Hyman demonstrated that animals, with induced cardiac arrest, could be resuscitated with electric current.

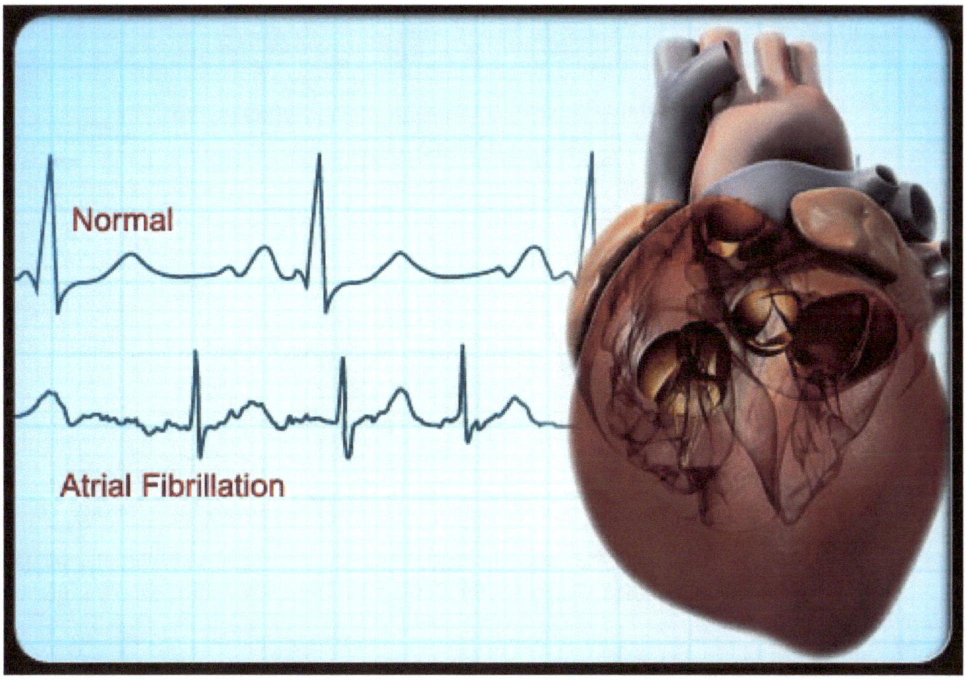

Fig. (4). Graphing of the rhythm of the heart, under normal and abnormal conditions. (With special permission of Hegda).

In 1952, Paul Zoll showed an artificial pacemaker that could be successful in maintaining a heartbeat for a limited period. Modern scientists have developed artificial hearts, currently being implanted. All sorts of electrical devices became a part of medicine, the electro phrenic respirator for spinal injuries, implanted and transcutaneous devices to treat chronic pain, stimulators to void the bladder and for paralyzed patients, urinary and anal incontinence. Stimulators became implanted in the brain to reduce spasticity and intractable epileptic seizure. Implanted electrodes and surface electrodes were used for scoliosis. Understanding improved with a more sophisticated electromyography which measures the velocity of nerve fibers over a constant distance, to determine the health of the nerve. Moreover, surface probes on the skull in separate places, give you reading of the activities of the brain, the electroencephalogram (EEG) (Fig. **5**). This will be discussed later but what we see is that the separate probes give separate readings which show that the brain works concomitantly or what we experience as dualism, being in one place but thinking of other things. These conditions show rapid brain waves (20-30 cycles per second) and under more meditative situations these separate waves become an aggregate wave, or alpha wave (7 cycles per second). The body is then synchronized and works as a whole. Healing occurs under this condition [2].

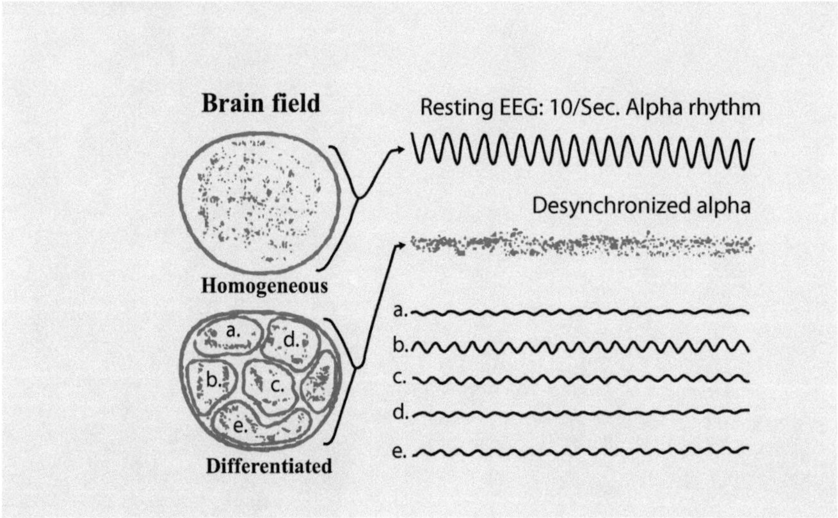

Fig. (5). Idealized: Alpha rhythm of EEG in state of relaxed wakefulness" and it desynchronization (After Lindsley, 1961 and Pribram, 1971). See Chapter 3 for Further Discussion. (With special permission of Genevieve Hogan).

The sophisticated understanding of the different muscle fibers such as the gastrocnemius with 1,000 to 2,000 fibers to maintain posture and only 2-3 fibers for laryngeal, pharyngeal and extra-ocular for finely controlled muscles, developed. The nerve cell and body of axon and dendrites compose the communication network [3]. Generally, there are motor and sensory nerves. The motor nerves, alpha and gamma go to the muscle and sensory nerves to the muscle spindle. Nerves are categorized according to the diameter, conduction velocity, spike duration, and refractory period. The sensory fiber nerves have five groups, proprioceptive, touch, pressure, vibration receptors, pain, hot and cold, and preganglionic and sympathetic. This is important because different frequencies and waveform excite these different groups. With this classification, scientists can determine the proper use of electro-therapeutics for the relief of pain. Later, these subtleties set the stage for artificial limbs with signals from the brain activity sent to the artificial limb.

Yet physicians stopped using electro stimulation for about 50 years since there was a lack of understanding of the nervous system, until, in the 1960's, Melzack and Wall published the "control gate theory". Non painful electrical stimulation was seen as blocking the pain signal to the brain and small portable units of "T.E.N.S." transcutaneous electrical nerve stimulators became popular. This led to a further understanding by Bruce Pomeranz M.D., Ph.D., (1987) who concluded that acupuncture (electro-acupuncture) activates small myelinated nerve fibers in the muscle, which send impulse to the spinal cord, and then activates three centers, spinal cord, midbrain and pituitary-hypothalamus to cause analgesia [4]. The spinal cord use enkephalin and dynorphin to block incoming painful information. The midbrain centre uses enkephalin to activate the raphe descending system which inhibits spinal cord transmission using monoamines (serotonin and norepinephrine). The third center is the hypothalamus-pituitary which releases beta endorphin into the blood and cerebral fluid to cause analgesia at a distance [5][1].

To activate the muscles, 4-7 volt impulses are needed to contract the muscles. Thus, if the body is subjected to T.E.N.S. and the muscles are in spasms, more volts will be needed until the muscles relax with stimulation. Even though the impulse amplitude voltage is not turned up after the start of stimulation it will be too much because the muscle is relaxed with less resistance. The current needs to be turned down. In electrical systems, there are series circuits like Christmas tree lights where the current flows through the system in one line, and in parallel circuits, each path is different, like home circuitry, with all the paths added up to determine total volts.

SAFE AND EFFECTIVE ELECTROTHERAPY

The waveform in a home is a sine wave since it is alternating current which flows in opposite direction continuously. In a battery, the direct current measurement is unidirectional since it flows only in one direction. Even with alternating current if the pulse width is over 500 microseconds, the patient will experience discomfort, below 100 microseconds the muscle will not contract. **200 to 400 microseconds are the best for therapeutics effects.** The muscles should contract without pain for 15 minutes and the polarity of the probes should be changed. Micro constant current stimulators have been developed where the current is constant as the resistance varies. There has been some success in this area over the last thirty years.

Electrical current, especially with acupuncture needles, without alternating (AC) pulsing from a generator, creates electrolysis with acid accumulating at one pole and alkaline in the other, thus acupuncture with direct current, besides being harmful to the tissue, can lead to the needle becoming rigid and breaking. It is thus necessary to specify safe and effective procedures for electrotherapy. This is the specialty of Dr. Omura. For the average person, the most important discovery is the simple TENS unit in which cost is minimal and if properly instructed can be one of the most effective self-healing techniques available, safe and effective. Since manufacturers produce many electrical instruments for use, the only way to judge its electrical parameters, is to connect it to an oscilloscope and examine the waveform. For the normal TENS unit, it delivers 120 peak volts but only for 15μseconds and 35 μseconds and has a sudden drop in phase and rise time thus, causing the muscles to contract at from 3.5 volts to 7 volts. The difference between the positive and negative phases time is determined but the area of the waves above and below the zero line. Omura showed that the frequency of the stimulator should be at the heart beat of the patient since the body accepts this frequency at the best. High frequency is used for acute situations where there is a need to relieve pain instantly. The effect only lasts several days, sometimes shorter or longer. Lower frequency creates a more stable and lasting effect.

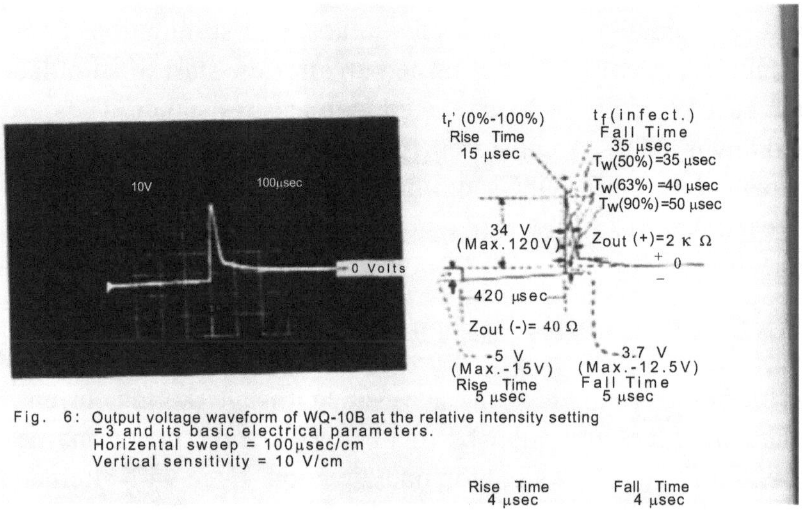

Fig. (6). Omura and Shinnick photographed with a Polaroid camera the WQ10 stimulator hooked up to an oscilloscope (Fig. **6**). One can see rising above the 0 line and dipping below the O line, a spike. The area under these spikes tells you the amount of current for both positive and negative, which is about 60% to 40%, thus one must change polarities after 15 minutes. (With special permission of Omura).

Yoshiaki Omura, is an electrical engineering (former member of the State Board of Medicine and Dentistry for Manhattan) who showed that blood flow increased with electrical stimulation or acupuncture. The experiment was simple, he looked at the finger nail with an intensified light and saw the vasodilation of the small capillaries [6, 7].

Diabetes has uneven blood circulation in different parts of the body which can be improved by acupuncture or electrical situation. Brain circulation is influenced by spastic muscles in the neck, and thus blood pressure in the brain can be high, and a favorable situation for a stroke to happen. It can be relieved by electrical or acupuncture stimulation [8]. Although the brachial artery may show normal blood pressure yet with spasms of the neck and shoulder muscles the person may be suffering from hypo-tension in the brain [9]. The symptoms are tension in shoulder and neck, depression, confusion, irritability, pain, short term memory loss, and insomnia [10]. He found that the frequency of the simulator must be near the heart rate for best results and done without pain. He previously showed that how direct current is harmful and creates polarity of acid and alkaline fluids, which blister and destroy tissue by electrolysis and in acupuncture can make the needles break. Never use electrical current without alternating (AC) pulse generator for electro-acupuncture treatment.

SUBTLE MEASUREMENT OF COULOMBIC, GAUSSIAN, AND PHOTONIC FIELDS

Robert O. Becker in the early 60's suggested that the body had a magnetic field outside the organism based upon the electrical current in the brain, used for internal communication and also with the earth's magnetic field [11]. This has implications like for example, exposure to electromagnetic fields from electrical motors, cell phones, power lines, TV sets, microwave ovens and any other pulsed generators of PEMFs. (Bjorn E. W. Nordenstrom, M.D. suggested a closed circuit in the body and provides evidence for this [12]). Discussion of this magnetic field outside the body was met with dubious laughter, then, but in 1970, through solid-state physics and electronics, the SQUID (superconducting quantum interference detector) could measure the magnetic field produced by the brains several feet away. Becker picked up faint electrical potential signals in wounds during healing. In fact, the stomach wall sends out infrared heat waves with the entire spectrum of light- "ultraviolet rays, x-rays, radio waves and so on. The fifty-foot aerial of the Naval Research laboratory in Washington can pick up radio signals coming from the stomach more than four miles away" [13]. The cell stomach lining is renewed every three days. This mitogenic luminescence or biophoton emission is essential for life and its origin is at the atomic level when the electron change orbits to emit a photon for information. Our physical nature, body, moves quite slowly. With this sophisticated system from radio astronomy, plant seedlings measurement of mitogenic waves showed that they communicate in red [14]. The Woods Hole Marine Biological Laboratory scientist, Brown showed that exposing simple organism to a magnetic field influenced their orientation to the earth. Also, pigeons were found to have magnetite in their brain to navigate [15 - 33].

Entropy cannot be seen, it is inferred primarily from inorganic experiments of pressure, volume and temperature in gases, as these variable changes, the system cannot go back to the original state without the loss of energy, and this phenomenon is called entropy. Negative entropy requires non-sine waves or harmonics. It means non-equilibrium (organic) by adjusting to conditions of life (all biological organisms exist in far-from-thermodynamic-equilibrium states) by getting energy from the earth's vibration, water atmosphere, food, and healthy behavior (meditation). According to the current measurement standards an ampere is defined as a unit of electric current depositing a unit of silver for a second, but this is incorrect. Experimentally, it deposits more than predicted. This electrolysis involves chemistry and reversible atomic time in which the second law of thermodynamics is erroneous and the speed of light is not constant.

In medicine, this flaw concerning entropy can be seen in ideas such as, "nothing we can do", yet life itself has this reversible capability, unlike inorganic gas experiment with dimensions of pressure, volume, heat, and entropy- where the system can never get back to the original energy. Earth itself gives life through negative ions and it pulse rate of 7.5 Hertz and octaves up. Humans all the time reverse their disease through certain practises. Also this bias can be seen in trying to explain disease by the DNA which is really a field that cannot be broken up to manipulate particular codes for certain diseases. Hans Peter Durr, Director of the Max Planck Institute points out that the "objectifiable world that exists continuously over time, seems so self-evident to us, and basically does not exist" [26 - 32]. The future cannot be predicted unequivocally over time, neither can disease.

Becker experimented in various frequencies of pulse generators and showed subtle electrical signals in wounds healing naturally. An extension of this phenomenon includes the disturbances from intense PEMF field approximate to individuals, like power line transformers, cell phones and electrical transmission lines. Discussing this, as high powered transmission lines were being built from Canada to the U.S., Becker was fired from his VA Hospital, his career was ruined.

In my clinical practise, over the last thirty-five years I have used both surface electrodes and/or electro acupuncture in 95% of my cases. The length of the success rate depends upon underlying infections, chronic or acute injury, and general health of the patient. The one-time success rate is high.

THE HEART HAS MEMORIES AND RETAINS MORE THAN ORGANS

The heart itself has pacemaker cells, the sinoatrial (SA) node and the atrioventricular (AV) node which are considered as the primary pacemaker cell groups in the heart. In the normal heart, the AV node follows the rhythm of the

SA node. During a heart attack the spread of these electrical impulses is disrupted. The EKG, which reflects the spread of the electrical impulse, is useful in delineating areas of cardiac damage. The purkinje fiber which runs across the front of the heart synchronizes the heart beats. Cardiac cells potentiate a charge and are synchronized for a healthy regulation of the heart. Omura was the first to measure the potential of a single cardiac cell. Simon Freed hypothesized that the conditioning of the body, accident, disease, can be found in the memory of the vascular fluids and purkinje fiber.

In the human organism circulation is continuous by the pumping sequence of the heart from de-oxygenated blood to oxygenated blood through the valves and pumping of the heart through the synchronizer purkinje fiber. Bykov, Gant and his associates have demonstrated that excitation of any of the visceral organs, even when weak, stimulates an increase in the rate and volume of respiration. Stimu-lation of the several types of interceptors found in the stomach, kidney, spleen, liver, secreting glands and pancreas affects reflex changes in respiratory activity and circulatory apparatus. A rise in blood pressure changes perfusates in the vessels of the spleen, intestine and kidney and provokes variations in the blood pressure. Rise in blood pressure or change in cardiac activity or breathing is caused by pancreatic glands and increased pressure of the perfusates. Experimentally, injections of acetylcholine (an excitatory neurotransmitter at neuromuscular junction) and nicotine into the spleen, intestine and kidney produced an increase in blood pressure and intensification of respiratory movement. Carbon dioxide (build up by shallow breathing) and adrenaline (stress induce) also produce the same reaction. The organs can activate archaic response yet fetal breathing (rising the abdomen on inhalation) can relax the organs.

The response between afferent receiving signals to the brain and the efferent response to the body through motor nerves has a whole collection of aggregate response as the internuncial or intermediary neurons. These areas of the brain have been identified between the hypothalamus and supra orbital region of the lateral hypothalamus. They have a relationship with the various effector organs of the automatic system. When stimulated, the breathing rate and blood pressure decrease and there is reduction of salivation and urination. This is a collective summation of the parasympathetic mediated function. Posture influences these systems. The posture of meditation creates a condition that affects reactivity, facilitating parasympathetic response to relax. Freed maintains that the organs are the reservoir of memory for trauma as in the phantom limb effect which is extinguished by both meditation and acupuncture. Acupuncture is a therapy for traumatic affective disorders such as the phantom limb pain syndrome. Freed also showed a possible physiological basis for effectiveness of acupuncture against other psychosomatic disorders. Gant and others found in animal experiments that the emotional component was as important for conditioning as the stimulus itself [33, 34]. Application of the heart's response to outside and inside stimulation is mentioned below. Shinnick, Omura and Blumenthal explored it in their monograph on the memories of the heart [35].

PULSE GENERATORS

The universe generates impulse energy from lightning discharge. The sun is photonic energy source reflected in the electromagnetic spectrum. Neutrons stars which spin at high speed and then enter a nebula creating gamma rays which are muted by our atmosphere [36]. (These frequencies are used for killing cancer cells). Other stellar energy sources, such as dying exploding stars, or the stars generally, whose light reaches us, have energy pulse signatures. In any space near us, if you visualize just a five centimeter area of space, to measure the different electromagnetic energies with an instrument, one can only find an average of several different types to get a wave form. This is not accurate but gives you some idea of the energy. In this little five centimeter space, waves from the whole electromagnetic spectrum could be found even if faint. The fact that it is being measured changes what is to be measured. As shown from the Wood's hole, even the body emits a variety of electromagnetic wave spectrum radiations.

The power grid in the U.S., generated by heat from fossil fuels, is like a railroad circular switchyard with the one polarity going to earth. This means that we are running high power voltage through the earth; underground organism has a unique frequency which has to be disturbed by this high voltage. Switzerland forbids the ground in the earth; instead ground runs high above the earth on poles. The earth itself has a pulsed frequency, trees have this, humans have this and organs in our body have this (the bases of the meridian theory of energy of organs which run on the surface of the skin and internally). Since we know that like waves forms can resonate, Omura and Shinnick showed that how organ pathways can be imaged on the outside of the body and compared against traditional Chinese understanding [37, 38]. Shinnick showed that how when the body is subjected to a toxin such as tobacco, the lung pathway deviates, that acupuncture points are really quite large and that when subjected to needles, mechanical pressure, Qigong, lasers, or other stimulation forms, the circles which surround an acupuncture point, invert and the bio chemicals displayed in the circle become its opposite [39 - 44]. Biochemical associated with pain instantly transform to opiate type receptors and become smaller in size.

Photonic Energy

These are several consecutive transaxial slices from single-photon emission computed tomography scans of a patient with baseline scan (top row) showing initial thalamic (arrow) asymmetry with the left activity greater than the right (Fig. **7**). The post acupuncture scan (bottom row) shows reversal of the thalamic asymmetry with the right now markedly greater than the left [45].

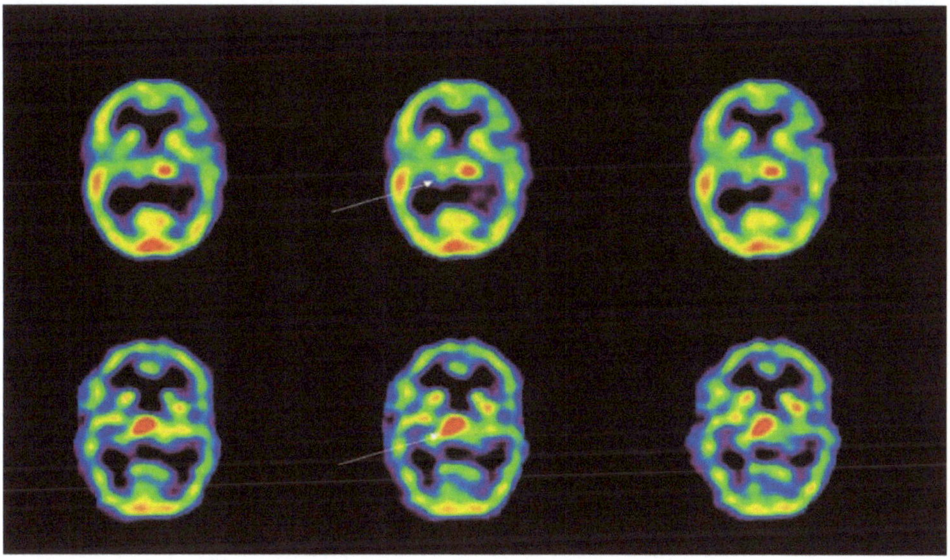

Fig. (7). Imaging the inside of the brain. (With special permission of Hegda).

Scientists from the University of Pennsylvania with Positive Emission Thermography saw that before acupuncture or electrical stimulation brain blood circulation was asymmetrical and afterwards symmetrical (Fig. **7**). Among them Patrick La Riccia, who received his physicians acupuncture certificate from Dr. Omura and urged that this study should be done [45]. Later, based upon this image, among other evidence, the National Institute of Health changed its mind on acupuncture supported by many physicians who urged its acceptance. This field showed great promise and still does. At the Rusk Institute of the New York Medical School, as a senior researcher with Dr. Mathew Lee, Director, we embarked on the use of thermography. This is computerized so that imaging of the surface of the skin could be coded in hot and cold and shown on a screen. One of the first uses we attempted was breast implant that had painful leaks down the arm but no evidence of this found. Thermography followed the leaks down the arm clearly, in hot red color, exposing the pattern. This proof leads to a change in the manufacturing of breast implants that did not leak.

The laser is an electrical current passed through a crystal, at first ruby (then Helium-Neon lasers and invisible infrared Gallium-Arsenide and Gallium-Aluminum-Arsenide), which translates the electron current into a coherent laser beam, does not disperse like a flashlight beam. Pekka J. Pontinen composed a comprehensive book on this bio stimulation using the knowledge from acupuncture stimulation to show these low level (8 Milliwatt) emissions are effective in pain relief, especially in auricular therapy (ear) or traditional acupuncture points [46].

THE HEART'S PULSE GIVES INFORMATION FOR HEALTH AND NOXIOUS CONDITIONS

In 130-200 A.D. European, Claudius Galen wrote about the pulse, which was very confusing, then, in 1484 Aegidiuscus Corbollensis, a Catholic priest, wrote in a great detail about the pulse, later Joseph Struthia started writing about the pulse in 1555, finishing in 1602. In 1630, Roberto Fludd integrated Chinese understandings while William Harvey wrote the classical work "Exercitatio Anatomica De Motus Cordis Et Sanguinis in Animalibus [47, 48]. Harvey's work more accurately describes the relationship between the lung and heart or venous and arterial blood flow, deoxygenated to oxygenated blood going through the lungs. Consequently, Europe has a long history of acupuncture and medicine. P.M.F. Nogier M.D., called as the father of auricular medicine (ear) showed different parts of the ear corresponding to organs and parts of the body, based upon clinical research [49] (Figs. **8, 9**). It looks like an upside down fetus in the ear. For neck and shoulder, the lower part of the helix lies on the top for lumbar problems and in the concha of the ear, the organs. Nogier also showed how when you take the pulse, in a certain thumb position while the subject holds a substance, the Vascular Autonomic Signal (RAC) on the pulse shows that the heart responding to the waveform of the substance. If not compatible, the pulse becomes rapid. He developed a set of frequencies or harmonics that correspond to wound healing, gastrointestinal and metabolic problems, locomotor problems, disorders of laterality, pain and nerve condition, brain and bone reconstruction and action on the cerebral cortex. He did this by developing frequencies for each of these diseases, for laser or electrical stimulation treatment. He understood that certain microorganisms have a certain color, such as bacteria, and develop colored lenses near the skin which the RAC responds to see if that substance is in the body from this colored compatibility wave from the microorganism has demonstrated that excitation of any of the visceral organs, even when weak, stimulates an increase in the rate and volume of respiration [50].

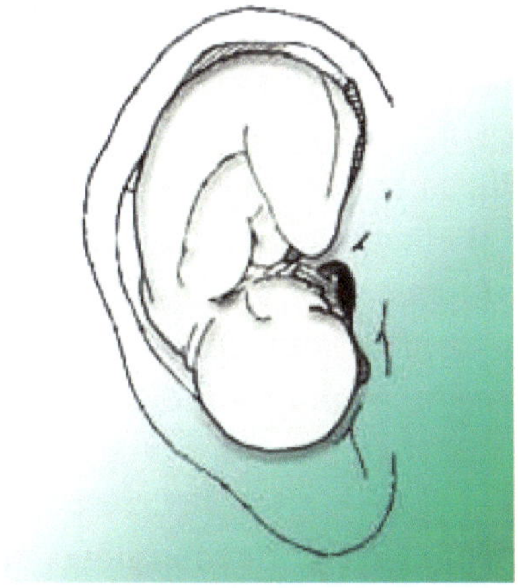

Fig. (8). Nogier's ear homunculus as an upside down fetus and representation points for treatment. These points can be stimulated for treatment, (Fig. **9**). http://sedatelec.com/english/acupauri.htm

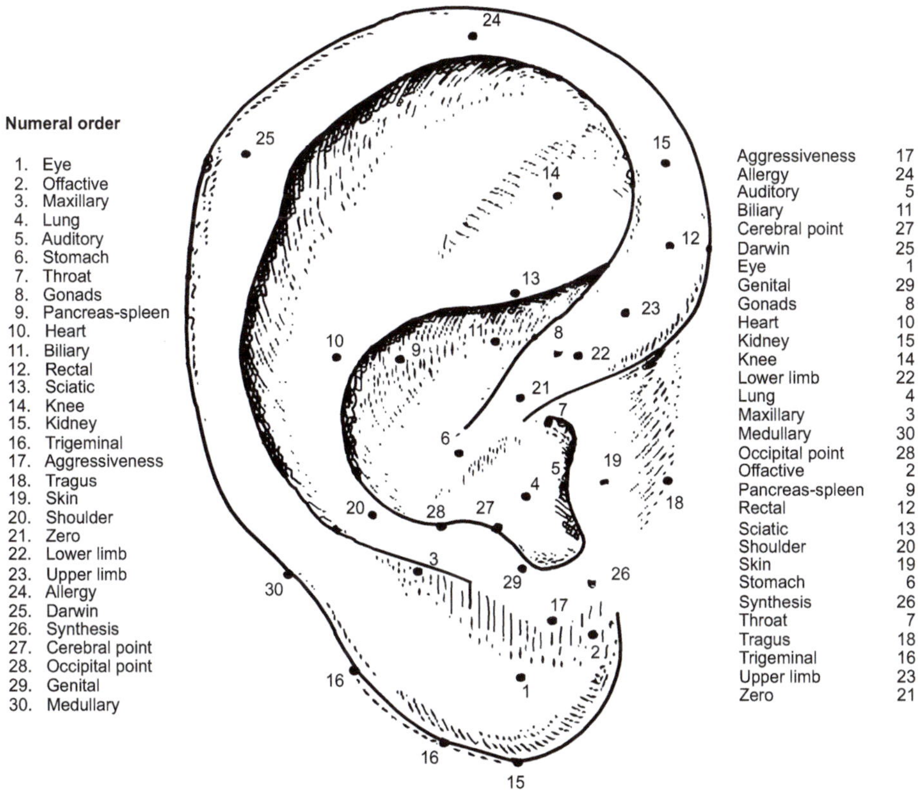

Fig. (9). The homunculus of the ear and the corresponding organs to locations in the ear. http://amine.rachidi.free.fr/Acu/Auriculo.htm

Considering one of the viscera, the heart, is a major organ of acupuncture. In the course of the classical Pavlovian paradigm, electrical stimulation of the hind leg of a dog is paired with the sound of a metronome of a given frequency [51]. Not only does the leg but also the heart responds to the shock and repeated sound. The conditioned cardiac reflect is elaborated more quickly (Gant) than the conditioned motor reflex. On pairing of the stimuli may prove to be adequate for the cardiac reflex rather than perhaps for the motor reflex. That is after one pairing of the stimuli, the metronome unaccompanied by the electrical shock, evokes a surge in the heart beat. What is meaningful for our study is the long retention of the conditioned cardiac reflex. Long after the response of the leg has been extinguished to the sound of the metronome alone, the heart will continue to equate the sound with electrical shock, Fear of shock, entirely unconscious, which is evoked into activity by the specific frequency of the metronome and, in states of mental distress by rough approximation to it. Freed showed a possible physiological basis for effectiveness of acupuncture against psychosomatic disorders [52].

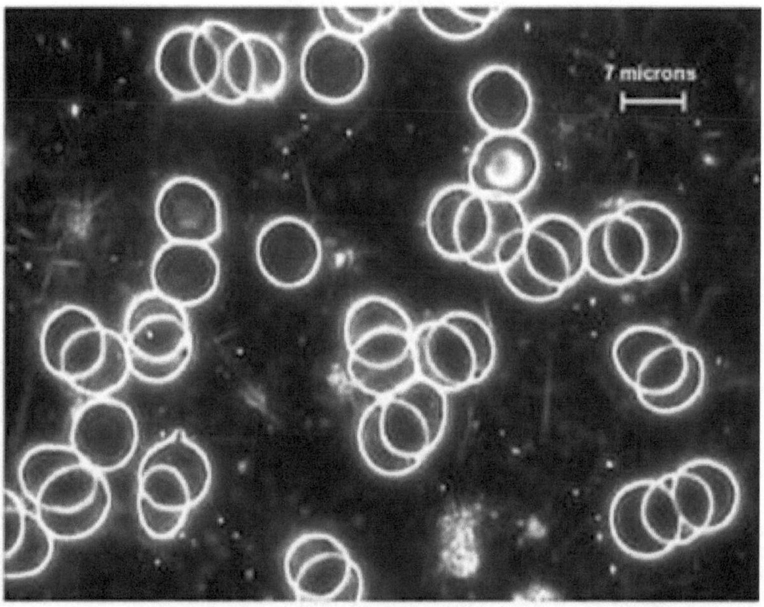

Fig. (10). Baseline condition showing normal, healthy blood from 75-year-old female subject [54]. (With special permission from researcher, Beverley Rubik).

The emission of light from cells found by a bio-physicist, Beverly Rubik, who measured this effect describing differences between the emission of cancer cells and ordinary cells [53] (Fig. **10**). More recently, she has taken photographs of cell structure exposed to cell phone Gaussian radiation before and after [54] (Fig. **10,**

11). This study utilized a custom-built, dark-field microscope attached to a digital video camera system. Omura also studied the effects of electromagnetic fields and electronic instruments in the home environment, TV, microwave oven, computer monitor and cell phones [55].

Blood from the same female 45 minutes later after using the cell phone in active communication mode is shown above [54] (Fig. **11**). Blood from the same female immediately after the carrying condition shows RBCs (red blood cells) which are entirely stuck together in rouleaux type aggregates, which look like rolls of coins [54] (Fig. **12**).

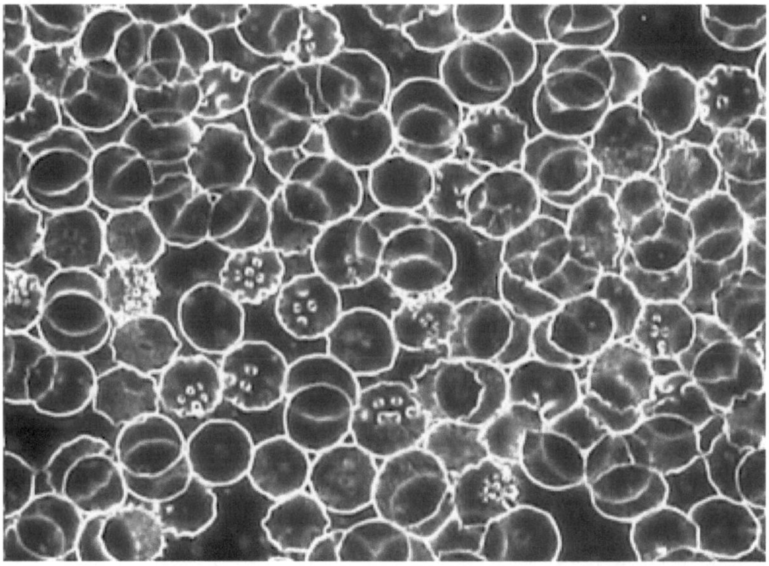

Fig. (11). Blood from 75 year-old female after active cell phone communication. (With special permission from researcher, Beverley Rubik).

Most RBCs are misshapen rather than round. Many RBCs show spiky projections on the surface, which are abnormal, spiculated RBCs called echinocytes. This particular subject, seventy-five years old and the oldest person in the study, showed the most characteristic changes in the blood following both exposure conditions. William Tiller in his work on "Science and Human Transformation" is much more inclusive of the different frequencies of different modern modalities and modern physics understandings [56]. One can see that creating graphs from Coulombic fields such as EEG, and EKG and using other measurement of global characteristics such as blood lactate and oxygen consumption during change from desynchronization to synchronization not on diseased people but those with higher synchronization has led to a better understanding of the states of the mind and body for healing. These state changes are tested in heart disease, spinal injuries, post-surgical care and meditative practices. It also gives us the capability to compare the highest states of synchronization in humans to inorganic matter, at different temperatures. This parallelism brings out properties of oneness or synchronization in both inorganic and organic matter. To be sure, we see a certain stability in disease, which pathologically reproduces itself in habituations but through synchronization of the activities of the mind and heart de-habituates into a more coherent physiology for healing. Furthermore, we will explore methods of meditation which strengthen negative entropy, or this synchronization, and a reversal of these pathological habituations which cause pain and suffering. What we see is that things get de-synchronized in organism without conscious control and changing desynchronization to synchronization de-habituates pathology. This is tested in clinical cases. The high costs of these technological tests without advancing or understanding treatment practices are the driving forces to examine diagnosis methods which are low cost. This is accomplished by understanding that the brain (finger strength) and the heart can recognize different waveforms and help test compatibility to drugs, test microorganism, organs for abnormality and vertebrae weakness.

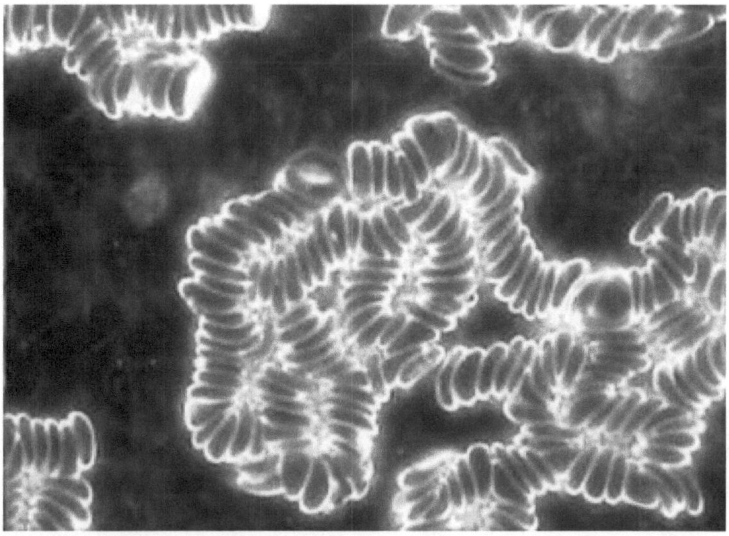

Fig. (12). Blood in same patient after carrying cell phone. (With special permission from researcher, Beverley Rubik).

Fields Notes: Conversations with Guy Obolensky 2003-2013 during Joint Research with the Natural Energy Institute, Inc. and Research Institute of Global Physiology, Behavior and Treatment, Inc. renamed Whole Person Self Healing Institute, Inc.

This book has been written for scientists, medical clinicians and lay persons. Using a multi disciplinary practical approach, its main concept is centered on negative entropy. The second Law of Thermodynamics states that the entropy of a system tends to get higher because disorganization increases as time progresses. Living things, however, behave in the opposite way. Erwin Schrödinger was the 1933 Nobel Laureate in Physics for his discovery that "matter is both particle and wave". In 1944, he referred to the concept of "negative entropy" in his popular science book, "What Is Life?" The 1977 Nobel Prize in Chemistry was awarded to Ilya Prigogine for his contribution to non-equilibrium thermodynamics, particularly the theory of dissipative structures. Organic beings are nonlinear, or reversible, and they are out of equilibrium. Inorganic matter is linear and in equilibrium. All living things are open systems. They preserve their natural state by using free energy, such as nutrients and sunlight, to create order and to maintain life. They also give an equal amount of energy back to their environment in the forms of heat and of entropy. Life thrives on negative entropy!

Bosons. Only non-gravitating magnetic bosom particles can congregate to affect long-range coherence and reverse their spin vector to negate positive entropy. Our sun is comprised of electrically charged and uncharged fermion particles, the evoke gravitating mass, angular momentum and RMS heat to affect irreversible entropy gain in dynamic time, whereas the sun's magnetic charged boson particles have no gravitating mass, enabling them to periodically reverse their spin vector to affect adiabatic entropy reduction in atomic time. This allows our Sun to perpetuate the life on the solar systems third planet. Boson particles can reverse their atomic time spin-vector to negate the positive entropy accumulated by fermion particles in dynamic times. Ilya Prigogine received the Nobel prize in chemistry for proving that both living and inanimate systems can circumvent the "fatal" entropy gained in dynamic time by simply employing the adiabatic-entropy-negating loophole existing in non -equilibrium thermodynamic illuminated by Prigogine.

Cavity of Earth: Schuman Resonance

The resonant properties of our terrestrial wave cavity are generally credited to the German physicist W.O. Schuman having experimentally detected by Schuman and Konig in 1954, the first spectral representation of this phenomenon was prepared by Balser and Wagner, in 1960.

There are about 1000 lightning storms at any given moment worldwide, each produces 0.5 to 1 ampere and these collectively keep the Earth's electromagnetic cavity circulating active. These so-called Schumann Resonances are quasi standing wave electromagnetic waves, like waves on a spring that have to be excited and need to be observed. They are not caused by anything internal to earth, its crust or its core. They naturally occur at specific frequencies between 6 and 50 cycles per second; specifically, 7.8, 14, 20, 26, 33, 39, and 45 Hertz, with a periodic variation of about 0.5 Hertz.

This daily variation appears to be a function of the height of the ionosphere and solar activity. As long as the properties of Earth's electromagnetic cavity remain the same, the frequencies will remain the same. Presumably, there is also variation due to the 11 year solar activity cycle.

The cavity is defined by the surface of the earth and inner edge of the ionosphere 55 kilometers up. At any moment, the total charge residing in this cavity is equal to 500,000 Coulombs. There is a vertical current flow between the ground and the ionosphere of 1-3 x 10^-12 amperes per square meter, The speed of light is 186,000 miles per hour per second and the circumference of the earth is 24,000 miles, which means that an electrical impulse from lightning strike will travel around the earth approximately 8 times per second, (186/24 = 7.75).

NOTES

[1]Ehrenprais showed how by introducing naloxone to a patient and then doing acupuncture or electro-therapeutics the effect of pain relief does not occur.

REFERENCES

[1] Shinnick PK. Historical Perspective China and the Olympics, (physical culture in China Pre-liberation and after liberation). New York: Far Eastern Reporter 1978.

[2] Shinnick PK, Freed S. A Case study of the synchronization of human energy in an acute condition of chronic heart disease through complementary treatment. Subtle Ener Energy Med 2003; 13: 3.

[3] Benton B, Bowman W. Functional Electrical Stimulation-a practical Clinical Guide. California: Los Amigo Hospital. Rehabilitation Engineering Center 1981.

[4] Stux G, Pomeranz B. Acupuncture textbook and atlas. New York: Springer-Verlag 1987. [http://dx.doi.org/10.1007/978-3-642-71742-0]

[5] Ehrenprais S, Balagot RC, Comaty J, *et al.* Naloxone reversible analgesia in mice produced by D-phenylalanine and hydrocinnamic acid, inhibitors of carboxypeptidase. In: Bonica JJ, Ed. Advances in Pain Research Therapy. New York: Raven Press 1979; Vol. 3: pp. 479-88.

[6] Omura Y. Basic electrical parameters for safe and effective electro-therapeutics [electro-acupuncture, TES, TENMS (or TEMS), TENS and electro-magnetic field stimulation with or without drug field] for pain, neuromuscular skeletal problems, and circulatory disturbances. Acupunct Electrother Res 1987; 12(3-4): 201-25.
[http://dx.doi.org/10.3727/036012987816358788] [PMID: 2895568]

[7] Omura Y. The effects of electrical and non-electrical acupuncture on cardiovascular & nervous system, and pre and post acupuncture evaluation of patients, including valuable visible diagnostic signs, such as the "abnormal cardiovascular sign of the ear lobules. Acupunct Electrother Res 1978; 3:

223-50.
[http://dx.doi.org/10.3727/036012976817553214]

[8] Omura Y. Simple and quick non-invasive evaluation of circulatory condition of cerebral arteries by clinical application of the Bi-Digital O-Ring Test. Acupunct Electrother Res 1985; 10(3): 139-61. [http://dx.doi.org/10.3727/036012985816714469] [PMID: 2866668]

[9] Shinnick P, Freed S, Blumenthal C, Omura Y. Heart. New York: The Heart Disease Research Foundation 1990.

[10] Omura Y. Non-invasive circulatory evaluation and electro-acupuncture & TES treatment of diseases difficult to treat in Western medicine. Acupunct Electrother Res 1983; 8(3-4): 177-256. [http://dx.doi.org/10.3727/036012983816714858] [PMID: 6145300]

[11] Becker RO. Cross Currents. the Perils of Electropollution. The Promise of Electromedicine. In: Becker RO, Selden G, Eds. The Body Electric. New York: Putnam Book 1985; pp. 67-81.

[12] Nordenstrom BE. Biologically Closed Electric Circuits: Clinical, Experimental and Theoretical Evidence for an Additional Circulatory System. Stockholm, Sweden: Karolinska Institutet, Nordic Medical Publications 1983.

[13] Pfeiffer J. The Changing Universe. London 1956.

[14] lifesciences.de/ib-003-.htm.

[15] Obolensky AG, Shinnick P. Coulombic, Gaussian and Photonic Measurement in Electromedicine with Links Between the Biochemical Processes of Neutrophils and Schumann Resonance. Blue Paper: A joint effort by Natural Energy Institute and the Research Institute of Global Physiology, Behavior and Treatment, Inc 2008.

[16] Longman GI. A New Dictionary of Physics 1958; 339.

[17] Obolensky AG, Shinnick P, Maize JP. . A New multi-disciplined approach to electro-medicine research. J Sci Heal Outcomes 2012; 14: 14-5.

[18] Flandern TV, Vigier JP. Experimental repeal of the speed limit for gravitation electrodynamics and quantum field interactions. F of Phy 2002.

[19] Ecole Polytechnique Federale de Lausanne. Public Release 41-21-693-4774 2010 Aug;

[20] Chang Kenneth. Wizardry at Harvard: Physicists Move Light. 2007.

[21] Zawada. Also see relevant patent revealing the critical wave numbers needed to achieve atomic-time reversal for aberrant living tissue. Violation of Time Reversal Invariance in Living Tissue US Patent 6.592,611,

[22] Obolensky AG, Shinnick P, Cathcart C. A Short History: Errors Stemming from Unidimensional Treatment of Time and Electromagnetic Phenomena. Blue Paper. Natural Energy Institute and Research Institute of Global Physiology, Behavior and Treatment, Inc. 2005.

[23] Schrodinger E. What is life? The Physical Aspect of the Living Cell & Mind and Matter. London: Cambridge Press 1969; p. 71. Schrodinger E. Statistical Thermodynamic. New York: Dover Press 1989

[24] Prigogine I. Time, Structure and Fluctuations Nobel Lecture. 1977.

[25] Prigogine I. From being to becoming Time and complexity in the physical sciences. San Francisco: W.H. Freeman and Company 1980; p. 123.

[26] Durr H. Sheldrake's ideas from the perspective of modern physics. Frontier Perspectives. 2003; p. 37. ISSN 1062-4767.

[27] Obolensky AG, Shinnick P. Electro-Magnetic Field Interaction: a Human Electro-magnetic Field (aura) Resonating with its Phase-Conjugate (time reversed) Replica can Reduce the Body's Mitogenic

Entropy; Summary of Recent Observation Related to Traditional Chinese Meridian Theory and Application to Healing and Disease. Proceedings of the Material Research and Living Systems. Boston. 2004.

[28] Shinnick P. The Science of Whole Person Healing, Electro-magnetic Field Interaction: A Human Electro-Magnetic Field (aura) Resonating with its Phase-conjugate (time reversal) Replica can Reduce the Body's Mitogenic Entropy; Summary of Recent Observation Related to Traditional Chinese Meridian Theory and Application to Healing and Disease. Proceedings of the Second Interdisciplinary International Conference;. Lincoln, Nebraska: iUniverse 2005.

[29] Obolensky G, Shinnick P. Electro-magnet. Shock Waves in a Controlled Non-linear Environment Create a Phase-conjugate (time-reversed) Replica Resonating with a Human Electro-magnetic field (aura). Its Use for the Body's Mitogenic Wave Entropy Reduction Has Implications for Medicine and Science. Proceedings of the Whole Person Health Summit and Second Qigong Summit 14-17th 2005 April. Washington D.C.: iUniverse 2005.

[30] Sharkey N, Haddad J, Obolensky AG, Shinnick P. Electric and electro magnetic field stimulation management of a complex ovarian cyst a case report. J Res Meth 2010.

[31] Haddad JB, Obolensky AG, Shinnick P. The biologic effects and the therapeutic mechanism of action of electric and electromagnetic field stimulation on bone and cartilage: new findings and a review of earlier work. J Altern Complement Med 2007; 13(5): 485-90. [http://dx.doi.org/10.1089/acm.2007.5270] [PMID: 17604552]

[32] Omura Y. Relation between transmembrane action potential of single cardiac cells and their responding surface electrogram *in vivo* and *in vitro* and related electro-mechanical phenomena Transactions of the NY Academy of Science Series, II. 32(8): 874-940.

[33] Gant WH. Cardiovascular component of the conditioned reflex to pain, food and other stimuli Phys Res 40: Sup #4, Phys Psy 1948; An Re of Phys. X. Gant WH. Physiological Psychology. Phipps Psychiatric Clinic. Annual Review of Physiology 1948; X. Gant WH. Russian Physiology and Pathology. Soviet Science 1948. A Symposium at the Philadelphia Meeting of the American Association for the Advancement of Science. Washington DC. AAAS Publication Review of Physiology 1952; X. Anoklin PK. Characteristics of the afferent apparatus, a conditioned reflex and its importance for psychology. In: Voprasy Parikholgie (problems in psychology) 1955; 6: 241-270.

[34] Bykov KM, Vladimirov GY, Delov VY, Konradi GP, Slonim AD. Textbook of Physiology. Moscow: Foreign Lan Pub 1958.

[35] Shinnick P, Freed S, Blumenthal C, Omura Y. Heart. New York: Heart Disease Research Foundation 1990.

[36] Shinnick P. Fields of Electro-magnetic Energy, Pulse Generators, Natural and Manufactured, Ways to Measure and Scientific Considerations. Proceedings of the Scientific Panel of the Third Science of Whole Person Healing Conference. Baltimore. 2007.

[37] Omura Y. Transmission of molecular information through electro-magnetic waves with different frequencies and its application to non-invasive diagnosis of patients as well as detection from patients X-ray film of visible and not visible medical information: Part I. Acupunct Electrother Res 1994; 19(1): 39-63. [http://dx.doi.org/10.3727/036012994816357394] [PMID: 7916176]

[38] Omura Y, Losco M, Omura AK, *et al.* Bi-directional transmission of molecular information by photon or electron beams passing in the close vicinity of specific molecules, and its clinical and basic research applications: 1) Diagnosis of humans or animal patients without any direct contact; 2) Light microscopic and electron microscopic localization of neuro-transmitters, heavy metals, Oncogen C-fos (AB2), etc. of intracellular fine structures of normal and abnormal single cells using light or electro-microscopic indirect Bi-Digital O-Ring Test. Acupunct Electrother Res 1992; 17(1): 29-46. [http://dx.doi.org/10.3727/036012992816357855] [PMID: 1351338]

[39] Shinnick P. The application of the bi-digital o-ring imaging test to toxic organ meridian and clinical medicine. Med Acupunct 2003; 14(3)

[40] Shinnick P. An Introduction to the basic technique and theory of omura's bi-digital o-ring test. Am J Acupunct 1996; 24(2 & 3)

[41] Shinnick P. Electro-magnetic Resonance: the Discovery and Use of the Omura o-ring Test (Bi-digital O-ring test); Implications for Traditional Chinese Medicine and the Meridian System, 400 Clinical Case Study and Important Omura Discoveries for Medicine and Science. Proceedings at the Second Whole Person Healing Summit and Second Qigong Summit 14-17th April. Washington D.C. 2005.

[42] Shinnick P, Borgna A. Electro-magnetic Resonance: The Origin and Discovery of the Omura O-ring Test (Bi-digital O-ring test), Which is a Non-invasive, Inexpensive Diagnostic Tool for Medicine; Important Omura Discoveries for Medicine and Science. Proceedings of the Material Research and Living Systems. Boston. 2004.

[43] Shinnick P, Blumenthal C. Application of the bi-digital o-ring test imaging method for acupunctur and electro-therapeutics in rehabilitation medicine. Abstracts of International Symposium of Acupunct Electrother Res. 13(4): 248.

[44] Shinnick P, Borgna B. Electro-magnetic Resonance Phenomenon: the Bi-digital O-ring imaging test; a non-invasive, inexpensive diagnostic method applied to medicine and science. Proceedings of the Society for Scientific Exploration. 22nd Meeting: Kalispell, Montana

[45] Alavi A, LaRiccia P, Sadek J, Newberg AH. Neuroimaging of acupuncture in patients with chronic pain. J Altern Med 1997; 3 (Suppl. I): 47S-53S.

[46] Pontinen PJ. Low level laser therapy as a medical treatment modality. Tampere: Art Urpo LTD 1992.

[47] Shinnick P, Omura Y. Difference in the location of finger placement on the radial artery for pulse diagnosis in the Orient; and, 15th to 18th century Occidental rare books on pulse diagnosis. Acupunct Electrother Res 1985; 10(4): 309-24.
[http://dx.doi.org/10.3727/036012985816714342] [PMID: 2871702]

[48] Shinnick P. Editorial: on contradictions between chinese and tibetan pulse diagnosis. J Altern Complement Med 2012; 18: 10.
[http://dx.doi.org/10.1089/acm.2012.1501] [PMID: 22236029]

[49] Nogier PMF. Handbook to auriculotherapy. auriculotherapy, electro-therapy association. Tulsa Oklahoma.: Acu Medic Centre London. 1969.

[50] Lacey J. Psychological approaches to the evaluation of psychotherapeutics process and outcome Research in Psychotherapy. Washington, D.C.: American Psychological Association 1958.

[51] Bykov KM, Vladimirov GY, Delov VY, Konradi GP, Slonim AD. Textbook of physiology. Moscow: Foreign Lan Pub 1958.

[52] a) Freed S. Possible physiological basis for effectiveness of acupuncture against psychological disorders. Acupunct Electrother Res 1987; 1(12): 113-123; b) Freed S, Acupuncture as therapy of traumatic affective disorder and of phantom limb syndrome. Acupunct Electrother Ther Res 1989; 14: 121-9.
[http://dx.doi.org/10.3727/036012989816358452]

[53] Rubik B. Life on the Edge of Science. Light from Organisms. Institute for Frontier Science; 1996: Oakland Ca: p.119-127. Rubik, B. Does short-term exposure to cell phone radiation affect the blood? Wise. Trad Food Farm Heal Arts 2014; 15(4): 19-28.

[54] Rubik B. Does short-term exposure to cell phone radiation affect the blood?. Wise Trad Food Farm Heal Arts 2014; 15(4): 19-28.

[55] Omura Y, Losco M. Electro-magnetic fields in the home environment (color TV, computer monitor, microwave oven, cellular phone, etc) as potential contributing factors for the induction of oncogen C-fos Ab1, oncogen C-fos Ab2, integrin α 5 β 1 and development of cancer, as well as effects of microwave on amino acid composition of food and living human brain. Acupunct Electrother Res 1993; 18(1): 33-73.
[http://dx.doi.org/10.3727/036012993816357601] [PMID: 7684553]

[56] Tiller W. Science and human transformation subtle energy, intentionality, and human transformation. California: Pavior Publishing 1997.

CHAPTER 3

Parallel Properties of Oneness in the Most Stable Inorganic and Organic States

Abstract: Enlightenment, physiological state of supreme Quiet, results abruptly from the Meditational state through unitization of fragmented physiology of ordinary man. Meditation has given long absorbing attention to actualities of the present moment. Subsequently Enlightened, all perceptions are of the total present, made possible by complete unresponsiveness to conditioned stimuli that had habitually reactivated residues of suffering. Tranquillity follows spontaneously, so does appropriate behavior, yet appearing "strange" to ordinary fragmented man. Despite extreme scientific disparities, a system parallel abstractly to Enlightenment appears abruptly at 2.17° Absolute, as superfluid in helium, ^4He II, a quantum liquid. Its background noise is virtually zero, its viscosity is zero; it flows without differences in pressure. Its strangeness transcends commonly-held dualities of opposites as does Enlightenment. Macroscopic motion is inherent in its most stable stationary quantum state paralleling most stable physiologic state of living man, when Enlightened. Is this existential energy of motion Qi, the 'life energy' of Chinese tradition?

Keywords : Conditioned stimuli, Enlightenment, Macromolecule, Non-reactivity, Now awareness, Parallelism, Physiologic state, Reactivity, Spontaneous synchronization, Stable stationary states, Superfluid helium, Transcends duality, Tranquility, Unresponsiveness.

INTRODUCTION

In the last chapter, we talked about organic and inorganic aspect of PEMF, pulsed electromagnetic fields which included photonic energy from light. This was not all inclusive since the purpose was not to study all aspects in detail, but only those aspects relating to self healing. In the same way we included Chinese medicine, acupuncture and electroacupuncture in our discussion, we now turn to Japanese methods of meditation namely Zazen. This is an involuntary method of meditation where you do not move, keeping the spine straight and becoming unfocused. This is similar to sitting on top of a walled in city watching below as people come and

Phillip Shinnick & Laurence Porter

go but not following them into or out of the city with curiosity. The advanced state is Fig. (**1**).

Fig. (1). The Vacuity. LP. 2009. (Special Permission of Laurence Porter).

We have shown the evolution of organic and inorganic science in PEMF. Now we want to manipulate temperature in the inorganic state of a gas since Nature seems to like low temperature away from the agitation of heat. In this chapter we will show how manipulation of temperature to near absolute changes the physics of this gas to a macromolecule which defies physical laws. In an organic being, the deepest states of meditation, the most stable (Bose-Einstein state) also create conditions which are not normal for ordinary humans. We present a parallelism between these two states which give us an understanding of Oneness in these inorganic and organic states. In this chapter we venture to discuss organic physiologic state of Ch'an (or Zen) Buddhism at its culmination, the awakening of Enlightenment. Also we present the shared properties of Enlightenment and quantum superfluid helium ^{4}HE II and juxtaposition parallel properties of Enlightenment and helium ^{4}HE II [1].

Enlightenment, physiological state of supreme Quiet, results *abruptly* from the Meditational state through unitization of fragmented physiology of ordinary man

(Fig. **1**). Meditation has given long absorbing attention to actualities of the present moment. Subsequently Enlightened, all perceptions are of the total present, made possible by complete unresponsiveness to conditioned stimuli that had habitually reactivated residues of suffering. Tranquillity follows spontaneously, so does appropriate behavior, yet appearing "strange" to ordinary fragmented man. Despite extreme scientific disparities, a system parallel to Enlightenment appears abruptly at 2.17° Absolute, as superfluid in helium, ^{4}He II, a quantum liquid. Its background noise is virtually zero, its viscosity is zero; it flows without differences in pressure. Its strangeness transcends commonly-held dualities of opposites as does Enlightenment. Macroscopic motion is inherent in its most stable stationary quantum state paralleling most stable physiologic state of living man, when enlightened. Is this existential energy of motion Qi, the 'life energy' of Chinese tradition?

PHYSIOLOGIC STATE OF ENLIGHTENMENT

According to Hui-neng (China, 637-713 A.D.) associated eminently with Ch'an Buddhism. Enlightenment is authentic only when initiated (awakened) spontaneously in a sudden unforeseeable experience. It is preceded by long practice in Meditation entered abruptly from ordinary life. We also think the opposite can occur; an abrupt awakening without long periods of meditation for example, in Hindu Shakti Pa from the Siddha Master [2].

A Master meditator's consumption of oxygen and blood lactate is characterized by an abrupt drop [3] (Fig. **2**). The low level of consumption remains flat, felt by the Meditator as a sustained Quiet. The unchanging consumption of oxygen suggests a prevailing single physiologic state. The low noise-level of the physiologic activities during this Quiet is viewed as of primary significance in the discussion that follows. It is taken to express exceptional coherence in structure and activity throughout the body-mind. We shall return to this in the discussion of the electroencephalograms of Meditators.

The goal of Meditation is Enlightenment. Its nature is intimated by Herrigel in the following quotation: "For the Zen Buddhist, everything that exists apart from man animals and plants, stones, earth, air, fire, and water exists demandingly from the center of being without having left it. For a Zen, he must not become as a little child but like forest and rock, like flower and fruit, like wind and storm. In the East this reversal (to the center) and homecoming is not left to chance, the approach can be prepared and methodically followed, above all, in Japan" [4]. The center becomes accessible spontaneously upon removal of the classically recognized obstacles: ignorance, delusions, and fears. They have fragmented man's perceptions, behavior, and correspondingly, his physiology. Obstacles surface in his Meditations. There, in the process of the Quiet they are changed to less threatening form and finally depart. The resulting void finally permits the spontaneous unification of the fragments.

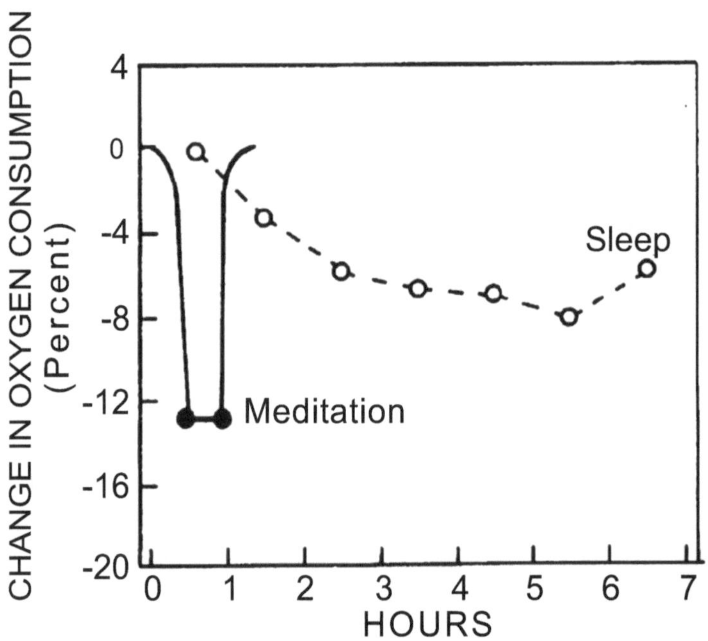

Fig. (2). Comparison of oxygen consumption during Meditation and during sleep (after Benson, 1975) with some modification at beginning and end of Meditation. (With special permission of Genevieve Hogan ISSSEEM).

Meditation is subject to many variations, personal and cultural. Most Meditations have one feature in common, total mindfulness of actualities of the present moment. Mindfulness was regarded by the Buddha as essential for effective Meditation. It involves total absorption of attention to the actualities while the Meditator remains completely relaxed physically. A form of Meditation, the Buddha is believed to have favored, mindfulness-of-breathing is somewhat as follows: with eyes unclosed, one starts by giving total attention to regular breathing as the air enters and leaves the nostrils and impinges above the upper lip. What is attended to can be greatly enlarged. Beginners are helped in maintaining unswerving attention against spontaneous distractions by mentally counting the breaths. Mindfulness must become so completely absorbing that the Meditator is unaware of the breather. The spontaneous distractions surfacing from the unconscious were named "obstructing devils" by the Buddha, translated by the

Japanese as "makyo" - not always an overstatement. The breathing, after an interval, which becomes shorter with practice (longer at first), experiences a sudden spontaneous reduction in volume and also in rate. A distinct Quiet possesses the Meditator, a new state of consciousness is attained. Following the termination of the session, some characteristics of the quiet persist (Fig. **3**). Further-on, we shall touch upon examples of Meditation free of methodology.

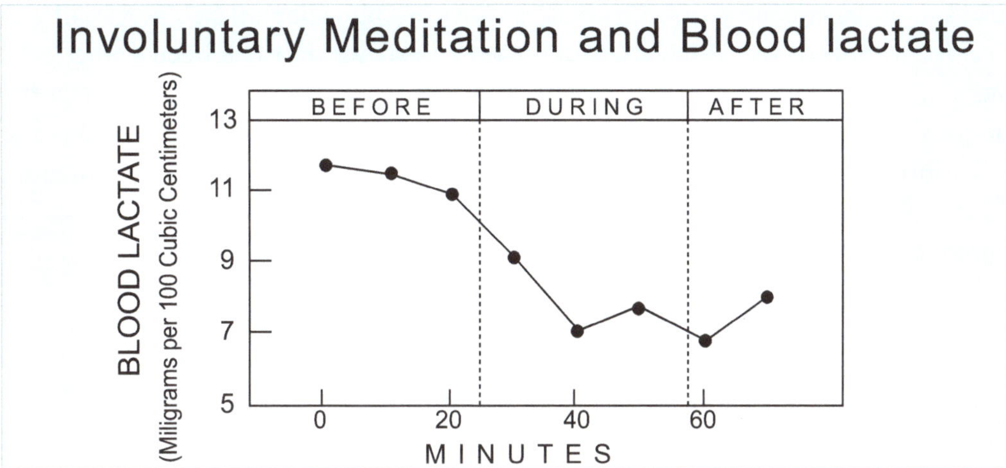

Fig. (3). Blood-lactate changes associated with Meditation. (after Benson, 1975). Before, During After the "Quiet". (With special permission of Genevieve Hogan ISSSEEM).

We take as postulate that the makyo-like obstructions, even when apparently trivial in content, occupy central importance as obstacles in the development required for reaching Enlightenment. Briefly, a major reflex of the makyo is "the I" and a major expression of the "I" is devastating emotion, noise throughout the body-mind. Makyo have been identified by Buddhists with visions, nightmares, hallucination, as distorted forms in dreams of events in childhood. Of course, these occupy central roles in Western psychiatry. The attitude toward them differs fundamentally in the Orient. During Meditation these phantasms are not to be dwelled upon, "interpreted". Instead they are, if possible, a struggle between forces of light and darkness [4]. This attitude leads in the course of Meditation to a reduction in the intensity and number of the makyo and conversely progress in unification.

What proves to have particular physiologic significance in the transition to the Quiet is the spontaneous appearance of prominent alpha rhythm in the electroencephalogram (EEG) of the Meditators. For controls, we first observe the EEG of ordinary man depicted schematically [5, 6] (Fig. **4**). Upper right is the resting EEG of these subjects with eyes closed, giving the alpha rhythm (about ten cycles per second) which disappears when eyes are opened. A very weak sensory stimulus, a faint noise, quickly (within 0.3 second) fragments the singly rhythm into superposition of many having low amplitudes. The "homogeneous brain field", at left of 'quiet wakefulness' is fragmented by the noise into components, a b, c, d, e (below), independent rhythms, ascribed by Lindsley to separate neural aggregates. He suggested that at desynchronization, neural elements in aggregates function independently as information-processing channels. The swift de synchronization of the alpha rhythm by very weak stimuli has been named, the 'alarm reaction'. This simple representation is not, of course, intended to cover the complex neuronal activities of alarm. This emotional surge of widespread nerve excitation jams information-channels, distorts communication into incoherent snatches, and renders neuronic messages indecipherable by the brain. In consequence responses that follow may be grossly inappropriate.

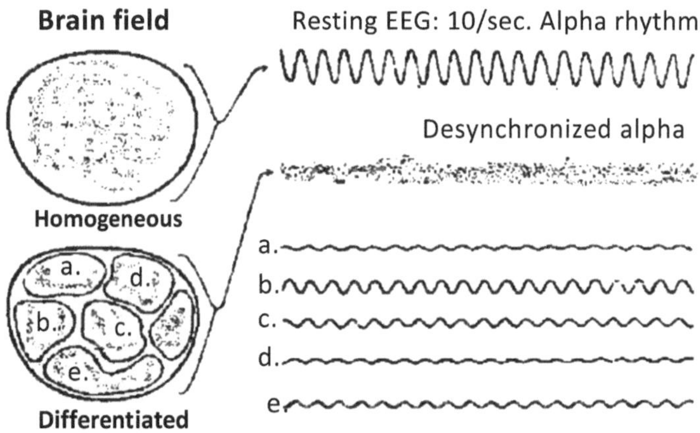

Fig. (4). Idealization: alpha rhythm of EEG in state of "relaxed wakefulness" and its desynchronization (After Lindsley, 1961 and Pribram, 1971). (With special permission of Genevieve Hogan ISSSEEM).

On the other hand, the alpha rhythm of the Meditators with eyes unclosed, under even stronger sensory stimulation, suffers no fragmentation and remains unresponsive to what ordinarily excites alarm. The homogeneous brain field is stabilized by the Oneness holding in Meditation. In contrast to ordinary man, Meditators despite stress, arrive at the "unification and tranquillity of mind", rather than the body-mind according to the unifying conception of Buddhists [7]. This tranquil state shows little disturbance in its alpha rhythm with its low level of background noise.

Bases for these observations is amply provided by studies of EEG of Zen Meditators [8]. Strong metallic clicks merely interrupted but did not shatter their alpha rhythms. Responses to the last click of a succession was as fresh as to the first in contrast to that of ordinary control subjects who became habituated, unresponsive to further clicks. Among Meditators no indications were evident of any residual influence of earlier clicks were evident. Only the present click, the Buddhist Now, was perceptible to the Meditators.

After several years in the practice of Meditation, a further sudden transition occurs spontaneously, the awakening of Enlightenment (Samadhi, Satori); in Chinese, Giu Xing, awakening of clarity- liberation from noise, confusion. Meditators have agreed; that they have experienced unification into a coherent Oneness (Fig. **5**). Similarly, experience through totally different modes of Meditation by mystics of the Middle Ages was perceived as profound unitization [9]. The level of background noise of this supreme Quiet makes possible super-vivid perception of faint signals and finer distinction between closely similar ones. This maximal sensitivity in the reception of information may reflect increased coherence through molecular relocation and reorientation within the former fragments. Thus a virtually homogeneous field of Quiet permitting a super-flow of clear information would be created globally.

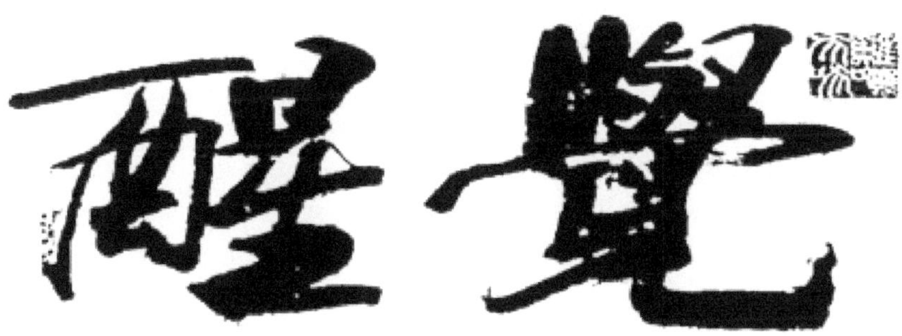

Fig. (5). Giu Xing-Awakening to clarity. (With special permission of B.M. Hegda).

Electro-encephalograms of the Zen masters are consistent with this approach. Particularly revealing and appropriate are simple statements of their experience: "The Zen masters more clearly perceived each stimulus than in their ordinary waking state. In this (quiet) state they cannot be affected by either external or internal stimulus, nevertheless they are able to respond to it and yet are never disturbed by it. Each stimulus is accepted as stimulus itself and is treated as such. One Zen master described such a state of mind as that of noticing each person one sees on the street but not looking back with emotional curiosity" [10].

The Zen masters "more clearly perceived each stimulus than in their ordinary waking state" since it was not blurred by the lower level of background noise during the state of Enlightenment or during the Quiet of Meditation. In their ordinary waking state the noise-level of background is especially high when the original neutral (such as visual) signal had been conditioned to represent an emotionally charged conditioned stimulus. A Zen master cannot be emotionally disturbed or "affected by either external or internal stimulus" since it had been conditioned in the past. An unconditioned component of the conditioned stimulus would not be responded to in the ever present Now of Enlightenment. Thus the conditioned stimulus had been deconditioned through the unresponsiveness. The master is therefore never disturbed by coupling of a chance neutral stimulus with a noisy emotional stimulus. This feature is confirmed by the last remark. The master "notices each person on the street but he does not look back with emotional curiosity". The visual signal he noticed was no longer conditioned as ordinarily to evoke the emotions and noise of unconditioned stimuli of the past.

ATTENTION TO THE PRESENT: LEARNING AND EMOTION

We have then empirical evidence that long practice in Meditation (when total attention is given to actualities of the present moment) had created awareness exclusively of the present, the Now. This state of awareness is made possible through the concurrently created unresponsiveness to conditioned stimuli.

Perceiving and responding only in the Now, how does the ideal Meditator learn or acquire information? The usual answer is, by observation in the momentary present free of specific earlier stimulation, without time - requiring processes of association. Let me quote a wish frequently expressed, "Perhaps we can break the power of thought and become free once again as we were at one time in our childhood before thought began to exercise its tyranny over us" [11].

How does the infant, the neonate, perceive and learn? According to contemporary studies, it is precisely by momentary observation uninfluenced by pedagogic preparation or effort. Rather, the neonate acquires information by assimilation into the totality of his development [12]. Similarly the eighteen month old learns to speak single words, pairs of words *etc.* Consequently learning as well as responses with what he has learned involves a measure of Oneness and may be regarded as *spontaneous and creative.* Because of similarities in behavior, we infer that ideal Meditation and Enlightenment provide conditions for "becoming free again as we were before thought began to exercise its tyranny over us".

Let us consider the destructive emotions: hate, fear, anger, envy, *etc*. They cannot be removed by opposing them with their opposites. They can be removed only by being brought to zero intensity. Krishnamurti, 1984 appeals not to distance oneself from them but to come ever closer. Observe oneself unrelentingly for the smallest sign of hate (for example) in all one's activities, no matter how irrelevant they may appear. "Pay total attention to uncover component of hate. In a sense you are possessed by hate, you are hate". Mindfulness in all aspects of the hate may lead if one is fortunately determined enough, to an equivalent of Meditation. Finally a Quiet descends, unresponsiveness to the conditioned stimuli involved takes over. The habitual reminding-stimuli, near-replicas of those that had surrounded the formation of the hate cease fueling the obsession. They are brought to zero. The door is actually open to love and instances are known for the complete reversal to occur.

Table I. Parallel properties juxtaposed (Extremely Low Noise-Levels).

Enlightenment	**Superfluid of Helium ^{4}He II**
Ordinary Temperature	**Below 1.2° A**
The extremely low noise-level of the Oneness (Enlightenment)is postulated as provided by optimal physiologic coherence. It would result from molecular structures in 'functional contact' extending to distant regions. Intrinsic motion within an active physiological state may be taken as axiomatic.	At virtually zero noise-level holding at lowest temperatures, oneness is uniquely expressed by the superfluid in ^{4}He II. It consists of macro-quantity of identical helium atoms occupying the single macro-cell of lowest energy in Bose-Einstein statistics. This the theoretical 'condensate' quantum liquid, possessing superfluity coherent and homogeneous, made so by collision and diffusion because of zero-point energy or operation of the Heisenberg uncertainty principle. Identification of the superfluid with the condensate has been amply authenticated experimentally [17]. The superfluid has no viscosity and its motion is intrinsic, requiring no difference in pressure. The motion constitutes a characteristic of the 'stationary quantum state' of the macro-wave function.
Transitions from the Meditational state to the awakening of Enlightenment occurs spontaneously and abruptly. Enlightenment becomes more coherent, subject to less spontaneous distraction the less the noise-level of background. Having been created in long practice through total attention exclusively to the present moment, Enlightenment limits awareness and responses exclusively to facts and events of the present, the classical NOW.	Therefore, superfluity transcend the duality: stationary/mobile. Spontaneous, abrupt transition at 2.17 ° A (the lambda $T_¡$ point) initiates (awakens) appearance of the superfluid component of ^{4}Helium II. The fraction of superfluid component in ^{4}He II grows with the decrease in thermal agitation becoming approximately 100% below 1.2 °A [17]. The superfluid because of its zero viscosity. Its inner super-mobility retains no structural impress from the past. Time is ever the present, the NOW.
Entire body-mind in state of Oneness possesses swift homeostasis--self therapy.	Any disturbance instantly permeates the entire superfluid. Its Oneness and restoration to homogeneity is also instantaneous. Homeostasis extends quickly over total system.

(Table 1) contd.....

Enlightenment	Superfluid of Helium ^{4}He II
Ordinary Temperature	**Below 1.2° A**
An instance of super flow of information in considered in the main portion of this essay. It becomes apparent in the sketched confrontation in Swordsmanship between a professional swordsman and an Enlightenment Buddhist. The superflow and quality of information mediated in the Enlightened state accounts for the Buddhist's superior Swordsmanship.	Compared with the flow of information above 1.2°A, super flow of information occurs below 1.2 °A in the superfluid. It would arise from a reduction in resistance to its transmission because of freedom from conflict of dualities, freedom from constraints such as narrow channels leading to receptors of the information.
Through unitization, Enlightened man transcends dualities (of opposite, of contradictions). It may take the form of unresponsiveness to the constraints, obstacles of ordinary man. Such unitization may appear as identification. When a bird sings, the enlightened Buddhist may sing with all his being. (Fowler, 1975) When above the peaks of the Himalayas, eagles soar, the Tibetan Buddhist soars with all his being. Far below are deep valleys. His swift effortless stride is leveraged from a mere touch of the earth. When he leaps at the sight of birds his whole being flies with them. Such a vivid experience has long been regarded by Buddhists as reality, direct realization of the truth. Similar realities have been experienced numberless times in different cultures by Enlightened man. We see them as confirmation among experience, clearly very different in nature from quantitative confirmation of events in space and time of science.	Unitization of fragments, here of helium atoms into a single quantum fluid and unification of dualities are also expressed in the behavior of the superfluid. An example is "siphoning-in reverse" which is spontaneously performed when an empty vessel is partially lowered into a superfluid with its rim markedly above the superfluid level. The outer wall becomes covered with a thick film of superfluid that moves over the rim to fill the vessel up to the same level that holds on the outside. Here the duality, inside/outside is transcended (ignored) likewise the duality, up/down. Another example where ordinary barriers to unification of spaces are overcome is the superflow of ^{4}He II through micro-channels of a vessel's walls so narrow as to block the flow of ordinary liquid helium above the lambda point, 2.17 °A. They strongly impede the flow of gaseous helium below 2.17 °A.
Clearly, one is inclined to transcribe the quotation on the right as a transition from ordinary agitated behavior to the behavior during Enlightenment, the Quiet without agitation.	The content of some "strange" behavior in superfluity may have behavioral correspondence in Enlightenment. "Observation of the liquid helium at the instant that its temperature is reduced below 2.17° A, reveals a remarkable alteration in its appearance. Liquid helium, He, is maintained below 4.2 ° A by lowering the vapor pressure so that boiling occurs under reduced pressure. Above 2.17° A bubbles of vapor form within the bulk of the liquid in the customary way and the whole liquid is evidently agitated as these rise to the free surface and escape. On the other hand, as soon as the transition point, $T_¡$ is reached the liquid becomes quite still and no more bubble are formed" [13].

The courageous all-out encounter with the hateful self is the creativity of Jiddu Krishnamurti [14]. The spontaneous direct action of his total attention makes unnecessary the classically prescribed methodologies of Buddhist Meditation.

Assimilated in the Now of Enlightenment are transcended duality between opposites or between contradictions as ordinarily accepted. Each member of the duality such as good-bad, subject-object, inside-outside, common sense-nonsense, expresses conclusions reached through habit or conditioning. What is left of the time-bound duality in consciousness is a generalization that the members have in common. The noise-level of the background generated by the generalization now free of conflict is lower than what ordinarily accompanies the separate members. Through its unresponsiveness, Oneness and Enlightenment have been maintained. Having negated potential resistance (noise) from conflicting duality, Enlightenment with its swiftness and precision of responses and its virtual "functional contact" of molecular structure may well be uniquely effective in a super-flow of clear information.

Factors erasing destructive emotions are liberating also in other circumstance. In the following they are expressed as spontaneous super-flow of information.

MASTER *VERSUS* TECHNICIAN

Swordsmanship of Zen masters several centuries ago surpassed what was displayed by the most skilled professionals in this dangerous sport [15]. The professional had learned his art and critical techniques from famous teachers. On the other hand, the Zen master as always gave "all absorbing attention to the actualities of the present moment" and thereby had attained all-important mindfulness. He acted from a Quiet in total body-mind creatively, effortlessly, without awareness of self. The professional's activity was essentially a performance of the habitual self, disturbed by the lightening, unprecedented strokes of the master's blade. Fearful of being cut to pieces, uneasily he faces the master who with undisturbed perception had instant, clear information of the initiation of his opponent's next move. This information without distortion in the prevailing low noise-level of background was transmitted swiftly and effectively to the unitized decision-making and responding physiology.

SYSTEM OF UNITY: SHARED AND PARALLEL PROPERTIES

Are there other systems with abrupt transitions from fragmentary states to a Oneness marked at its appearance with extremely low noise-level of background, with wide deviations from ordinary properties, "strangely" different from the familiar ones holding before the transition? One such parallel system presents itself despite that it is 'worlds-apart' in conventional science. However to those unitized into Oneness who see all nature as ONE un-analytically, un-fragmented. The proposed parallel is not disturbing but rather added evidence of the universal ONE.

SHARED PROPERTIES OF ONENESS

Enlightenment and the quantum superfluid of Helium ^{4}He II share the following properties:

1. State of Oneness of high stability and coherence
2. Extremely low noise-level.
3. Result from abrupt transition between states.
4. Active solely in the present, the NOW free of reactivation from the past, free of memory
5. Transcend duality between opposites.
6. Respond as Oneness and appropriately to stimuli and pressures.
7. Transmit information of exceptional clarity.
8. Display behavior to 'ordinary' man as "strange", generally expressing liberation from ordinary constraints.
9. Basic states (at 'zero' noise levels) consist inherently of both stationary and moving aspects.

Is this basic existential energy of Enlightenment identifiable with Qi, the "life energy" of Chinese tradition?

The listed basic properties shared by Enlightenment and the quantum superfluid of helium, ^{4}He 11 below 1.2 ° Absolute are listed below. Following the list more specific characterization is presented in two columns of juxtaposed correspondences.

REFERENCES

[1] Freed S. Chemical-biochemical signal and noise. 21st Annual Meeting University of Virginia. 576-84. Freed S, Induced specific immunological unresponsiveness and conditioned behavior reflexes in functional isomorphism-meditation and specific unresponsiveness. Inter J of Neuroscience; 1988: 44 275-283. Shinnick P, Freed S, Life energy in physiologic states of chan (or Zen) Buddhism and inorganic analogous states of superfluid helium liquid. JSHO; 2011: 3:12. Shinnick, P. Parallelism between physiology state of enlightenment and Analogous inorganic states. Presented at the Society for Scientific Exploration, 21st Annual Meeting University of Virginia, May 30, 2002.

[2] Blofeld J. The zen teaching of huang po. New York: Grove Press, Inc. 1958.

[3] Benson H. The relaxation response. New York: William Morrow & Co 1975.

[4] Herrigel E. The method of zen. London: Routledge and Kegan Paul 1960.

[5] Lindsley DB. The reticular activation system and perception integration. In: Sheer D, Ed. Electrical Stimulation of the Brain. Austin: University of Texas Press 1961.

[6] Pribram KH. Language of the brain. Englewood Cliffs, New Jersey: Prentice-Hall 1971.

[7] Kapleau RP. The three pillars of zen. New York: Anchor Books Doubleday 1989.

[8] Kasamatsu A, Hirai T. An electroencephalographic study on the zen meditation (Zazen). Folia Psychiatr Neurol Jpn 1966; 20(4): 315-36.
[PMID: 6013341]

[9] Underhill E. Mysticism. New York: E.P. Dutton 1961.

[10] Kasamatsu A, Hirai T. An electroencephalographic study on the zen meditation (Zazen). Folia Psychiatr Neurol Jpn 1966; 20(4): 315-36.
[PMID: 6013341]

[11] Fowler J. Stages of faith: the psychology of human development and the quest for meaning. New York: Harper Row 1981.

[12] Fantz RL. Early behavior development approaches. New York: John Wiley & Son 1967.

[13] Tilley DR, Tilley J. Superfluidity and superconductivity. 3rd edition., New York: Adam Hilger 1990.

[14] Krishnamurti J. The flame of attention. San Francisco: Harper & Row 1984.

[15] Suzuki ST. Zen and Japanese culture. Princeton: Princeton University Press 1959.

CHAPTER 4

A Meditation on Meditation for Beginners: A Creative Odyssey from Years of Practice

Abstract: This chapter is written for beginners in meditation. Using an experiential approach, it exploring a variety of meditation concepts, which include the time of day one meditates, colors or vibrations one might experience and breathing techniques, such as alternate nostril breathing and fetal breathing. The author explores a meditation technique that helps one be able to perform under stress and tailors it for various mind/body/spirit disorders and conditions. He also shares the meditation techniques he developed during his 10 years of experience as a world class athlete.

Keywords : Beginning meditation, Behavior, Body/mind/spirit, Brain blood-flow, Breath, Color, Depression, Disease, Earth vibration, Entropy, Expanded awareness, Hysteria, Organic/inorganic, Immune response, Interceptors, Jaw relaxation, Lungs, Micro reductionist, Non recognition, Number awareness, Olympic team, Oneness, One-pointedness, Siddha yoga, Subject object, Vibration, Weight lifting.

A PERSONAL INTRODUCTION TO MEDITATION

When I asked a lay person to read this chapter on meditation, his question for me was, "How did you get there?" Let's find out.

Starting as a teenager -- and through my 20's -- my world revolved around athletics. From being a star football, basketball and track & field athlete in high school to competing in several Olympic games, I spent more than a decade achieving many successes as an international athlete. While most spectators might believe that world class athletes are in glowing health, the fact is I was constantly experiencing debilitating injuries that impacted negatively on the quality of my day to day life and on my ability to perform on the playing field.

In meditation, when we close our eyes and focus on the center of this space, we are brought to our third eye. Focusing on that point can manifest an eye looking at

Phillip Shinnick & Laurence Porter

us. The eye might become a bird, which emerges from space, transforms itself from no form into form, then returns to no form (Fig. **1**).

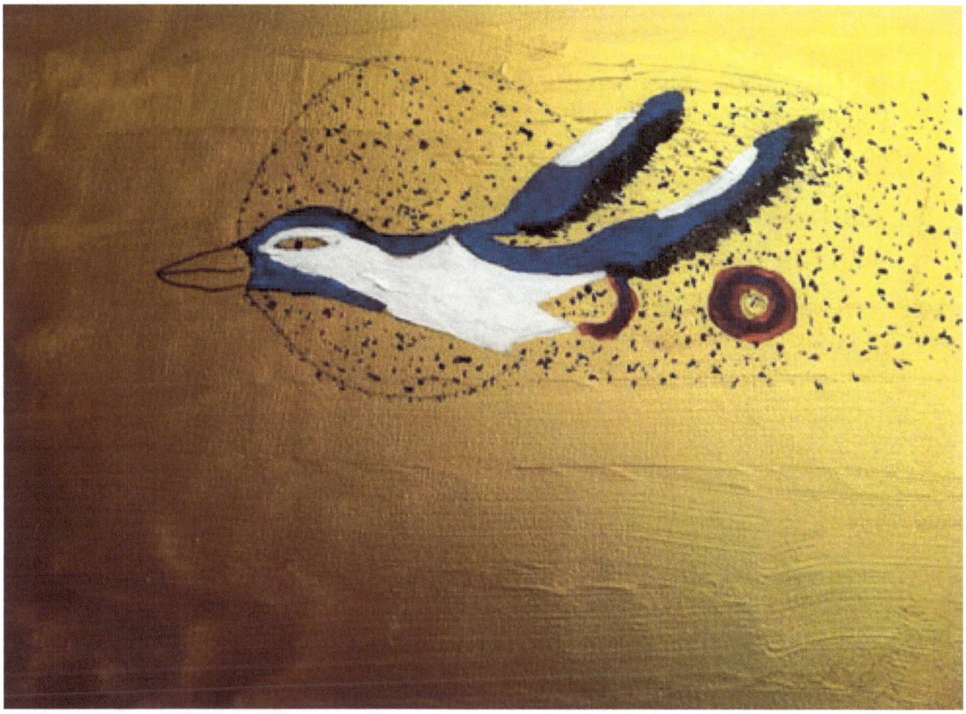

Fig. (1). No form to form. PKS 2011. (This figure is reproduced from his original painting with special permission of the artist, Phillip Shinnick).

When nursing my injuries, I would ask every friend, mentor, teacher and fellow athlete for help finding remedies for those afflicting ailments. Even the most prominent doctors and physical therapists could not offer me proper assistance in the alleviation of pain. Since I couldn't stomach drugs, and surgery seemed like a shortcut to disability, those were never viable alternatives for me.

Being in pain, I feared for my career. If I could not figure out how to heal myself properly, my quality of life would be threatened. That was when I radically changed my focus. In 1968, I totally revamped my training methods; I started going to Yoga and dance classes. What began as a desperate attempt to fix myself, became my lifelong practice of learning from research.

My unique perspective comes from years of experience as a world class athlete. I discovered that the body is not a machine, and that healthy living requires more than merely fixing mechanical problems. Our bodies are sophisticated organisms with chemical, electrical, energetic systems that require integrated forms of treatment. This radical idea is in direct opposition to the current trend of highly specialized medical practices, which rely too heavily on drugs and rush too quickly to surgery for expedient solutions.

My work and my life are one. That is a natural way of living that began with my pioneer ancestors, a family with a deep reverence for nature.

One of my grandfathers was a surgeon. When he graduated from Rush Medical School in Chicago, he got on a train to Lewiston, Idaho near Lolo Pass, the pass the Lewis and Clark expedition went through to reach the West coast. With pack mules and a horse, he rode up to Elk City in the Selkirk Mountain Range. My grandfather found miners from China, who had sailed to Portland, Oregon from Canton, mining gold, quartz and other minerals in those mountains. He settled in Grangeville, Idaho, where he founded the local hospital and had a Chinese cook.

My other grandfather was a horse rancher on the Snake River. Fleeing the snakes, he went up on the Camas prairie to raise sheep but switched to wheat when the railroad arrived. He founded the Grange Growers Association to store wheat until prices would improve. He served as head of the Fisheries and Game Department, regulating hunting and fishing in the Rocky Mountains and became a governor of Idaho. With his pack mules and horses, he would stay up in a high mountain camp and hunt elk for weeks. He took me fly fishing on the Little Salmon River there, and he once arranged for my brother and me to drive his pickup truck. We spent four days alone up in the high meadows when I was only 12 and he was 14.

By nature and by heritage I am a pioneer. Even before I made the Olympic team and traveled the world in competitions, I hitchhiked through Europe with only a knapsack at the age of 19, sleeping out in the open air under the stars every night. At 20, I went to Alaska to help build a church and hitchhiked alone, with no money, down the Alcan through the wilderness for five days. I fought forest fires in the mountains, rode round-up on ranches and worked as a farm hand doing heavy manual labor.

In the pioneer spirit, I was inspired to organize and lead a trip to China in 1976, a time when Westerners were not even allowed to be there. I travelled through Africa and Russia, crossed the Caspian and Black Seas, spent time in Eastern Europe during the Cold War and played baseball in the Nicaraguan war zone.

I have a natural impulse to protect myself from myself and from outside tragedies. My pathway into medicine came through meditation, and I dealt with my sports injuries the same way. I just rested. Once I understood how I had gotten there, I made the necessary corrections. Preserving my health through meditation or prayer started at the age of 12. I have always been aware of what I call "the other" in the universe. This other presence I find in myself as well.

During graduate school, I worked as an intern in the office of the mayor of Seattle while earning my Master's Degree in Public Affairs. It was there I met Henry Jackson, a US Senator from Washington. When I talked to him about the Vietnam war, he told me we needed the war so we could test new weapons. I wanted to be elected to Congress, to earn my fame and express my political instincts, but Henry Jackson's comments discouraged me from going in that direction. It seems Washington was just too much of an anti-communist, warmongering state for me.

When I met New York Senator Robert Kennedy in the mayor's office, we hit it off right away. Like me, he was ready to see the Vietnam war come to an end. He invited me to sit next to him on the podium when he made public speeches. It was wonderful to make a friend whose politics were similar to my own. Nevertheless, I lost my political interest in getting elected since Washington's politics were more like Jackson's than they were like Kennedy's. That's when I made the commitment to fight for social justice rather than pursue personal ambition. When Kennedy was assassinated, I moved even further away from public life and more toward being an organizer for peace and justice. I never looked back.

While writing a paper on the unconscious for a graduate course in psychology, I had an intellectual epiphany. Doing a philosophical historical analysis, I found that "will" was a factor in understanding unconscious impulses and behaviors. The two other factors were knowledge and action. Will manifests itself at the beginning of any action or process and channels knowledge into action, causing changes in behavior. Once I understood this, it changed me radically. Knowing there is the possibility of uncovering my deepest impulses is still compelling to me. When I calm my mind and create an environment without static, I hear things other than my own ego. That is when my inner self and the outer universe are exposed to my consciousness, and I am able to perceive more information. Years later, I realized that Abhinavagupta, the 11th century Indian philosopher, had already expressed my discovery so beautifully when he stated that any action of any being is subject to three fundamental energies: the energy of will, the energy of knowledge, the energy of action.

Doing my scientific inquiry and research does not require a grant or anyone's approval. I do it with the understanding that possibly nothing may come of it. I have little interest in the outcome. I just do what feels natural to me. It has sometimes taken 20 years for my work to have exposure. It is accepted only when the time is right. When others see value in my work, they help me. Since my work flows from my own natural impulses, it is mostly easy for me to do. This is who I am. In Kung Fu we say that the mind is a drunken monkey not to be trusted. The three natural expressions of Kung Fu are the Warrior, where I fight for justice and offer protection, the Scholar, which is the work I enjoy doing and the Monk, my love for meditation. I find great comfort in living these ancient ways that fit me so well.

A BASIC PHILOSOPHICAL APPROACH

Scientific work today must include the best information that can be gleaned from all branches of Eastern and Western knowledge. It is imperative that we develop the connections between our body/spirit Self and the outer world of organic matter, inorganic matter, space and energy.

To connect our lives to the universe, we will have to subjectively and objectively incorporate our personal experiences into whatever work we are doing. In this book, personal experience is always intertwined with the research and experimentation that is presented. According to Quantum physics, the observer and the instrument used by the observer cannot be separated from the experiment. They all merge into one totality. Therefore each of us affects reality. Meditation is a useful tool to reconcile how we perceive the world and how we experience the reality of the outer world. It is a bridge between the objective and the subjective. It helps us to see that duality is an illusion. When we misperceive duality as the reality, we are seeing the world in black and white, and we lose the true depth of the Oneness of reality.

A micro reductionist approach relies upon numbers, technology, and technical diagnosis. It makes no attempt to understand or solve the problems of disease and suffering. By observing our own physiology and our own behavior patterns, we will come to understand how to modify our behaviors, and we will learn how to help ourselves. It is urgent that we make necessary changes in our behavior if we intend to survive.

Our meditation practice will eventually connect us to the Oneness of all phenomena. My early years were spent discovering my body/mind/spirit connection. I challenged others to become more conscious of themselves, to explore the strength and enrichment we receive by connecting with natural forces. Let us begin this part of our adventure with a close look at the breath.

BEGINNING WITH THE ESSENTIALS: THE BREATH FOR BEGINNERS . . . APHORISMS ON MEDITATION

Having meditated for most of my life, I have often been asked what meditation is, what I do, how it applies to my life and where it fits into science. There is no short answer to any of these questions.

To be a success in sports, in intellectual work, in organizing activities -- for almost any endeavor at all -- a clear head, a relaxed body and one-pointed attention are essential.

I first experienced breathing meditation in South Lake Tahoe at 8,000 feet while training for the 1968 Olympics. In 1963, I broke the world's long jump record and qualified for the 1964 Olympic team. Because we competed in a rainstorm on a muddy runway, I was unable to hit the take-off board. Now I was being given a second chance to succeed. If I could make it to the 1968 Olympic finals, I felt confident about doing well. The US Olympic committee hired a consultant to help athletes deal better with lower air pressure and oxygen levels while we trained at a high altitude. Participating in this meet was the only way one had a chance to be selected for the Olympic team that year. Our consultant had taught techniques to emphysema patients that had improved their breathing capacity. From him I learned to lower my level of stress with long exhalations and by relaxing my mind.

The essence of meditation is comprised of the movement of the breath, of the mind, of the body, the use of will and opening ourselves to the space beyond sense stimulation.

Since it happens automatically, we are usually not even aware of our breathing. Conscious breathing -- becoming aware of the breath -- is a first step when we begin to meditate. It is good practice to become aware of the movement of the breath through meditation. This awareness can help us reduce stress, which constricts our lungs. The oxygen we inhale is pumped by the heart into the bloodstream. It circulates throughout the body, bringing healthy energy and a vitality that is the source of aliveness in the body. The synchronization between the heart and the lungs is a wonderful example of the life process.

When we pay attention to the breath, we might realize that our breathing is limited mainly to the chest. If we pay closer attention we will notice that the breath really starts in the lower abdomen. By placing our hands just below the navel, it helps us feel the movement of the breath there. This is where our energy reservoir resides.

When our focus is placed there, we are in the actual experience, no longer in our head. This center is where we ground ourselves in all the forces of the universe. After breathing from there for a while, we might feel heat in our hands, and throughout the body. Sometimes the hands start to tingle as we feel that charge of energy in both hands. The space between them becomes more dense and alive.

Because we breathe in and we breathe out, there is duality in the experience of breathing. To achieve one pointedness, pause between breaths. Pause before inhaling. Pause before exhaling. This practice will help alleviate some of our pain and suffering by synchronizing mind and body.

Practicing too many complicated techniques brings confusion. Although it might not feel easy to do, it helps us be more at ease with ourselves when we simplify. By thinking less, we have a clearer, more direct experience of reality [1].

Conscious breathing slows us down. When not centered in the breath, we spin too fast, and we can be thrown off, like the horses, from a merry-go-round spinning out of control. When we are centered, we are still. Then we will not be distracted by the static around us.

To sustain life, we must breathe the air and drink the water. Both interact between inner space and outer space. We breathe in. We breathe out. Drinking is an outer to inner experience. Sweating and urinating are inner to outer experiences.

Simply resting our consciousness on the upper lip is a good meditation. After focusing on the upper lip for some time, one becomes aware of the texture of the breath and its temperature. If the breath is hot, you probably need water.

Focusing on the difference in the sound between inhalation and exhalation, we become more aware of a subtle flow that connects us to a deeper perception of the life energy.

Being in a one pointed state when we pause between inhalation and exhalation opens us to another dimension. There we observe, listen and watch, but we no longer participate. This kind of focus leaves no room for thinking. Enslavement to our thoughts distracts us from perceiving our life force. This meditation synchronizes us with the outer and inner flow of reality. Practicing it requires time and patience, but it can be very rewarding. After a while, when we begin to perceive the qualities, such as the warmth, force, flow -- or resistance to flow -- of our breath, we can get helpful information about the state of our health.

That pause in the breath between the inhale and the exhale is an arc of transition, a rainbow in the empty sky. It is the pause before the space beyond duality comes alive, where change can occur. Movement and stillness dance together. We experience movement and see transition all the time: night and day, in and out, thoughts rising and falling. Movement, which comes out of stillness, is everywhere. The space between two breaths is eternity, the here and now where we can rest.

All of creation is One, yet it expresses itself through an infinite multitude of processes. They all exist for a while, but, eventually, they all come to an end. It is the transient nature of life. Our awareness of the transience can cause much pain if we desire to be immortal. It is out of our control, so it can bring fear to our heart. Over time, we learn to give up the attachment to our ego through meditation. Then it will be easier for us to accept that when we cease to breathe, breathing itself will continue to be expressed as it always has.

We know we will die. But we are in denial of death. Afraid to live fully, we reduce life down to what we think we can control. In childhood, we build defenses that are useful and necessary. As adults, we find it difficult to let go of our defenses. We harden ourselves, cutting ourselves off from the flow of life, and we create a limbo in which we are afraid to live, afraid to die. Fear causes us to tighten. Then we become less conscious of our breath, and our breath gets more mechanical.

Proper breathing techniques can be learned; they require some understanding and experience. A tight, stressed torso constricts the lungs. By raising the abdomen, the diaphragm moves more freely, allowing greater amounts of air into the lungs. Long exhalations are important to empty the lungs of used oxygen.

We need less oxygen when we are in a stable state, so during the deepest meditations, oxygen consumption drops rapidly. Quietness of the breath can be found in the transition arc, beyond the duality of the breath, revealing a fourth dimension, a state free of habituation, thoughts, bodily functions and sensation.

Fetal breathing regularizes variance in body blood pressure caused by stress and tension. In fetal breathing, the stomach relaxes on the inhalation, while the jaw relaxes on the exhalation. This breath is good for those suffering from organ stress. Extend the exhalation twice as long as the inhalation, while directing the mind toward the painful area. Wherever the mind goes, energy goes. Relaxing the jaw releases the neck and shoulders, allowing a better flow of blood to the brain through the arteries on the back of the neck and under the jaw. Poor circulation in the brain can result in hypotension, fatigue and insomnia. It is possible to have low blood pressure in the head even while high blood pressure is found in the arm. Fetal breathing reduces activity in the mind and decreases the intensity of emotions caused by trauma, anxiety, fear and pain. Drugs for high blood pressure, based on brachial or arm measurement, can have unanticipated consequences for the brain, which might be suffering from hypotension, usually produced by a stiff or spastic neck.

Alternate nostril breathing has shown me that if my left nostril is blocked, it means I am hungry, deficient in energy or digesting food. When the right nostril is clogged, it means that I am either thirsty or too hot. Living and training for many years in smoggy Los Angeles, I suffered from sinus congestion. To rectify this problem, I had a saline solution with strong antihistamines injected directly into my sinus cavity. My sinuses emptied. That worked for a while, but it did not address the underlying problem. I later discovered, through alternate nostril breathing, the problem was food. When I drank beer or ate cheese, my left sinus would get clogged. For four months after giving them up, I was resentful because I liked beer and cheese. After a while, beer tasted so awful that I stopped drinking it for many years. Today, I have no clogging in my left sinus with moderate usage. Habits are hard to break, but to have a stuffy head motivated me to find a solution. Almost three decades later, I usually wake up with a clear head. When I don't, I simply look at what I had the day before to realize the cause.

I practiced Zazen sunrise meditation for years. After a while, if I did not wake up at dawn, my meditation would start anyway, even as I slept. As soon as I woke up, I got right into position so the flow of the meditation would not be interrupted. Since then, my meditations have undergone many changes. Now I place my mind in my lower body. In yoga, my mind focused on the third eye. In Zazen, my mind did not focus at all. Sometimes, I simply watched as my breath wafted over my upper lip or entered the left nostril and went out the right one [2].

Alternate nostril breathing creates a circle that goes in two directions. A halo might appear around the head after practicing this breath for a while. Very few people can see this halo, sometimes shown around the heads of religious figures in paintings. This halo is typically found in both the Yogin Vedic and Christian traditions.

In Siddha Yoga, the emphasis is placed on inhalation and exhalation of the breath. The inhalation makes one sound, the exhalation another. This is the universal mantra: in and out. The breath goes in, then out. We see when practicing that the inside is not separated from the outside. We are in a continuous process that connects us to the vibration of the whole universe. When we become conscious of the movement of the breath, we transition from duality to Oneness.

Timeliness: When we start a meditation practice, it is best to meditate at the same time every day. Regularity helps create a good space for meditating and its results can be measured (Fig. **2**). Over time, it is essential that we watch how we react and respond to our own habits and feelings. Become mindful of things you do every day that might cause bodily damage like often carrying a heavy bag on one shoulder that will cause the body to go out of alignment after a while. Do you sleep well? How is your posture? Do you digest your food easily? How often do you find yourself feeling angry or fearful? What is the impact on you of the heat, the cold, dampness, dryness? When you answer these and many other questions, you become aware of yourself in new ways. You are beginning to bring your unconscious processes up out of the darkness into the light of your conscious awareness.

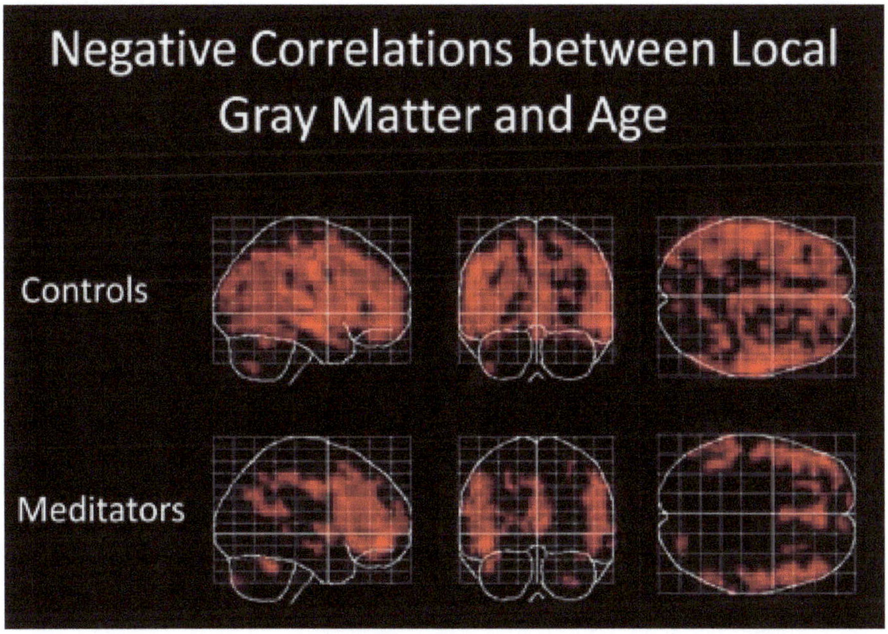

Fig. (2). More grey matter is better. One can see that with meditation there is more grey matter (fewer areas of red) [3, 4]. http://www.huffingtonpost.com/2015/02/06/meditation-brain-aging_n_6629858.html

When we examine ourselves, becoming more mindful of that which goes on inside of and around us, we come to realize that all experiences are actually processes, and processes only happen over periods of time. We need to be aware of the outer processes as well as our own inner biological responses to them. It is helpful to see the influence our mind has upon our inner reactions. As an athlete, I kept a daily diary, recording my heart rate, moods, strength, injuries, and training results. Once we develop a deeper understanding of how the body and the mind work, our meditation will have a more timeless quality.

More Awareness: We are generally as unaware of our own internal processes as we are of the outer world of reality. Meditation helps us access natural phenomena and increase our perceptions. Even before that first breathing experience I had at Lake Tahoe, I was already doing meditations that heightened my senses. Meditation helps us experience the world more creatively. Through meditation, we can find space beyond memories, beyond personal history. Meditation reveals dimensions where we might find solace. When the mind quiets down from the kinds of distractions caused by too much thinking, our fear of death and other anxieties dissolve. Instead of everything being experienced as separated in time and space, all things appear as a continuum. Life is seen from above, as if from a greater distance. In that space lies the opportunity to reside more in the here and now, no longer dwelling in the past nor projecting into the future.

Where? Meditating next to a calm lake, near a rushing river, in a forest or a park, has natural quiescence. Country people are lucky to have this experience, but these idyllic conditions are not required for good meditations. One can meditate in a dark room or a bright room -- any place will do. It is good to have a space that grounds us in our meditation. Ultimately, it is in our body and mind that the meditative state is always present. It is important that we learn to meditate wherever we find ourselves. For example, walking in a crowded city for hours can be an eye opening meditation. All rules must be abandoned.

Position: When you are ready to meditate, sit with your legs crossed in an upright position for a chosen length of time -- 10, 20 or 30 minutes. Breathe . . . relax . . . sway naturally between earth and sky, from left to right. Balancing the spine and opening the hips are necessary parts of the process. At the beginning, these practices may be painful -- particularly for men. To be in a good position with the spine erect helps us connect lower and upper energies. It also helps us stay alert. Practicing yoga will help create a more limber body and a flexible spine that will be capable of sustaining long periods of seated meditation. Standing and walking meditations are also advisable.

Mostly I meditate with my eyes closed. I stay one pointed inside myself, away from the cerebral cortex. The brain is a center for feelings. It receives signals from and reacts to the outside world. Getting out of the brain, into the lower abdomen, brings internal perception, and, slowly, the body's vibration is activated. When I meditate outdoors in a natural environment with my eyes open, I see the outer vibration.

Expanded Awareness: Meditation has shown me ways to dance with life, expand my consciousness and find creative solutions to complex problems. In the vast expanse of consciousness, suffering appears as only one of many possibilities. We can see reality from many different angles, but we never see all of it at once. We can be blind to the nature of the mind, which we see as fragmented, not whole. Suffering occurs when we focus on only one aspect of life. We contract around it as it becomes the self-created reality in which we live, but when we stay in the flow, we move from one experience to another without attaching to any of them. The sequence of these possibilities seems random, but each of us is different. Every person has her or his own sequence of pain, pleasure and suffering. Consequently, there really is no choice. We must each work with whatever is there before and within us, our own unique mixture.

Here to Stay: How do we get to our good senses? Where do we go? Our spirit will protect us from agitation, but we have to get to a quiet place where it can be heard. Our birth and creation hold us between the tension of being alive and the letting go of ourselves to embrace a deeper reality. When we are confused, let us find the way to put our mind at ease. Let us rest on the blue sky of awareness so that we can see the wonders before us. My experience shows that it takes one to two weeks of morning and afternoon practice in a contained environment for things to settle and for the void to appear.

No Formula: When we obsess over meditation, we lose its essence. Being at ease, natural, spontaneous requires presence. When we are present, we just forget about all we previously learned in order to have a direct experience of reality. We let go of that which has already passed. We let go of that which might come. We even let go of that which is happening right now. By not attempting to figure anything out, without trying to make anything happen, we can relax into ourselves and have greater clarity.

We are conditioned by the beliefs we've been taught to cherish, by the type of schooling we received, by the place where we were born and by many other factors as well. Because we see them as real, these conditionings bring us suffering. We defend our actions, our countries and our religions, which often results in violence. Our work is to free ourselves from all these conditionings so that we might see our true nature, which lies like a jewel kept deep down in darkness.

NUMBERS . . . FOR GOOD AND FOR BAD

Belief in numbers works in many ways. It can be limiting or it can be liberating. When I was in high school, I attempted to jump over a bar set at seven feet, which was the world's record in high jump at that time. Four years later, I succeeded. By then, the record had gone up to seven feet, six inches, and everyone seemed able to jump seven feet. In 1965, with the second highest jump in the US Nationals, I jumped six feet, eleven inches. In 1966 I jumped seven feet, half an inch in Seattle. When I looked up at that high bar, it seemed insurmountable. In order to reach ever higher heights, I had to overcome my fear of the bar and my fear of the number.

At the moment I planted my foot, I would freeze. My right shoulder was back, and I would let my leading leg propel me into space. That was the one pointedness I used to help me overcome my fear of the number seven feet. A performance can be severely limited by feeling fearful of or having superstitions about a measurement, a number or a height.

Judges use numbers to determine the winner of any match. The natural process of moving through space in time is compromised when there is a preoccupation with numbers. In competitive sports, beautiful movements are reduced to numbers. The most complex gymnastic moves are judged and given scores.

There is something perverse about obsessing over numbers. It can obscure a deeper appreciation for sports. Numbers tend to focus on goals. Then the goals become more important than the process. Using numbers and focusing on goals can be helpful while training and conditioning, but obsessing over numbers can distract from the beauty of the moment during competition. Thinking too much about numbers, goals or points limits performance and creates negative feelings.

Numbers played an important role during my years as a career athlete. Breaking records is based on numbers. From ancient times to the present day, sports contests might be held at dawn or dusk. They can be played to commemorate a birth, mark the memory of a death, celebrate a harvest or holiday. Events were timed to synchronize with natural cycles. Obsessing over numbers does not prepare one for unexpected circumstances. That became painfully clear to me during the 1964 Olympic games in Tokyo, when I had to face the most horrendous weather conditions. Nature caused failures that year, not losing to competitors.

Counting might be helpful when meditating. Be conscious of the breath. Pay attention to the length of the inhale and of the exhale. When treating patients, I often ask them to count to four on the inhale and to eight on the exhale. Our brain grasps numbers and intervals.

Keeping records is an ideal way to track the mind. I once did that to help improve my golf game. At one time, I was distracted by a series of events that were interfering with my life. I could not bring my mind's activity to consciousness, even with my 40 years of meditation experience. While playing golf one day, I could see that my game was way off. When I started to take a swing, thoughts would arise, causing the shot to go awry. I put a writing pad in my golf cart the next time I played, and I recorded the flashes of thought that distracted me during my swings. Thrown by the distractions, I was unable to recognize any subject. Once I started paying attention, the subject came to me in a flash. I recorded 76 distractions during one 18-hole game of golf. Out of 76 occurrences, I categorized eight subjects, all of which were troublesome for me. Now, what was most needed was patience. Once I was conscious of what was happening, the demons were easily flushed from my mind. I developed a clear strategy to deal with each subject after it appeared, and I simply let go of those that had no solution. After that, my game improved by one or two strokes per hole.

In ancient Egypt, the person who wrote down the number of bushels of grain going in and out of storage was the one in control. He held the power. Business and commerce all revolve around numbers. When numbers are off, it can lead to the loss of business, of jobs and of fortunes.

After many years of training for track, I could run 220 yards three times at about 21 seconds per run with a three-minute rest between runs. It exhausted me, causing me to throw up. Over time, I built my confidence through conditioning. Obsessing about the right amount of time for the interval can ruin an athlete. It is distracting to meet the number. Focusing on numbers in competition does not make for a great performance. When an athlete is in the moment, in a timeless state, a world class performance is far more likely. For keeping the mind more attentive to a workout and less aware of the pain of conditioning, applying numbers can be helpful.

Around my 60th birthday, when injuries prevented me from running, I began swimming with a tri-athlete swim team. Our workouts were timed. At first, it made me too tired to think about time as I swam. The fatigue slowly receded as my mind focused on the number of laps and the pace. Jim Bolster, my swim coach, instructed me to switch from one stroke to another in a complicated matrix.

This was good training. It was as helpful as counting the breath in meditation. At first, my mind could not retain the full workout. After a while, I was able to keep track of each lap, relating it to the whole range of sets. Then I knew just where I was, and I was aware of how many strokes I was doing in each lap. When I relaxed and rotated more, it began to require fewer strokes.

Scientists like numbers. So do sportsmen. They elevate numbers to a realm that approaches animism, even believing that numbers might have a life of their own. Compulsive gamblers often become entrapped by this same belief. Numbers symbolize increments of reality, but they hide the subjective nature of life and the world. Numbers crunchers hide behind symbols to simplify things, thereby eliminating the dialectics and subtleties of nature. People working in finance create great stress by filling their heads with numbers. The pleasure that could be derived from playing with the numbers or from having an adequate amount of wealth, cannot overcome the amount of anxiety caused by living in an uncertain world where the numbers constantly rise and fall in value.

To distract myself from pain and fatigue, I consciously counted each stride, every lamppost, during the last miles of the several marathons in which I ran. Once, when I sat in the dentist chair to have a tooth filled, I sank backward, counting slowly, as I withdrew from the sensation of pain and the noise of the drill. Using numbers to hypnotize myself helped me feel no pain.

The numbers 135, 185, 205 and 225 are increments weightlifters use when bench pressing. One must get used to the feel of heavy weights. In 1965, I bench pressed 185 pounds. That was as much as football players were doing in those days. Lifting weights with fellow Olympians in Los Angeles later, I increased from my then 185 pounds to 285 pounds with practice. In leg press, we went up to 600 pounds. Someone always stood next to whoever was lifting to assist in case of a collapse, which most often happens on the first attempt.

At UCLA, I trained with Russ Hodge, a fellow Olympian. He held the world's record in the decathlon. He told me he had just lifted 1,200 pounds on a leg press. Until that time, I had matched all his lifts, up to 600 pounds, but I found it impossible to imagine how he could have lifted a weight that heavy. Russ said he was using a new method. Before he attempted the lift, he would concentrate. First, he would think, push fast and go all out for 15 seconds as if sprinting. Before if the lift did not happen by eight seconds, he would give up on it. I trusted Russ, so I tried what he recommended. At first, nothing happened. I thought, weight go up, and I thought of sprinting. Suddenly, after about thirteen seconds, the weight moved up quickly, effortlessly, and I lifted 1,200 pounds that very day. If you have an urge to lift heavy weight, by all means, give it a try, but don't give up if it feels too heavy. Just stay focused.

Sri Chinmoy, a great yogi I knew and loved, used his mind to perform powerfully for peace and love. He lifted astronomical weights, which damaged his joints and caused disintegration in his organs, tendons and joints. In old age, he continued, even in his deteriorated state. His actions demonstrated so beautifully that One Pointedness commands gravity. Nature's forces bowed before his power. He taught that mind surpassed pain or fatigue. Some of his disciples, ordinary people, swam the English Channel or ran around the world. At his gathering with Carl Lewis and Roberta Flack, I saw people who seemed perfectly happy limping around. They had met their number [5].

ANOTHER ASPECT OF NATURE: COLOR & VIBRATION

To have a deeper understanding of Nature, watch the space between objects. Synchronize the mind with the body through voluntary movement, such as Tai Chi Chuan and Kung Fu, or through involuntary meditation, such as Zazen. When we come to a quiet place, we begin to experience the unity of the vibration of the body and the vibration of space. This will open us to the Oneness of All, where wondrous things happen.

Changes occur to the physiology of the brain during meditation which not only bring a state of relaxation, but also create a certain stability throughout the day and later [6] (Fig. **3**).

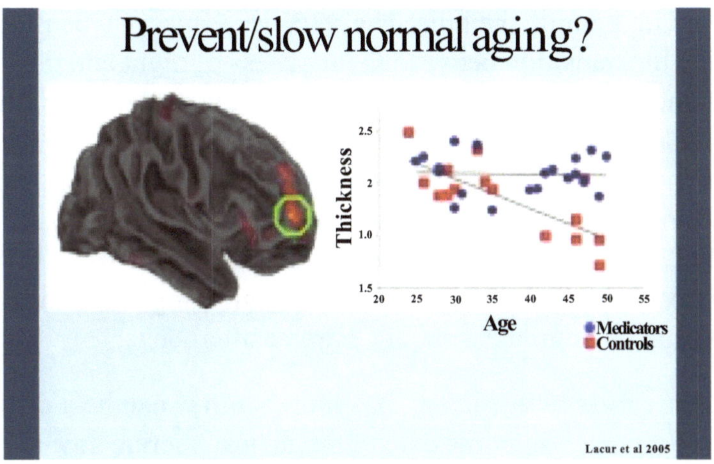

Fig. (3). Controls and meditators aging meditators. https://blog.bufferapp.com/how-meditation-affects-y-ur-brain

After decades of practice, I experienced my inner vibration by placing my hands on my abdomen. Men place the right hand over the left hand. Women place the left hand over the right hand. The web of the hand is placed over the umbilicus with thumbs crossed so the web is interlaced. Reaching the lower part of my body was difficult. I devoted myself to this practice for about a year, but I only got down to my throat. Every time I tried to go deeper, a ring of energy around my throat seemed to expand like Saturn's rings. He Ben Hui told me to go to my third eye, since it had been my yoga practice for years. From there, I could go backwards into the Dan Tian, or red field, in the abdomen. My third eye meditation had resulted in outer space experiences as well as many flashes of pure color, such as blue Saktipa from Siddha Yoga. Eventually, when the yogic third eye and Taoist Dan Tian are in harmony with each other, they connect us to all that is as well as the top to the bottom in our bodies.

Meditation changes according to our moods, surroundings, time of life and improves over time (Fig. **3**). We all have a favorite time to meditate. Mine is sunrise, but sunset is equally enlightening. To perform when the sun sets is supreme. At sunrise and sunset, the lights of the zodiac appear. Highly charged particles from the sun scoot into our atmosphere. They loop around Van Allen's belt, which protects us from harmful sun rays. The sky is electrified, colors dance in the air, a feat for those who can see space.

Ten days before the 1964 Olympic trials began, I would finish my officer training at Hamilton Air Force Base in Northern California. It was difficult to train for both at the same time. I would wake up at 4:00 AM, put on combat boots and fatigues, and go for a run in the hills. The stars were shining when I left the parade ground. During the transition between the darkness of night and the light of dawn, the space around me vibrated. It slowly became electrified with blueness and a sparkly spot, colored red, that resembled plasma. I was blessed by nature. I bathed in its natural energy. Afternoon workouts were quite different. I ran fast -- 300 meters three times in a row -- and lifted weights under the hot sun. At the same time, I fulfilled the obligations for my officer training. Now I believe that the Earth's naturally supportive energy early in the morning was probably better for me than the torture I endured during my extreme afternoons.

Language and numbers both convey meaning, but they can be a distraction when practicing meditation. Sometimes, I prefer to just vibrate my voice, avoiding language and numbers altogether. The sound of my vibration, which I feel in my lungs and chest, has gotten deeper over time. My voice becomes a musical instrument in harmony with a primal sound. I like doing Kung Fu animal forms --

the crane, tiger, leopard, dragon or snake. They require me to hiss, growl, yelp or roar, depending on what is appropriate to each animal. It allows me to escape from language, numbers and meaning. I love making pure, natural sounds.

Our blood rushes to the head, causing it to heat up, during any intellectual or mind focused activities. To create a balance, we bring our full attention down inside the body. It is not a matter of controlling. We just center ourselves in the lower abdomen. One reward of this practice is to feel the internal vibration of our body. After some time, the body's center will connect with the third eye and with the crown of the head. Now the heat will be uniformly distributed throughout the whole body, no longer centered in the head [7].

We see outer vibrations when there is a resonance between inside and outside. That is the source of life. Each human being is a microcosmic version of Earth and it's energy, which vibrates in octaves at about seven to 15 cycles per second. When we wander too far from this optimum resonance, it is harmful to our health. The brain is out of synch with Nature when it vibrates at 30 cycles per second. Meditation helps recalibrate the mind and body. After about 30 to 40 minutes of meditation, oxygen consumption and blood lactates drop abruptly, a sure sign of stress reduction. Meditation can help get us through intense suffering and pain because it reveals the Oneness of body, mind and will. Though meditation does not cure our ills, it can bring us hope and be a comforting respite from our pain. Those benefits we derive from meditation and right thinking will prevail until another wound from the forgotten past surfaces or a new injury is sustained. Peace and suffering are woven together like threads in a tapestry. Let us learn to keep sight of the whole design.

The Schumann resonances define the Earth's vibrational frequency. Negative ions create the positive vibrations of life. A meditation practice moves our mind through space, creating the interaction between the outer vibrations of Earth and the inner vibrations of our bodies. We start our practice by moving the mind out of the head and into the body. Then we continue by moving the mind outside the body without returning to the head.

As we now know, the Earth vibrates in octaves at a frequency of about seven to 15 cycles per second. The living body emits a certain vibration. The arteries pulse with the heart as it beats, but we are generally not even aware of this constant background vibration. We rarely recognize the most elementary movements of the body, like our breath moving in and out. According to traditional medicine, each organ has its own vibration signature, its own color and pathway, and each organ activates at certain times of the day. This system was discovered by ancient clinical observations that we have continued to watch and track for many years. The result of research I did, which has been published in another book, showed that there are energetic pathways on the outside of the body, which are influenced by organ changes. They vary according to the amount of disease or health found in the body. These organ energies bifurcate to the left or right side of the body, but when the body is in a synchronized state, they come together at the center.

In the state of Oneness, space is creativity. This place beyond suffering is fun and spontaneous. When awareness of the inner and outer vibration of space develops, we might look there for a sense of stability. When doing Qigong, we can choose to direct our creative, healing energy through our hands into our body. Our mind can be used to heal others. We can use outer ethereal connections to energize the spirit.

Immersing ourselves in the beauty of natural surroundings brings ease to our spirit. In Spring, the vibration is strong and hard to miss. A communion with Nature sets us to a frequency that can heal any sort of disease, but it works best when we return to Nature over and over again.

Regulation of breath and relaxation of muscles that came from running through the woods helped create an ideal way for me to connect internal and external space. It was a wonderful way for me to quiet my busy mind and tight body. When we are in a one pointed state, movement has many benefits, but it can be destructive to push the body too far when attempting to calm the mind. It can take hours to relax the mind if it is in knots, and injury might occur by then. There are no rules. Self knowledge and understanding the forces at work are what matter here.

Taoists love a full moon, which is at its most sacred when directly above the head. Meditating at midnight under a full silver lunar light is a natural phenomenon that calms and cools the impact a hot sun and intense passions have on our daily lives.

Is it possible to synchronize ourselves? Yes, it happens when all the aspects of our being vibrate in unison. What is this vibration and how can that happen? The vibration reveals itself to us when we seek it. There are various techniques that will help in our quest to experience the vibration. Yoga has been one traditional way. Though I have tried many, the best way for me to see the outer vibration is to spend half an hour, several days in a row, peering into space. Slowly, while we are attentive, the phenomenon of space appearing as movement can be seen by us in the distance between our eyes and an object. It can occur, as it has for me, while gazing across a lake. One day, it might look like it is raining. On other days, it could reveal different possibilities. A closer look will show us that vibration has form. Tiny pulsating dots electrify space. It has movement and non-movement like a vibrant field of plasma.

Language is necessary to communicate with other human beings. Silence is required to communicate with Nature and its multitude of different vibrations.

The Earth is currently rotating at about 1,040 miles per hour, while it is orbiting around the Sun at a speed of about 66,000 miles per hour. Meditation invites us into the realm of singular creation, allowing us to be at one with such mind-boggling forces. From there, we observe that things move fast in a synchronized, coordinated symphony. Nature's child becomes Nature itself in this silent meditation of one-pointedness.

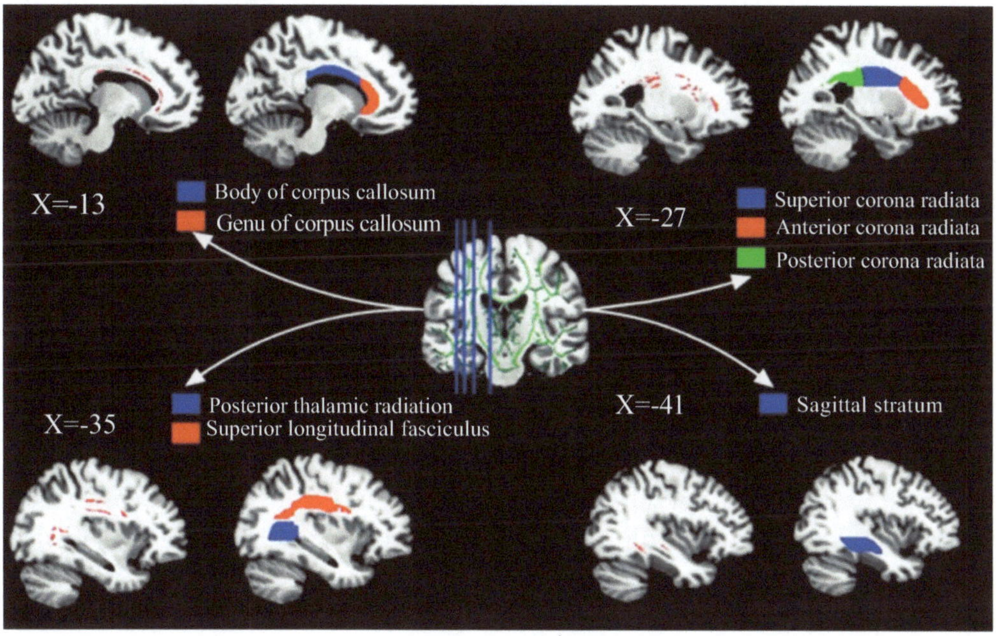

Fig. (4). Dr. Chen mentions a study conducted by Dr. Tang and Dr. Posner that involves diffusion tensor imaging technology. It reported that training in meditation can induce changes both in specific networks of the brain and in the state of the brain itself. In both cases, the efficiency of white matter when it is being measured by diffusion tensor imaging, is often increased after only a few hours of meditation training (Fig. **4**). This dynamic pattern of change in white matter involves the anterior cingulate cortex. This part of the brain network is related to self-regulation. This discovery could lead to an improvement in or the prevention of mental disorders. The research hypothesized that when frontal theta is induced by meditation, it produces a molecular cascade that increases myelin and improves connectivity. An earlier study by Dr. Tang's group reported that short-term meditation training could produce a significant change in the brain's attention networks that are related to alertness and conflict resolution [9] [DOI: 10.1073/pnas.1207817109] [PMID: 22689998].

Language can save, enslave or liberate. Some who have heard Huang Po speak report they have been enlightened by his words [8]. Reading sacred texts can infuse the reader with light. In the Bible, the Word of the Lord and Christ's teachings help many people endure suffering. Believing that if we are righteous we will go to Heaven shines like a beacon of hope in an ocean of despair. Yet this belief might cause rigidity, which can result in even greater despair. Sometimes, we feel we have entered a state of grace from just hearing the right words at the right time. Non verbal blessings are also manifested through the natural powers of those who have mastered internal and external prana, Qi or energy. The Master transfers an emanation of energy by placing hands upon a person.

While meditating, I have experienced that outside space encompasses everything and is always new. It manifests itself through various forms of consciousness. Though outer vibrations explode, get still and fuse the microcosm with the macrocosm, the singular consciousness of the self continues to be experienced.

Awareness of the lack of differentiation between the subject and the object dissolves the subject/object into a field of emanation. The Self is aware. The ego has dissolved. With intention, we can navigate through this newly found space. We all have the singular power to connect with the Oneness that brings us to the Here and Now when we recognize it. The Self can conduct the forces that magically synchronize space-time with the present moment.

In a state of Oneness, a flash of light may illuminate the inside of our mind. After I had been meditating for three or four days in the classic sitting position at a yoga retreat, a young man asked if he might place his hands on my head. It was fine with me, and when he did, it felt really nice. I thought I had fallen asleep with my eyes open, looking at a clear blue sky, but my eyes were closed. To my surprise, when I opened them I saw a cloudy horizon. When I re-entered the space inside, I was enveloped in blue. Upon reflection, this phenomenon seems quite natural since we live in a blue atmosphere. The mantel holder of the Blue Medicine Buddha says, "There is no Medicine Buddha". What we call Medicine Buddha is really the healing blue mantle of Earth, which is available to nurture all of us when we are receptive. Several times I have also experienced my mind flushed with green, yellow or red. For people on Earth, colors are natural manifestations that nourish the heart and infuse us with pure joy.

Flashes of color can occur while doing Qigong or Siddha yoga. They can also be transmitted to another person during healing through the energy of the hand. According to ancient healing traditions, each color is associated with an organ, but my experience indicates that colors can be felt throughout the whole body.

In Tibetan Buddhism, Taras are female Bodhisattvas. In Hindu mythology, they are feminine archetypes. Green Tara is compassion. Red Tara is fierce and magnetizes all good things. Black Tara is power. Yellow Tara is related to wealth and prosperity. Blue Tara is the incarnation of the transmutation of anger. And White Tara heals. She is compassion, longevity, serenity. For me, they are glorious emanations of natural vibrations. When we pay homage to the forces of creation, they might appear in response to our deep appreciation of them.

Colors that are experienced in yoga come from activity in the third eye that occur when we are one pointed. In Japanese Zazen, we rest at ease and wait for the mind to settle while maintaining correct posture. This practice may reveal a stream which flows to nothingness. The great Void may feel like a grayish expanse that stretches in all directions. In that state, one might sense a great Presence that is basically stable, though it is in stillness and in movement at the same time. This is a basic property of Oneness.

White light is the light of our consciousness. It is rare. It can emerge unexpectedly in the recesses of the mind. People who see this white light of consciousness feel they have been awakened.

MEDITATION, ILLNESS AND DISEASE

Meditation helps us connect to our vibrational being. It can be a useful tool for people who are sick, and it can be a major force in deconditioning ourselves from deep rooted habits. We tend to identify with them as if our habits were really us. Meditation creates a path for letting go. By expressing the truly spontaneous that is appropriate to each moment, we are alive to the now, and we do not attach to the outcome of our actions, which will always be fresh. Illness often comes from physical, emotional or psychological habits that are detrimental to us. When we meditate we see our patterns more clearly. We will start to break away from them by recognizing the signals that indicate there are problems that need our attention. Knowing what is necessary at any moment, and letting go of what is unnecessary, frees a lot of energy for healing ourselves.

I have researched reactions shown by a master and a novice in deep meditation. Though the novice is able to reach a deep meditative state, it is not as deep as that of the master. While they are meditating, a bell is rung. The brain waves of the master show a slight change when he hears the bell. When the novice hears it, he comes out of the meditative state, immediately returning to his normal state. When the bell is rung a second time, the master recognizes the sound, and he reacts as he did the first time. The novice has no reaction, but his situation is different from that of the master. He is not present. This is a classic example of non-recognition. It is a similar story to that of a person who does not not want to hear something and, therefore, does not hear it. The master hears the sound but as if for the first time. He is not attuned to non-recognition.

Be observant. Observe everything, become aware of what is around, and practice observing without reacting. The power of observation, the ability to look at oneself through the eagle's eye, lies within all of us. I know people who misplace things all the time and can't find them. Others I know keep rigidly perfect homes and can't tolerate anything being out of place. Both are extreme behaviors that derive from the problem of habituation. They are not present, aware, alive to the moment, nor following energies as they arise. They don't see that everything is constantly changing. Though the world sleeps, we must awaken. When we are endlessly distracted by an overactive mind or burdened by frequent memories, our senses grow lazy. When we attach ourselves to old habits and patterns, we get trapped in the past. We are too enslaved to our old ways, leaving us no room to be creative.

Impulses Come from Deep Seated Habitual Happenstance Propensities and Not What We Think We are Rationalizing

Depression weakens the immune system. It can lead it to not recognize the self from the non-self. Microorganisms may invade the body. Depression lulls it into not recognizing these non-self bacteria, fungus, parasites and viruses. Meditation makes internal signals more accurate, like sending the right immune response to the right pathogen. The immune response is very particular to the type of pathogen and subdivision [10 - 13]. When a pathogen enters the body, an immune response is triggered. Under an imprecise response, the immune system may be fooled into non- recognition. The pathogen is a non self and the immune system should react to the non self. Next time the pathogen enters the body, it is free to proliferate because the immune system has been conditioned for non-recognition.

What is good on one level can be bad on another. Non-recognition is good for not reacting to the past and remaining in the present. It is dangerous when the immune system does not recognize a pathogen, or when we ignore what is around us, putting ourselves in a vulnerable state. In some cases, the immune system reacts to the self as if it were the non self. An autoimmune disease can be deadly because the immune system attacks the self or body and self-destructs.

Conditions like depression cause the immune system to not work precisely. If bacteria, parasites, fungus and viruses are allowed to invade us, our internal space can be dominated by the non-self. When we are de-synchronized or in a differentiated state of being, we start to fall apart. Our relationship with the outer world affects us greatly on a micro level.

Chronic infection weakens organs and muscles where blood circulation is poor. I have done research with other scientists, which shows that even antibiotics, when taken to fight infection, will have no effect in an area of the body where blood flow is not good. The immune system cannot reach the restricted area, even though it knows it has created the right amount of antigen. And because it has already produced the antigen, it will no longer react to signals from a persistent infection. This is the way destructive downward cycles can begin in the body.

How can we manage our inner demons? Meditation is an important way to help us maintain mental health. Once we realize that we are obsessing over something or find ourselves acting out against problems from the past, when we feel insecure or unworthy, meditation helps us find a quiet space. There we can face our demons and recognize them for the ghosts they are. Meditation can ease the traumatic biological effects triggered by fear, anger, depression and anxiety in our body.

Modern medicine uses expensive diagnostic technology, which particularizes and isolates each part of the patient's body as if it were some separate entity. Doctors regard only body chemistry, often failing to look at the whole person. The amount of time doctors are allowed to spend with patients is dictated by insurance companies. Their fixation on already established statistics, and on the importance of numbers meeting certain pre-determined norms, does not take into account the specific uniqueness of each person. Medical sociological models, based on norms, ignore those who are at either end of the bell shaped curve. We are faced with a limited, mechanical system that rarely works because life is not mechanical.

It is vital that we bring to our consciousness an awareness of the complexity that makes each of us a unique, living organism. All of us embody multiple layers of comprehension regarding the state of the human condition. Finding out what type of meditation is best for us and establishing a practice will connect us to ourselves and our natural inner wisdom. Illness must be responded to directly from an alive place, not from language, nor from a logic skewed by narrow views of medicine and life. Connecting to life and to what maintains life will reset and synchronize the whole organism. Obsessions in the mind will recede, creating space for new possibilities. Meditating brings about shifts in old patterns. It opens us to a deeper understanding of how to protect ourselves from recurring trauma.

Though few scientists actually apply it, observation is considered the gold standard of scientific research. Simply observing the facts that do not fit our beliefs, without dismissing them, is a hallmark of genius. In medicine, exceptions to the rule are ignored. Or they are seen as aberrations instead of merely differences.

Doctors recommend prescription drugs, technological diagnostic tests or invasive surgeries for all our ills because those are the routine procedures used by the practitioners of modern medicine. Today, in-depth, hands-on treatment is rare. Though this reality seems hard to accept, most people will blindly follow doctor's orders. Patients believe that doctors hold the knowledge and have the authority, so they trust them without a second thought, thereby selecting the other to be in charge of the Self. Yes, doctors have studied medicine for years, but we must begin to take responsibility for our own mental, physical and spiritual health and for the quality of our own lives.

Calming the mind is a good place to start helping ourselves. Calmness will open some space where we can quietly begin taking notice of our patterns and observing the relationship between cause and effect in our countless daily activities. When something does not make sense to us, we can slow down our brain activity. When we are calmer, the possibility of making sense from confusion is more likely. This is the meditation of making sense out of no sense.

It is easy to be oblivious to even our most oft repeated behaviors. When we stay in one position, for example, like sitting at a desk for too long, it leads to tight muscles, which cause poor circulation. Illnesses begin with that sort of detrimental habit when we repeat it over and over for prolonged periods. We can choose to clear the mind of extraneous activity by meditating upon our habits of thought and behavior and by observing many of the aspects of our lives without making any judgment. These are healthy first steps toward change.

The back pain I used to have can serve as an example of what we might learn by being attentive to cause and effect. Since no doctor was able to help me, I finally started to pay closer attention to the pain in my back. I soon realized that it hurt more when I had been driving. After sitting in the driver's seat for 15 minutes, my back started to hurt, so I placed a level gauge across my lap. It revealed that the seat was not level. When I looked under the seat, I found a broken spring on one side. Over a period of time, pain settled into my asymmetrical body, which had become that way from tilting to the left. Once the broken spring was fixed, my body sat more upright when I drove, and eventually the pain just vanished.

The ability to reach a meditative state can be easier or more difficult depending upon the degree of each person's pain. Human beings have spasms and seizures; we suffer from deep aches, acute pain and intestinal irregularity. We have headaches, earaches, toothaches and many other aches. Pain confuses, distorts and distracts the mind, but relieving our pain with recreational or prescription drugs can be dangerous, even deadly, as unanticipated consequences can occur at any moment. When we are in pain, but it feels outside us, it might be a challenge to feel the Oneness of Being. On the other hand, opening to our pain might be the very thing that will connect us with the Oneness of Being. Eradicating a symptom without addressing its root cause only perpetuates the problem. It may be part of life to suffer, but we are not powerless in the face of it. Suffering is not our enemy. When we open to it, suffering can be useful. When we examine how we fear our own mortality and vulnerability, we learn to accept the human experience, which helps us find the way out of our pain. One intention of this book is to demonstrate how to alleviate pain.

In order to see things as they are, we must observe and become aware of the effect old memories and sudden feelings have on us when they get triggered. We begin to move away from reacting to events like we did in the past as we recognize the subtle, destructive impact stress has on the body. Once we realize that emotional states are not from the present but rooted in past experience, we can let go of them.

Dr. Chen shows that a group of neuroscientists from Seoul National University in Korea also applied MRI technology to examine the brain structure differences between a well-matched sample of long-term meditators and non-meditator controls [14] (Fig. **5**). Whole-brain cortical thickness analysis based on MRI imaging, and diffusion tensor imaging to quantify white matter integrity in the brains was compared between 46 long term meditators and 46 matched non-meditation volunteers. They found that the 46 long-term meditators showed significantly greater cortical thickness in the anterior regions of the brain, located in frontal and temporal areas, including the medial prefrontal cortex, superior frontal cortex, temporal pole and the middle and inferior temporal cortices. Significantly thinner cortical thickness was found in the posterior regions of the brain, located in the parietal and occipital areas, including the postcentral cortex, inferior parietal cortex, middle occipital cortex and posterior cingulate cortex. Moreover, in the region adjacent to the medial prefrontal cortex, both higher fractional anisotropy values and greater cortical thickness were observed.

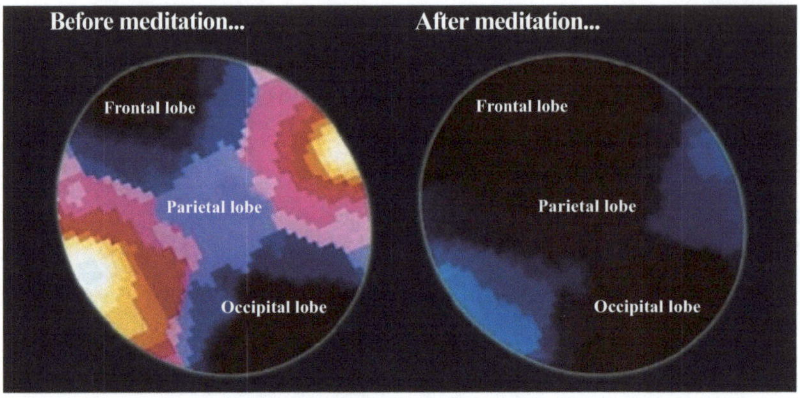

Fig. (5). Long term meditators show differences in gray and white matter. http://www.collective-evolution.com/2014/06/15/a-neuroscientist-explains-what-happens-to-your-brain-when-you-meditate/.

Negative and positive ions influence our health. We feel energized when we are at the beach, in a forest, near waterfalls or after a storm because the air is charged with negative ions. A negative ion is a molecule that has gained one negatively charged electron. On the contrary, when we are exposed to too many positive ions, our health is compromised. We can feel tired or depressed, and we lack energy. Positive ions are massively present when it's humid or before a storm. Pollution, office air conditioning systems, fluorescent lights, computers and printers generate positive ions. A positive ion is a molecule that has been stripped of one of its electrons.

Out in the real world, we begin to be more in touch with ourselves and with our experiences. As our perception gets clearer, we see what is happening in the moment as it happens, and we recognize it for what it is. We stop reacting from deeply buried, unconscious, emotional states that are rooted in the past. Being alive and aware in the flow of the present allows us to see that each moment offers fresh solutions, and the moment feels more stable.

He Bin Hui taught me a type of mind power called Nian Li, which uses language to transmit energies. As the healer, I mentally enter my heart and describe in thoughts what I am doing. Then I point my finger at the troubled organ, and in a clear voice I command it to heal. There is a concentrated electromagnetic field at the end of the finger. A signal, which tells it to heal, is transmitted through this field to the organ. Energetically, it is almost the same as talking with a stern voice to a young child who is misbehaving.

Hypnosis works in a similar way. Freud realized that hysteria impacted negatively upon visual, sensory and motor functions. Implementing a different idea or thought into a patient's mind through the use of hypnosis has worked for the relief of hysteria. Hypnosis has also shown positive results when practiced on people affected by extreme forms of paralysis. Many medical miracles can be understood in the context of treatment for psychosomatic illnesses, which have responded amazingly to suggestion and to belief.

When a person loses a limb, the space previously occupied by the missing limb can continue to hurt or itch. It has been demonstrated that acupuncture can cure the phenomenon known as phantom limb syndrome. This indicates that the effect of physical or emotional trauma from events that happened long ago continue on, much like the sensations still felt in the phantom limb.

While receiving Nian Li treatment, the patient concentrates on the solar plexus, the center of the unconscious in Taoist tradition. For treating a patient with diabetes, I used the Nian Li technique on his pancreas. "Make this patient's pancreas normal", I said, speaking to my heart from within my mind. Then I pointed my finger at his pancreas and commanded aloud, "Get normal". It did so immediately. Sadly, he was addicted to substances harmful to his pancreas. His behavior didn't change, but his insulin injections were moderated for several days. The state of another person can be influenced by a mind manifested through will. This technique is more powerful than external Qigong. A reservoir of energy, accumulated through meditation, can be transmitted from one person to another. The Qi that people feel on another's body may be simply that person's defense to keep out.

We can use our mind to go through space, being attentive to the lower part of the abdomen. Space becomes the medium that helps us to connect to another person's body. If you can rest in your lower abdomen, you can transmit energy or Qi to a person that is next to you. Commanding nature is a power we all have but never use. It is mostly lost to us but was known to the ancients.

If we stray too far from ourselves, illnesses, injuries or accidents can be wake-up calls. Painful as that might be, when we listen to the pain, we find new openings. By protecting our physical, mental and spiritual health, we might manage to live longer instead of succumbing to afflictions we have brought upon ourselves. The longer we live, the more time we have to develop wisdom that will help us maintain the delicate balance necessary to navigate our way through life in a compromised world. Our life is a dance. We are all playing hide and seek.

There is nothing mechanical about the quietness of meditation. What we seem to acquire during one moment of meditation can drift away at another, and what we find, we lose, only to find it again, but this time it is different. We forget to be present; then we remember. Again and again we get distracted. Although the mind might want to attach to a previous meditation experience, it is not likely that it will reproduce itself a second time. Let us remember -- even when we forget or find ourselves in a dark shadow -- that we are still in the Oneness. Practicing long meditations on a two-week retreat will bring us back to stability. When we experience the essence of creation directly -- by seeing colors, feeling the depth and subtlety of the energies of inner and outer space -- we connect to the healing forces of life.

The dance that occurs between being present and non present is natural. It does not rain on a tree every day. Yet, if we look at the tree over a period of time, we will see that it is growing. The same phenomenon applies to us. Nothing can be forced when it comes to being present, here, in the Now. We just need to be attentive to the nonlinear nature of forgetting and remembering. When we observe, we recognize that duality is actually two parts of one movement. If we do not get stressed about it, we either naturally evolve toward being in the present or we remember to bring ourselves back to it. There is such a thing as spiritual greediness. When we get to be obsessed about our progress, we lose the very essence of being present.

The body is a web of interconnected non-local energies, and there are always benefits to connecting with it. Getting to know our body is another major step along the path as we learn to help ourselves. Touching it can be healing and beneficial. There is a cardiovascular point on the back of the neck, for example, and on the left shoulder off the scapula, which, if stimulated, can relieve heart tension. Running or swimming can release tensions in the neck. After a while, the body gets into a rhythm and relaxes into it. Simply rubbing the back of the neck until any tenderness there is gone can be efficient. Paying attention to our feelings will guide us toward knowing better what we need. When we touch one part of the body, we might release some tension or the damage from an old wound that has remained trapped in some other part of the body. The more time we spend with our body, the more we send it our love and the message that we care about our life.

Pain often strikes quite suddenly. You just pick something up, and BAM, you feel a sharp pain in your back that came out of nowhere. Experienced healers know that pain was just waiting to happen. The stress and the tension were already there minus the pain. The incident triggered the pain. The restricted motion of the body, once it experiences the pain, often protects the body from further damage.

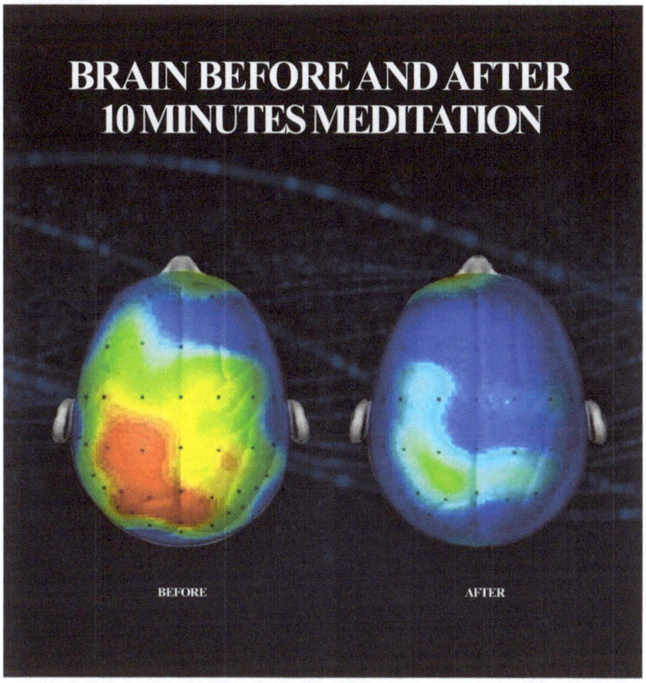

Fig. (6). In 2009, Yang-Sheng Chen revealed that Vestergaard-Poulsen and his colleague from Aarhus University in Denmark, using MRI imaging, found a higher density of gray matter in the lower brain stem regions of those who practiced long-term meditation than they found in age-matched non-meditators (Fig. **6**). Their findings show that long-term meditators actually have structural differences in their brainstem regions, which are concerned with cardiorespiratory control. This could account for some of the cardiorespiratory parasympathetic effects and traits, as well as the cognitive, emotional, and immunoreactive findings reported in several studies of various meditation practices [15]. http://www.lovethispic.com/image/176518/the-brain-before-and-after-meditation

Back pain, which is usually caused by stress, is quite a common problem for those of us who are living in modern times. Becoming aware that pain is a signal to change emotional and physical behavior is crucial. One might have a bulging or herniated disk, for example, without even knowing it. A stressful situation could cause the disk to suddenly have a reaction. Vertebrae are held in place by tendons and muscles that are subjected to a lot of stress. When they become too stressed, the body responds by protecting the area, inviting us to pay attention to what is happening there. The condition will naturally improve over time, as the tension and stress recede. Most people suffering from back pain make the unwise choice of having surgery and taking drugs, which might cause the condition to get even worse. A better solution would be to identify the source of our stress and find out what is causing the imbalance in the body. We can then proceed toward changing any unhealthy behavior so the healing process can begin.

We experience pain as a cruel hoax played on us by unfair forces, and we take no responsibility for it. Instead of recognizing pain as a manifestation of the body, designed to protect us, or experiencing it as a reminder to pay attention to our behavior, we blame external causes and look for external remedies. We ignore warning signals that tell us something is wrong and end up feeling like victims of arbitrary events that have nothing to do with us when we find ourselves in pain.

Surgery attacks the spinal disk as if it were the culprit. But the actual culprit will not be found under the surgeon's knife. The problem might be lack of flexibility, weakness, tension or stress in the body. Exogenous drugs or opiates are prescribed for the relief of pain, but they cloud the mind, which loses focus. When we keep a clear head, we can correct the condition ourselves by reducing our stress and by paying attention to the predicament we are in because we created it. This power that we all have is given away by us when we believe that only the doctor has the knowledge. When we accept that the doctor is the only one who knows, and is always right, we lose our connection to nature and to ourselves.

It is important to have an intimate relationship with our body, to spend time with it and see from our deep experience of it how it works and how it sustains our lives. Many of my women patients have a posture that indicates discomfort with their own bodies. This might reflect how our male-dominated society sees and treats women. The pelvis is either too far forward or too far back. The shoulders are caved in, and the neck is very tense. Over time, maintaining these postures causes problems in various organs.

Good posture is not merely the "Stand up straight!" command we were given as children. The body holds ancestral knowledge we can use to heal ourselves. As a species, we evolved through many different stages until we reached our current upright position. To have good posture it is necessary to understand that the body is three dimensional. Our skeleton, which may be the most primal part of our body, holds us up. It gives us the ability to move through space, which is a real gift. It is important to understand how the articulations of different parts of the skeleton resonate throughout the whole body. When deformation occurs in the skeleton, all the systems of the body are affected. For example, the rib cage will be compressed on one side from scoliosis. This might cause lung or heart problems. A tense spine can create distress in the digestive system. Since a spinal cord nerve passes through a vertebra to reach each organ, tension compromises the signal to the organ and prevents it from functioning properly.

Being in our body literally means going inside of ourselves, into our bones and into our organs. The body is our home here on Earth. We live in it. It embodies a collective as well as a personal memory. When we start this journey we might find ourselves going back and connecting with more primal forms of life from which we have all evolved. When we connect the body to our emotions, thoughts and sensations, we will realize that they are all part of one movement. A change in the body will affect the mind the same way that a shift in the mind will affect the body. We will connect with the natural forces of Earth, space, the sky and the breath, which will naturally help the body to find its own alignment and its proper place in the universe. The body will no longer be enslaved to the many societal rules it has to endure.

Whether we sit, stand or walk as we meditate, our posture is important. The body needs to be relaxed and present at all times.

Experience shows us that right thinking, proper practice and meditation are antidotes to harmful habits and promote longevity. Insights gained with age can help us to see the real nature of things, to understand the relationships we are in, to improve upon them and to find inner peace.

In order to heal ourselves, we need quiet to hear the wind, feel the sun, smell fragrances, hear subtle rustlings in the trees or see zephyrs waft about in the reeds. Taking time to turn inward each day, away from daily struggles, may open a window for us into another space. A thirty minute meditation is enough time to teach our consciousness to not see things that are not there and to realize that our life is not limited to our thoughts or our conditioned experience of life.

THE SELF IS OUR TEACHER . . . AND NO PARTICULAR FORM OF MEDITATION IS THE WAY TO GO

Life is difficult. We build armor to defend ourselves against its arbitrariness. To appreciate our worth in a world that is hostile and seems against us is not easy. Depression and disease can result [16]. In meditation, we have a partner, one that is always there and never fails us. When we meditate, we find a space where we can melt into a larger world, the entire universe. Looking with the naked eye, we see ourselves as we truly are. For the time when we meditate, at least, we feel our power, the aliveness of creation in the Self, and we are at One with All.

As part of the human condition, we protect ourselves from realizing that death awaits, but that leads to suffering and misery [17]. We can be overwhelmed if we recognize our individual existence in a world full of violence, suffering, injustice and natural catastrophe. In fact, it terrifies us. One day, our body will die, and the mind will go with it. Virtuous thoughts, good behavior and spiritual beliefs might soften our stark awareness of existence. That sort of cover up could lull us into believing that we are all right. Behaving well can bring us a certain amount of peace, but it is no antidote to the primal understanding of "I Am".

With meditation, we shed the armor that protects us from seeing that which we are, the I Am, and we start to see things as they are. Any overt attempt to eliminate the armor directly could lead to mental instability. Attention to the now, without memory deforming the present moment, is a meditation. Accepting our condition is essential. See the world, without experiencing the sense of a me-other dichotomy, where the other is a threat. This otherness might be the result of a misguided belief we hold that separates us from others.

Our feelings are deeply rooted, and we have many ideas of why we should hold on to them. We all fear the great mysteries we call life and death. When we couple those fears with an ego-armored defense against them, we suffer. Ironically, this delusion about our own mortality could bring about a premature death.

Meditation loosens the grip that real or imagined, often irrelevant, experiences hold on us. The protective shell we have built over the years was once useful, even necessary. It has become an integral part of us, but when we fail to recognize it is no longer needed, it becomes hardened and rigid. It stunts our growth. It creates stiffness, illness and regression. When we lose the armor, we have access to clear information that will help us manage stress and better solve complex situations.

Our true nature, deeply buried inside us, can be released [18]. The deeper Self can be ignited if we allow it to come to the surface. Scary, antithetical thoughts can go against our best self-interest, or distract us from reaching a deeper understanding of reality, but meditation creates the quiet that lets us be in the moment. Stillness is required to reach our depth and truly know what we need to do. Let us feel heavy, like a stone, a big stone that is falling, sinking to the bottom of the ocean. We become so heavy that stillness occurs, followed directly by a wonderful sense of lightness.

The Self is the teacher, but we must quiet the mind to hear desires and directions from our own depth. The Self speaks in another voice. It is often unheard because background static and unconscious behaviors caused by past traumas, emotional stress and our repetition of parental neuroses keep us distracted. Being fearful, we respond mechanically to present experiences and remain trapped in the darkness of our past [19].

Consciousness, perceptions, feelings and thoughts do not bring peace, but any attempt to stop the movement of the mind will cause even more movement. Contemplation of impermanence is a good mental discipline. Being free does not mean forgetting injustice; it does mean not participating in it. Paying attention and observing closely can wipe away hate and hurt. Meditation is silence without cause. It releases creative energy.

Attention is different from concentration. When we concentrate, we are not relaxed. Concentration limits the mind. Based on memory, it creates a partial view, prevents receptivity and narrows our ability to have direct experience. Attention is not based on memory. To be attentive is to be completely absorbed in the present moment.

Our desires, our cravings and our greed cause us confusion when we impose our will in pursuit of material -- or even spiritual -- gains. If we pay attention to the nature of the ego, we will see that when it takes over, we are deluded into believing we can possess whatever we want. The ego is a necessary part of ourselves when it is healthy. Since what we want to possess is viewed as external to us, we lose the natural connection between what is internal and what is external. Attention to our true Self, beyond our fragmented desires, frees us from our enslavement to the will and the ego. When we are at ease, relaxed and being natural, we find ourselves in harmony with the world.

A quiet mind is beyond subjectivity and objectivity. This mindlessness is unmovable; it is beyond duality; it leaves us free from the blockage of the mind. By looking outwardly for realization, we never really free ourselves from obstructions. What we need to uncover always lies within. When we shroud ourselves in cloaks of perception and cognition, it prevents us from seeing the real luminosity of the mind. As Ts'ao Tung said, "Neither subject nor object, no direction or location, no form or appearance, no gain or loss" [20].

The ideal form of my meditation is no form. The surroundings suggest the right form in each moment. A strong will is required to learn the proper form of swimming, golf, tennis, baseball, yoga, Kung Fu. It requires concentration, which distracts from attention. Concentration is scripted learning. The mind imposes the form onto the body. When I stopped learning and quit pursuing proper form, my natural form came. It had nothing to do with classes or games. Attention to the moment is the true form of no form. Improvisation is in the moment, away from the tyranny of mechanical movement.

Many people cannot sit and "do nothing" for long. Meditating on "nothing" does not give us back nothing. After a while, we experience the void, the great Abyss. It is beyond the ego, memory perception and feeling. It opens a vast expanse of silence, the awareness of a gentle vibratory movement. The mind stands still. It happens in the present, the Now, free of the past and the future. It can be a fleeting experience, but it is enough to have had it. In the state of Oneness, a flash of light may illuminate the inside of the mind. There is no need to force it. Opening ourselves to sitting still will happen gradually. Sitting to meditate for extended periods of time will happen.

TRAUMA, OPPOSITES, EMOTION, FEELINGS

How can we see things as they are? It is humbling to accept ourselves as merely one individual among billions of people. Our humility is well founded, but it can leave us stupefied. In the face of this predicament, meditation gives us hope.

Our emotional life is complicated. We each follow a unique set of patterns due to our own individual life story. When we are not aware of our emotional state, we attach to it. Then our reactions are mechanical, not alive in the here and now. We do not judge our emotions when we are totally aware of them. Being present to what we feel will allow us to be truly alive, but it is always for the best to simply observe as we detach from our feelings.

Take anger, for example. When we get angry, our physiology changes. The blood rushes to the head, which gets hotter. The heart beats faster. The eyes bulge. The circulatory system constricts. We are ready to explode. This intensity can wake us up to the Oneness of our emotional state and the body itself. Now there is no separation of subject and object. In a flash we see that anger is an energy. As with any energy, anger can bring us to our center. Anger can be useful in certain situations if we don't separate it from the whole of our experience. When the anger drops, our physiology returns to its normal state. If we are not present to the anger, it will take over. It can consume us, and it might cause us to act out. Anger, when cut loose from our consciousness, can only be a destructive force. This realization might occur to us when we are feeling our anger. It could present itself when we are not trying to control anything, as our emotions rise to the surface while we are meditating. In the meditative state, we simply watch our emotions as they come and go like clouds in the sky.

When our anger, or any strong emotion, rises up, we might deny it or try to justify it by blaming someone else. "Look what you made me do", we often say to others or think to ourselves. Trying to control our anger creates perversions in us that are far worse than the anger itself. Repressed, it attacks the body like a malignant tumor [21]. Yoga describes anger as the dance of Shakti in the face of Shiva's tendency to expand. Reason wants to rationalize the strong emotions and find a way to place the cause elsewhere. It is natural and it is human to feel angry, so instead of blaming others or rationalizing, it is best that we take full responsibility for our anger. A good meditation technique is to calm the mind from arising thoughts, which refuel anger.

Because children have not yet built any armor around their feelings, it is enlightening to watch their emotional fluidity. They flow from one emotion to another without attachment. They are whole and pure at each moment.

Dance, or any type of movement, can be a medium through which we might expel demons from within ourselves. They are demons, of course, only because we fear them and try to keep them imprisoned. The battle between our fears and the liberation of ourselves from our fears will go on until the moment we face the trauma that caused us to become frozen in the first place. To dance with every aspect of life, whether we find it good or bad, is essential. It is powerful to fully express our sadness, anger or shame through the body. It releases memory from cells that have been keeping stress inside to protect us from the shock until we are ready to confront it. We empower ourselves when we freely feel and fully express our emotions. A reservoir of energy, trapped in the darkness, gets released when we feel the anger. Remaining present to these emotions creates an acceptance of life and the possibility of moving forward. We can liberate ourselves through body movement in sports, dance, yoga, martial arts, *etc*.

The compulsion to discharge emotional tension by overdoing physical exercise at the gym or when playing sports is a socially accepted form of addiction. Through meditation, being in the form and relaxing are more important than the sport itself. It is essential to be free, natural and at one with water when swimming. This is the meditation of sport. When pressure to succeed is applied, we get distracted from any natural process that might be unfolding and from the love of the game we are playing. To coordinate and synchronize, we must fuse with the natural process, especially in form related sports, and Be Here Now.

Meditation develops our ability to be more adept at non-reactivity. Attention to the breath is the best way to recognize what is happening right now, free from past memories or future concerns. Breathing is usually an involuntary activity, but it can become voluntary. As we become more conscious of the breath, the external world appears to be more stable. At first, we watch the inhale and exhale. Then we extend them for the breath to quiet down. As our mind and body become more at one, more whole, the intensity of past experience becomes more muted. When we meditate, our breathing slows down; it becomes less intense. The mind/body is a more whole entity. Feeling less disturbed, it dissociates itself from archaic fluctuations of energy.

When you begin meditating, watch thoughts as they arise. Note each thought and its general content. Then let it go. In mere moments, a new thought will appear. Just sit and watch the thoughts come and go, one after the other. The next time you meditate, just let go of the thought without looking at its content. At first, you might find it difficult to not look into a thought or to ignore its content. The second phase of meditation could be more like shooting ducks at a penny arcade. When the duck pops up, shoot to get rid of it. Then wait for the next duck to pop up. This may seem impossible, but be patient. After several meditations, the mind begins to grasp this new experience. Thoughts arise more slowly. They will become clearer, have more substance, less fragmentation and there will be fewer snippets of memory, even when we are not meditating.

The first phase, where we recognize our thoughts but don't hold onto them, will transition into the second phase after ten breaks. A break is when we become absorbed in a thought and forget to let it just drift away. That shows how much we are enslaved to thoughts. This allows the mind to see how thoughts block the will. When the will asserts itself over random thoughts that creep into the mind, we are all better off.

In the second phase, not recognizing the content of thoughts slows down their frequency. It is still not easy to let go since the thought process is so real to us. Memory wants to assert itself and take over the moment. When the mind slows down, ideas are more complete, more consistent, and awareness is deeper. The mind will fight back. It wants our attention, and it seeks to be comforted by the familiarity of the past. Meditation is a way to free ourselves from the past. It allows us to reveal a more authentic person.

I once believed I could expose the unconscious by asserting my willfulness. Now I see that meditation is the way to break the yoke of servitude. It is possible for us to be free from unconscious impulses and to reach enlightenment. Throughout history, others have held similar beliefs.

After years of practice, I am still amazed when a favorable meditation shows me glimpses of celestial experience. The energy descends through my body, the top of my head is beaming, my third eye pulsates and spaces open. Since life always brings new problems, unexpected stress, pain, suffering and mental instability, those uplifting experiences fade away. Even so, things do tend to get better over time. Glimpses of great forces outside ourselves reassure us and bring hope that there is much more to life in this universe than just pain and suffering.

The body is the host for our physical and our emotional pain. The mind is crowded with obsessions, regret, disappointment, depression, fear of life and fear of death. To bring ourselves beyond the dual state of suffering, we must be in the moment to find inner peace.

In Yogic terms, Samadhi is the state of higher meditation, the non-dual state of consciousness. Satori is the Hell on Earth we go through in this life. At first, while meditating, it is possible to experience both Samadhi and Satori. In the great Abyss of Oneness, which we may come to enter through our practice, I found stillness and movement. In the vast space, a voice arises, as though another is speaking, yet it is our deepest impulse speaking to us. We can only know what to do through clear language when we can listen to our Self.

The state of Oneness can be experienced during highly intense competition. When I sprinted, I felt a vibration in my mid-section that was stable. It did not move. My extremities, detached from internal one-pointedness, still rotated effortlessly. There is not just one true way to greater stability. Following mechanical ways of meditating will not enable us to respond as accurately as we could to negative stimulation or stressful situations.

Let go of what has passed, what may come, what is happening right now. Do not try to figure anything out, or make anything happen. Relax right now and rest in your natural state without thoughts, analysis, intentions and let things just settle by themselves [22]. This Mahamudra is music beyond words and symbols. To do nothing might be the most difficult challenge we all face to realize our true nature.

In Zazen meditation, maintaining correct posture, while letting go of thoughts and not interfering, is a way to get the Makyo (Japanese devils) to dance their dance without entering the body. That way they play out their rituals without doing us physical harm. The mind sees there is no sense attaching energy and feeling to the Makyo, and things calm down after this meditation. We all need quiet time in order to tame our ghosts, whether they are real or imagined. For the beginner who thinks meditation is all fun, waiting patiently for things to die down a bit could be difficult. In a similar way, proper yoga is painful as we slowly open our joints and relax our muscles.

Meditation is not a visualization technique. It is not about imagining colors or energies that we direct toward the body with our thoughts. These meditations are not mind exercises. They are a way to cultivate energy, which is an actual experience. Visualizing is done in the head. It is not the direct experience of feeling Qi or other energies.

I have experienced a Qigong master, who got into a front forward stance with his face forward, his shoulders parallel to the floor, his mind focused. He sent Qi right through his outstretched finger, pointing it in front of him, like he was shooting a pistol. Scientists stood six inches apart in a circle that was 15 inches away from him with the palms of our hands perpendicular to the Qigong master's pointed finger. I was the seventh person. When he focused his mind, I felt the Qi pass through me like a wind that penetrated my flesh.

FOOD AND OUR EATING HABITS

Shopping for food, preparing and eating it, can be meditative experiences. Food is essential to life, but our relationship with it is often complicated. It can create all sorts of emotional and physical ailments, so examining this aspect of our lives is very important to our well being. Food and eating can be highly charged emotional issues in many of our lives. How we eat usually originates with our relationship to the mother's breasts and the degree to which we were, or were not, nourished by our mother or other caretaker.

Are we aware of what we eat, of what we put into our bodies? Do we eat to nourish or do we eat to destroy ourselves? Do we please others by what we do or do not eat in our attempt to satisfy their ideas of how we should look? Do we eat mechanically? Do we eat consciously? Do we connect to the value of food? Do we realize the many steps that have taken place in order for food to be available for us? Do we appreciate that someone had to grow and care for the food we eat?

Food is energy. It contains energies that are necessary to life. It is essential, not only to our bodies, but to our more subtle energies as well. That which fosters a healthy body fosters a healthy spiritual life. If we want to take responsibility for our thoughts, our feelings and our actions, we must also be responsible for what we put in our mouth. These choices will have a big impact on our health and on the health of our whole society. When we connect with our food, we are paying homage to our Earth, the Sun and water. It is a humbling experience. When we truly love ourselves, we treat our food with love and feed ourselves accordingly. Shopping at the green market, or a farmer's market, we can choose fresh foods that vibrate with a wide range of beautiful colors. While cooking, we can pay the utmost attention to what we are doing, as we enjoy the vibrant colors, smell the inviting odors and taste the yummy flavors as we chop, slice and cook our special combination of ingredients. Eating can always be done with a conscious reverence for the food. All these activities will contribute to the elevation of ourselves to be more at one with Nature. In today's world, this is something we have to choose to teach ourselves because eating natural foods has become unnatural to us.

Healers who work with other people's energies have to ground themselves. They often need to eat the types of food that replenish their energy.

TOWARD A MORE TRANSCENDENT SEXUAL UNION

The union between two human beings is beautiful (Fig. **7**). Once the layers of confusion have been removed, its simplicity sings like a cascade of fresh water on a radiant Spring day. Such an experience is within reach for everyone because it is right here inside of us. All we need is to just open to it. Although it is a simple thing to do, it is not easy.

Meditation is usually practiced individually or in groups, but it can also happen when two people engage in a sexual union. The true meaning, the real beauty, of sexuality, has been lost due to widespread puritanical religious propaganda that spreads moralistic fearfulness. When we pay attention to it, sexuality reveals that opposites melt into each other, dissolving into the Oneness of the Shiva/Shakti Nature. It requires being present to the breath, to the creative forces of Nature and to the emptiness from which they spring. We must move beyond fear and realize that any kind of possession is an illusion. Letting go of primal fear, we access the Primal, which is the Divine.

This union transcends any one single individual, and making love this way becomes universal, a feat where lovers, in ecstasy, are vibrating with the whole. As they transcend to a higher consciousness, the ego that separates us from reality dissolves. They enter the Realm of the Infinite by committing to the beauty and creativity of the present moment. Bodies are vessels to be cherished. They can transport us to our center and to Pure Love. This is a realm beyond morality. It is pure, alive, uncontaminated by the ego, a place where there is no right or wrong.

As with any process, this process involves suffering. Letting go is not easy. Making a commitment is difficult. But as we open to suffering, we see it as part of the process, which helps to loosen its grip on us. We sense that above the clouds the sky remains blue and space is vibrant. The Supreme Lover becomes a gateway to the blue sky of pure consciousness, and the journey continues until there is no longer any differentiation. There is only consciousness. Tantric yoga, a pure form of yoga, takes us to the depth of this exploration.

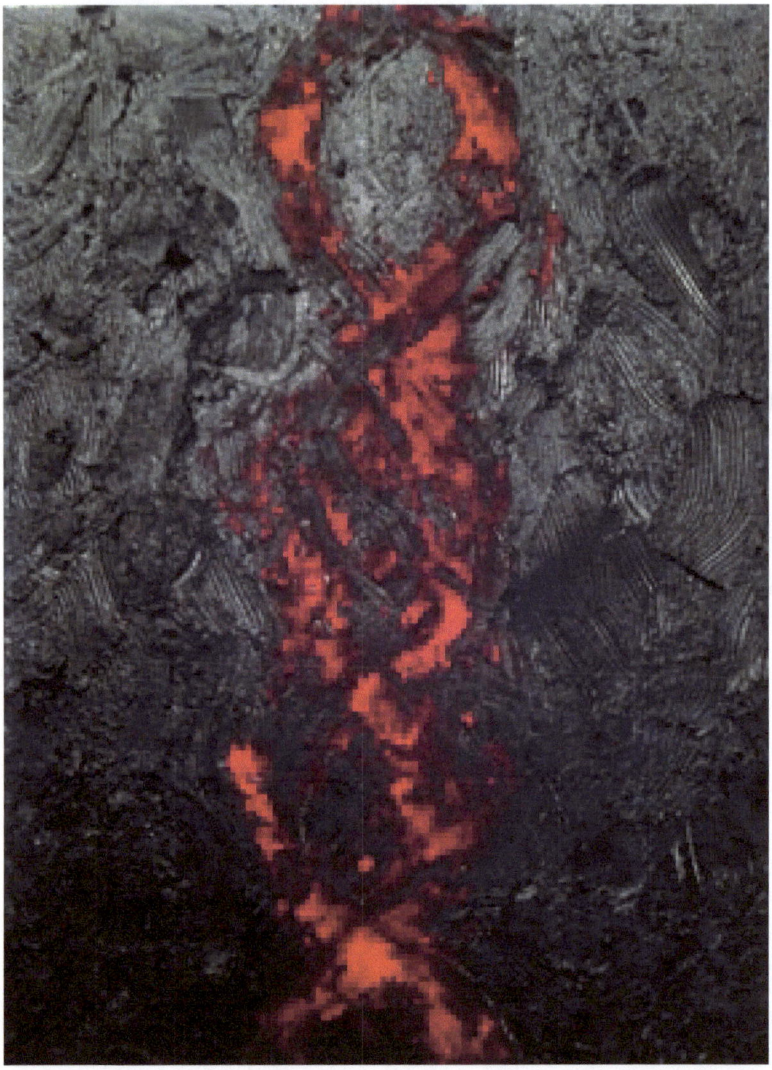

Fig. (7). These are zoomorphic exercises based upon five animal forms introduced by Shiva/Shakti rising Kundalini. (With special permission of Porter).

This initiation requires the guidance of a master because energy is being moved from the bottom of the spine to the top of the head. Kundalini energy is the coiled Shakti serpent asleep at the base of the spine (Fig. 7). Once awakened, the snake begins its journey upward until it is united with Shiva at the crown. The journey is perilous. Nevertheless, in the same way we become aware of our physical, mental and spiritual health by paying attention to ourselves and to our actions, we can start looking carefully at our sexual behaviors, habits and patterns. By the simple act of us paying attention to it, the threads of our sexuality will begin to unravel and guide us on our journey. Whatever needs to will manifest in order for us to grow. When the student is ready, the master will appear. If the Path of Kundalini is not our intended destiny, we can still choose to evolve toward a richer, more fulfilling sexual life.

NON ATTACHMENT TO LIFE AND TO DEATH

Our fragmented society believes there must be a cure for each ill and problem. Lots of time, effort and money are spent on finding those cures. We put more energy into defending ourselves against death than we do into valuing life. It is difficult for us to accept that death and life are two sides of the same coin. In this chapter, we have explored the attachment to our thoughts, feelings and actions. We do not even see how addicted we are to our thoughts. Nor do we see that this addiction rules our lives and the world in which we all live. Thinking is a constant activity. It continuously distracts us from ourselves and our intense fear of death.

Our inner eye opens to the Oneness beyond duality when we meditate. We see that life and death or illness and health are two parts of one movement like coming and going are. In the Wholeness of the meditative state, we are perfect. We do not try to change, to grasp or to attain anything. We just are. We stop attaching to our thoughts as though they are real. We see that our actions are as innocent as those of a child at play. Children do not attach themselves to their playing. They are simply alive to the moment. This aliveness can be as intense as if it were a matter of life and death, but they still do not attach to it. They are not yet fragmented and not yet afraid to die.

When we open to our deep nature, we see there is nothing to fear. When we cling to our perception of ourselves, we want to protect it, which causes us to be tense and to suffer. We can heal ourselves, but we cannot actually cure anything. When we take a pill, we are merely suppressing our symptoms, not addressing root causes. In Wholeness, we accept disease and death as just two of the many parts of life. We open to them as natural parts of ourselves, not as enemies. This is what it means to be healed. We can have fun being children again, and we can enjoy being actors in the play of life. There is no need for us to attach to the different roles we will have to play during our lifetime. Meditation helps us return to our Natural state.

REFERENCES

[1] Dyczkowski M. The aphorism of siva the siva sutra with bhaskara's commentary, the varttika. New York: State University of New York Press 1990.

[2] Pine R. The zen teaching of Bodhidharma. New York: North Point Press 1987.

[3] Chen K. Meditation can change your brain for better and longer. Yang-Sheng: Research Updates 2015; 5: 1.

[4] Hölzel BK, Carmody J, Vangel M, *et al.* Mindfulness practice leads to increases in regional brain gray matter density. Psychiatry Res 2011; 191(1): 36-43. [http://dx.doi.org/10.1016/j.pscychresns.2010.08.006] [PMID: 21071182]

[5] Singh J. Spanda Karikas. India: Indological Publishers & Booksellers 1980.

[6] Chen K. Meditation can change your brain for better and longer. Yang-Sheng: Research Updates 2015; 5(1): 11.

[7] Singh J. The doctrine of recognition. New York: State University of New York Press 1990; p. 75.

[8] Hsiu P. The zen teaching of huang Po. New York: Grove Press 1958.

[9] Tang YY, Lu Q, Fan M, Yang Y, Posner MI. Mechanisms of white matter changes induced by meditation. Proc Natl Acad Sci USA 2012; 109(26): 10570-4. [PMID: 22689998]

[10] Stein M, Schiavi RC, Camerino M. Influence of brain and behavior on the immune system. Science 1976; 191(4226): 435-40. [http://dx.doi.org/10.1126/science.1108202] [PMID: 1108202]

[11] Weigle WO. Self-nonself recognition by T and B lymphocytes and their roles in autoimmune phenomena. Arthritis Rheum 1981; 24(8): 1044-53. [http://dx.doi.org/10.1002/art.1780240810] [PMID: 6169351]

[12] Greaves MF. Cells surface receptors: a biological perspective. In: Quatrecasas P, Greaves MF, Eds. Receptors and recognition Vol one. London: Chapman and Hall 1975.

[13] Mitchison NA, Rajewsky K, Taylor RB. Cooperation of antigen determinants and of cell In the induction of antibodies. Proceedings of Symposium Prague. In: Report of Immunology. Czechoslovak Academy of Science; WHO, Int Atomic Energy.; Academic Press: London 1970.

[14] Kang DH, Jo HJ, Jung WH, *et al.* The effect of meditation on brain structure: cortical thickness mapping and diffusion tensor imaging. Soc Cogn Affect Neurosci 2013; 8(1): 27-33. [http://dx.doi.org/10.1093/scan/nss056] [PMID: 22569185]

[15] Vestergaard-Poulsen P, van Beek M, Skewes J, *et al.* Long-term meditation is associated with increased gray matter density in the brain stem. Neuroreport 2009; 20(2): 170-4. [http://dx.doi.org/10.1097/WNR.0b013e328320012a] [PMID: 19104459]

[16] Becker E. Angel in armor a post-freudian perspective on the nature of man. New York: Braziller 1969.

[17] Becker E. Denial of death. pulitzer prize. New York: Braziller 1973.

[18] Lacey J. Psychological Approaches to the evaluation of psychotherapeutics. process and outcome. In: Eccle C, Ed. Brain and consciousness. New York: Springer-Verlag 1966.

[19] Cleary T. Classics of Buddhism and zen. London: Shambala 2005; p. 328.

[20] Cleary T. The five houses of zen. London: Ts'uo Tung 2005; p. 307.

[21] Dyczkowski MS. The aphorisms of siva. New York: State University of New York 1990.

[22] Tantra the Supreme Understanding: Tilopa's Song of Mahamudra of Meaning. Available from: http://www.osholula.com/poetry/tilopa.html. 1971.

CHAPTER 5

The Scientific Measurement of "Qi": Techniques for Qigong Beginners and for Qigong Addiction Therapy

Abstract: Where does Qigong fit into the science system? Qigong is both physical and mental exercise; it does not have a religious component. It differs from psychology because it is both mind and body. Theoretical knowledge has an understanding but has no practice. Religious worship may develop the mind but has no body practice. At its core Qigong is the manipulation of the regulation of the body, breath, and mind into an integrative whole, with the breath as the key regulator practice to make this happen. Measurement of Qigong is provided with a variety of measurements to chemical process, electromagnetism, and cellular pathogens. Research on Qigong, a term used for a variety of traditional Chinese energy exercises, cultivation and therapies (Chen 2003), has occurred primarily in China. A summary of scientific approaches and measurements to Qigong is provided and a reference to the Qigong Institutes' database of scientific studies. Definition of Qigong and Methodological Restrictions.

Keywords : Addiction therapy, AGA thermogram, Chemical reaction, Diseased states, DNA synthesis, GE micro-pressure detector, Infrasonic sound detectors, Liver cancer, Microwave radiation meter, Qigong definition, Physical/signal.

INTRODUCTION

Our created geometric world of planets, various forms of stars in the aging process, and diffuse plasma gases and matter, make up our universe. So the painting above reflects geometry and matter interacting for creation which is the foundation of Qi which will be discussed and measured in detail (Fig. **1**).

According to ancient literature study, the term Qigong first appeared in Jin Ming Zong Jiao Lu by the Taoist priest Wun Xu (239-374) in the Dong Jin dynasty but was not widely adopted in thousand years of dynasty changes until the Qin dynasty (1616-1911). Recently, it has been found that this term is used in health and medicine books in the Republic of China (1911-1949) [1 - 3]. It formally came into use in the 1950s after the foundation of the People's Republic of China,

Phillip Shinnick & Laurence Porter

especially after the establishment of the Tangshan Qigong Sanatorium in Herbei Province. Since then it has been used in Chinese medical clinics and practiced generally. Its development was diverse and expressed as Chan Ding in Buddhist deep mind meditation concentration, Zuo Wang in the Confucian tradition, Dao Yin in medical breathing exercise, and Nei Gong in the martial arts internal techniques. All mean inner cultivation. Even in Taoist tradition Qigong became internal elixir, heavenly cycle, or fetal respiration. In modern times. Wu Shi, Qigong, Taoist Qigong, and Zangmi Qigong all taught particular methods, especially through these schools these techniques have spread throughout the world[1].

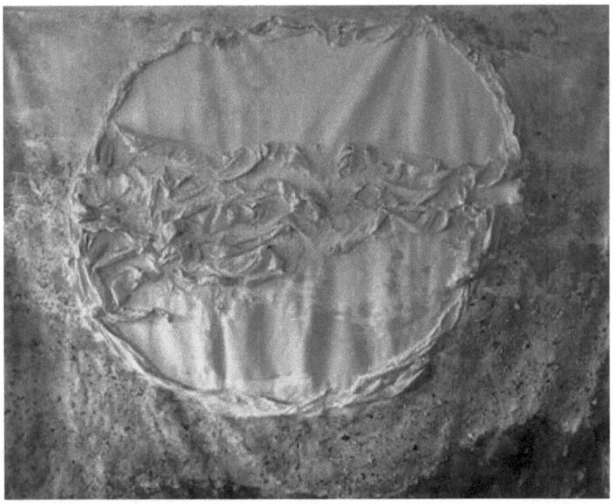

Fig. (1). Creation. LP 2010. (This figure is reproduced with special permission of Laurence Porter). Photo Herman Costa.

In the future, even modern techniques should not be seen as different from Qigong if they fall under its definition. How can it be possible that modern techniques come under the title of Qigong if they are not familiar with it? This can happen because Qigong techniques are available to anyone at any age who watches the breath and the reaction of the mind and body to disease because this is how they were originally developed. Also, submitting to a master's direction is not comfortable for Americans. Yet many will submit to brutal coaching techniques but it is true that Chinese and American women are more receptive to Qigong training [4]. Many masters do not understand medicine and science, and so are unable to comprehend the language of modern medicine and do not integrate modern advancements. Learning Qigong cannot be done without practice otherwise the theory of Qigong does not convey anything. The regulation of San Jiao (the three regulators: mind, breath, and body) is an individual experience, and each individual does this through individual practice. Learning the thousand techniques is not possible or recommended; therefore, practicing one or two methods is the best. Also, doing movement or voluntary Qigong is not the same as involuntary (sitting and forgetting).

Focusing on a formal form and getting the right form from modern techniques, especially after more ancient texts are translated, will find similarities with ancient techniques. To develop as part of modern medicine theory and science, all the mind-body sciences-psychology, physiology, biology, physics, biochemistry, and so forth-need to be used to see Qigong effect on the mind, breath, and body. The Chinese and Americans respond differently to internal Qigong, presumably because of cultural differences. The Chinese have a more accepting response to Qigong's philosophical basis that a person can heal herself or himself, or that it is possible to understand disease by watching the natural process of cause and effect. A practice for all is not necessarily the best practice; it should be based on the individual personality and state of health or disease and not prescribed apart from the person. Qigong incorporates moving meditation, standing meditation, sitting meditation, and varieties of mind involvement and noninvolvement (Zen).

External Qigong is limited by the number of its practitioners. Excessive external Qigong can weaken the practitioner; therefore, an understanding of the variety and effects of external Qigong on the practitioner and patients is important and is being researched [5].

Traditional Chinese Medicine and Qigong share the same classic philosophy, worldview, methodology, and aims. Scientists in the U.S. are attempting to prove to other scientists that Qi exists and devising ways to convince other scientists to study this phenomenon. Other cultures, like China, have studied Qigong since the late 70's resulting in a proliferation of studies after early pilot studies showed qi can be measured. The summary of Qigong research from 1977 to the present was made available through the Qigong Institutes' Database compiled by Dr. Sancier and available for researcher at the Qigong Institute website http://www. Qigonginstitute.org [6 - 10]. Dr. Chen used this database and presented many studies translated from Chinese.

DEFINITION OF QIGONG AND METHODICAL RESTRICTIONS

First, we must come to an understanding of a definition of Qigong. Qigong is a term used for a variety of traditional Chinese energy exercises, cultivation and therapies, as suggested by Dr. Chen [11].

The Lin definition of Qigong is a good start for as a way for a template of common understanding.

Qigong is the self–training method or process through which cultivation of qi (vital energy) and yi (intention and consciousness) can achieves the optimal state of both mind and body [12]. Furthermore, the Chinese Society of Qigong Science defines Qigong as: The distance and directional effects produced by well-trained Qigong practitioner under the Qigong state. Internal qi is for self-help and health and external qi is for healing others. This external qi implies three characteristics, qi exists only when a practitioner enters into the Qigong state of mind, the qi can travel a distance (affecting heat, light, electricity, magnetic waves, radiation and other signals), and qi is directional depending upon the intention and focus of the practitioner.

Certain methodological restrictions result from research experience. Not all Qigong practitioners can emit qi and few may not at certain times. Qigong practitioners can affect the instruments of measurement, so a certain understanding of the research design may be important for the practitioner but not necessarily where or how the measurement instrument works. Repeated trials are important because of inconsistencies [13].

MAJOR METHODS OF MEASUREMENT EQ (EMITTED QI) AND RESULTS

Physical Signal Detectors

The major methods of measuring external qi effects according to Chen's research are the following detectors, 1) physical signal detectors (light, electricity, heat, sound, magnetism); 2) Chemical dynamics methods (reactions); 3) biological materials detectors, such as *in vitro* cells, DNA synthesis, Vitamins, cancer cells, organic matter such as a leaf, *etc.*); 4) animal studies (because of psychological factors) in diseased states (*i.e.* changes in cancer cell growth rate) and healthy states (lifespan); 5) human studies in diseased states and detectors for the repair of tissue, bones, *etc.* and the qi affect.

Utilizing a Far-Infrared Detector (8-14 mμ)

A modified far-infrared radiation was detected at a distance of 50 cm from the palm of a Qigong practitioner, with modification as high as 80% at the frequency of 0.3 Hz. This contrasted with the control group (non-Qigong subject) which showed almost no difference for the infrared radiation itself in wavelength or intensity. The specificity is in the modification of frequency. The results of similar tests to another Qigong healer showed that there was no difference in the amplitude modification, but a difference in frequency modification, reflecting the different characteristics of EQ frequencies emitted by practitioners trained in different Qigong methods.

AGA Thermo Gram

An AGA thermogram can display the entire procedure of Qi emission by reading the thermal flow moving from the arm to the palm and finally to the fingertips. Then, the surface temperature of the patient's afflicted area, although one meter away from the healer was raised by 3°C. Meanwhile, when a control subject was introduced in this study, they found that correlated changes could be induced on the corresponding parts of a non-Qigong practitioner when standing next to the Qigong healer, but not without the Qigong healer present.

GE Micro- Pressure Detector (Placed from 0.5m to 2m)

Ge micro-pressure detectors were placed at the distances of 0.5, 1.0, 1.5, and 2.0 meters from the Qigong practitioner. The Qigong practitioner emitted *qi* toward the target (Ge germanium detector) through two of his fingers. At first, there was no recorded signal and the Qigong healer reported some mental difficulty in pinpointing the target for *qi* emission. However, after some practice, he could pinpoint the target and repeatedly produce some signals on the micro-pressure detectors. They recorded many micro-pressure signals from the Ge detector at all four distances mentioned above with a little time lag, which they explained as the reflection of the unspecified particle flow from EQ. There is a possibility that a Qigong healer might get tired after a number of *qi* emissions and the signals might then become weaker and weaker in this situation. Supporting this idea is the fact that when the Qigong healer eats adequately, the signal would again be strong.

8 mm Microwave Radiation Meter

With an 8 mm microwave radiation meter, they used the near field (20-40 cm to antenna) to test the EQ and the far field (4 to 5 meters to antenna) as the point of reference. They conducted 50 trials, 28 of which have formal records of radiation curve. Twenty-two of these trials have significant increases in the wavelength to above 10 mm during the period of *qi* emission.

Infrasonic Sound Detector (Denmark B-K Corp's Infrasonic Sound Detector 1,3,5,6,10 or 40 cm Distance)

The subjects included 10 Qigong healers (aged 28-61) and 10 controls (non-Qigong practitioners, aged 17-41). The test was performed in a soundproof lab with baseline noise less than 40 dB. The testing equipment was Denmark B-K Corp's Infrasonic Sound Detector. During the test, each subject was required to sit in a comfortable position, relax, and slightly close his eyes. The distances between the sound sensor and the testing point were at 1, 3, 5, 6, 10, and 40 cm. The tested acupoints included "Laogong" (on the palm), "Baihui" (on the top of the head), and "Mingmen" (at center of the back near the waist). The subject was instructed to focus his attention on the tested acupoints during the examination. The test results were derived from testing each point at all the specific distances. The Qigong group recorded significantly higher infrasonic sound pressure than the control group ($p < .001$). The range of infrasonic sound pressure detected for the control group was between 40.6 and 43.6 dB, decreasing as the distance increased, while the range of infrasonic sound pressure detected for Qigong group was between 48.8 and 54.7 dB, and was not affected by the distance to sensor. This study provided some support to the Qigong theory of "Where the intention goes, the *qi* goes".

Chemical Dynamic Methods Using Qigong with Yi or Intention and Directionality

Glucose Oxidase luminal

Glucose $+O_2$ -------->Glucose Acid + H_2O_2 [→ Fluorescence →Photoelectron Current]

Glucose consists of a 5 hydroxyl group and 1 aldehyde group, after oxidizing reaction, aldehyde group becomes carboxyl group (organic acid). The reaction speed is accelerated after Qigong by 400%. The photoelectron current and the reaction speed can be measured when luminal is mixed with hydrogen peroxide.

$$H_2O_2\text{----}H_2O + O_2$$

Hydrogen peroxide is an oxidizer and under the influence of EQ decomposes, only the oxygen is measured.

Strong Light

$$C_6H_{14} + Br_2 \text{------------} C_6H_{13}Br + HBr$$

Under a strong light Hexane and Bromine will produce bromohexane and hydrogen bromide. Bromine has a deep blood red color with similar properties as Chlorine. The reaction is accelerated after Qigong, with no strong light, becoming normal brown (fading from deep blood red color) after the reaction results in greater fading [14].

Detector Using Biological Materials

Biological materials, such as individual cells (*in vitro*) and biological tissues, are assumed to possess vital energy and are especially sensitive to the EQ emitted by Qigong practitioners; the concept of a biological detector has been existed for a long time [15].

Liver Cancer Cell and Lung Cancer Cell Cultures, DNA Synthesis and DPPC Liposomes

Chinese researcher reported a strong effect of EQ on the liver cancer cell (BEL-7402) and the lung cancer cell cultures (SPC-A), on the cells of living organisms, on the blood plasma eAMP, on the structure and pharmaceutical characteristics of Vitamin C, on the DNA synthesis and living cycles of liver cancer cells and that EQ, on structural changes in water and aqueous solutions, on the phase behavior of dipalmitoyl phosphatidylcholine (DPPC) liposomes, enabling the growth of Fab protein crystals. Similarly, it effects on the inhibition growth of the microstructure of E-coli bacteria and tumor cells in mice, on the inhibitory growth of hepatitis B virus and on human liver cancer cells.

Using tree leaves to detect the effect of EQ is one of the classics, well-known and simple studies. It uses a fresh tree leaf as the sensor, with two extra-fine probes inserted into different veins of the selected leaf, and then connects them to an electronic signal amplifier to adjust the amplification. During these experiments, they were able to detect field potentials from the tree leaves before any external intervention. When the Qigong healer emitted qi to the leaves at a distance of 50 cm, the observable field potential was several times stronger. When the qi emission was stopped, the signal strength returned to its baseline. In the control group, where a 35°C heating device was used at the same distance, the leaves showed no response (to exclude the possibility that the detected change was due to the body temperature of the Qigong healer). When a non-Qigong person treated the leaves, there was no effect. These "tree leaf sensors" can be used continuously for eight hours, and then they need to be replaced with the new leaves. From the viewpoint of traditional science, these "tree leaf sensors" do not truly meet the conventional standard of a detector, nor do they have perfect reliability of performance; however, they became a classic biological detector in the study of EQ.

Detectors Using Living Sensors

There has long been skepticism about the therapeutic effects of Qigong, and the effects of Qigong are often attributed to psychological suggestion (*e.g.*, Lin *et al.* 2000). Researchers shifted their focus from Qigong studies to living organisms that closely resemble the bio-characteristics of humans. It seems that almost all conventional animal or biological models used for research could become suitable biological sensors for detecting EQ

Effect of EQ on Cancer Growth

In the studies examining the effect of EQ on cancer growth, metastasis and survival time of the host, tumor models were formed in 114 mice by transplantation of U27 or MO_4 cells into their subcutaneous tissues. The tumor-infected mice were randomly divided into two treatment groups for three separate studies – Qigong group (exposed to EQ 10 to 30 minutes daily for a period of time) and control group (no treatment). In study 1, mice in both groups were sacrificed on day 20 after the transplantation. The average tumor volume in the Qigong group was significantly lower than in control (2.2 *vs.* 6.3 cm^3; $p < .001$). In study 2, the mice were sacrificed on day 23 and all axillary lymph nodes and the lungs were taken out individually to be examined histopathologically for metastasis. The metastasis rate in the EQ group was significantly lower than the control group (1/16 *vs.* 6/15; $p < .05$). In study 3, the mice were not sacrificed but were allowed to live their lives and the time of death was recorded for each. The average survival time in Qigong groups (n=10) was significantly longer than that of the control group (35.4 *vs.* 30.5 days; $p < .01$). The same authors performed similar studies in different settings and they all reached the same conclusion.

Effect of Qigong on Anti-Cancer and Anti-Tumor Effect of EQ on the Immunologic Functions of Tumor Bearing Mice (TBM)

The anti-tumor efficacy of EQ emission on transplanted hepatic cancer in mice was investigated. In this study, 30 nude mice that had been injected with transplanted hepatic cancer cells were randomly assigned to one of the three groups: (1) the control group (no-treatment); (2) the imitation group (sham healer imitated Qigong healer's movement); and (3) the Qigong group (treated by a Qigong healer). The Qigong or sham treatment included emission of EQ towards the mouse cage at a distance of 8-10 cm for 10 minutes every other day for a total of four sessions or 40 minutes. The results from three repeated experiments were found to be similar: compared with the control group, the tumor growth-inhibitory rates of the Qigong treated group were 70.3%, 79.7%, and 78.7%, respectively ($p < 0.0001$). The inhibitory rates of the imitation treated group were 9.5%, 2.6%, and 2.5%, respectively ($p > 0.05$). An electron microscope showed that the morphological alterations in the Qigong-treated mice included decreased cell volume of most of the cancer cells; nuclear condensation, nuclear fragmentation; decreased ratio of nucleus and cytoplasm; swollen mitochondria with poorly organized mitochondrial cristae, some vacuolated and many apoptotic bodies in extracellular space. These results indicated that EQ of a well-trained Qigong healer could inhibit the growth of transplanted hepatocarcinoma in mice.

The Effects of EQ on Human Bodies

Reported benefits of Qigong therapy include degenerated disc disease, rheumatoid arthritis, myoma of the uterus, shoulder peripheral neuritis, fractures, cataracts, cardiovascular disease, irregular pulse, hemiparesis, and asthma [16 - 21].

We do not have to conjecture about the existence of Qi, since now it is measurable in a variety of ways--- for light, electricity, heat, sound and magnetism (magnetism needs more study) and is shown to affect chemical molecular changes, biological materials, and living organisms. The inhibition of cancer cells, speeding up or slowing down the biological and chemical processes require directionality with intention. This has been shown and is the yi part of Qigong.

MAJOR TECHNIQUES OF QIGONG PRACTICE ACCORDING TO HE BIN HUI[2]

Adjusting the body, the breath and the mind, usually referred as 'three adjustments', which are the three basic techniques or maneuvering contents in Qigong practice. Every form of Qigong is invariably composed of all these techniques, although the arrangement or compositions varies. In fact, they are important not only in Qigong practice, but are indispensable in all daily activities, since the three adjustments cover almost every aspect in human autonomic conditioning system. From the standpoint of operational process, Qigong techniques can be regarded as such skills that are intended to maximize the body's potential into full play and enhance the physical and mental health by regulating human autonomic conditioning to an optimal state. Figs. (**2** & **3**) are some forms used.

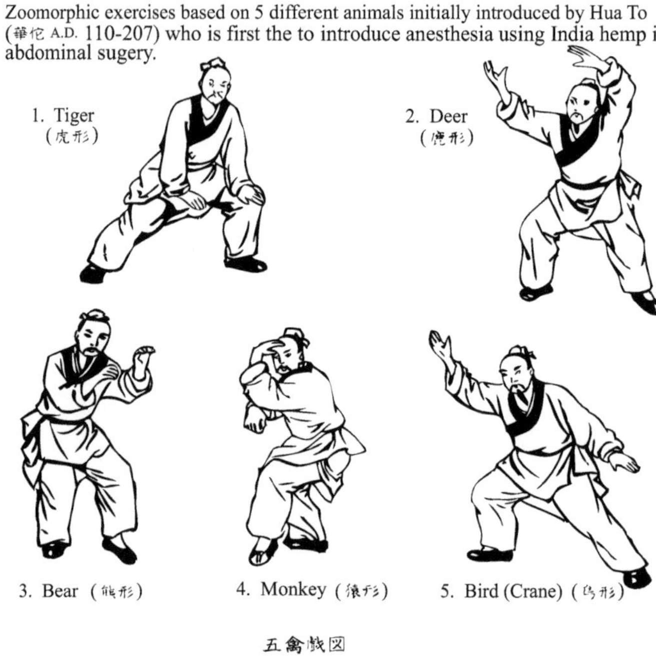
Zoomorphic exercises based on 5 different animals initially introduced by Hua To (華佗 A.D. 110-207) who is first the to introduce anesthesia using India hemp in abdominal sugery.
1. Tiger (虎形)
2. Deer (鹿形)
3. Bear (熊形)
4. Monkey (猿形)
5. Bird (Crane) (鸟形)
五禽戯図

Fig. (2). These are zoomorphic exercises based upon five animal forms introduced by Hua Tuo (110 to 207 A.D), and also surgery performed by using Indian hemp for breath and spirit of the body. Eyes half closed, standing straight, eyes straight ahead, arms relaxed, legs at right angles, mind empty of thoughts, concentration below the navel all promoting breathing and the flow of internal Qi. Moreover, most postures and movements have certain health preserving and therapeutic effects (Fig. **2**). (With special permission of Hegda).

The Qigong state pursued by Qigong practice refers to the state in which the three adjustments are integrated into oneness. Consequently, the process of Qigong exercise may involve practicing each of the regulating techniques separately at the beginning and then gradually reaching the state of three-adjustments integrated into oneness.

Adjustment of Body Posture

Adjustment of the body, also known as posture training (Lian Xing, 炼形) or body movement skills (Shen Fa, 身法), refers to the maneuvers used to adjust the body posture both while at rest (static) or in motion (dynamic). It is intended to position the body posture according to the requirements of Qigong state. For example, in practicing static Qigong, the body must assume a fixed posture in order to reach mental tranquility and composure; and in practicing dynamic Qigong, physical movements are applied to smooth meridians and to induce the internal Qi. These are used to mobilize essence.

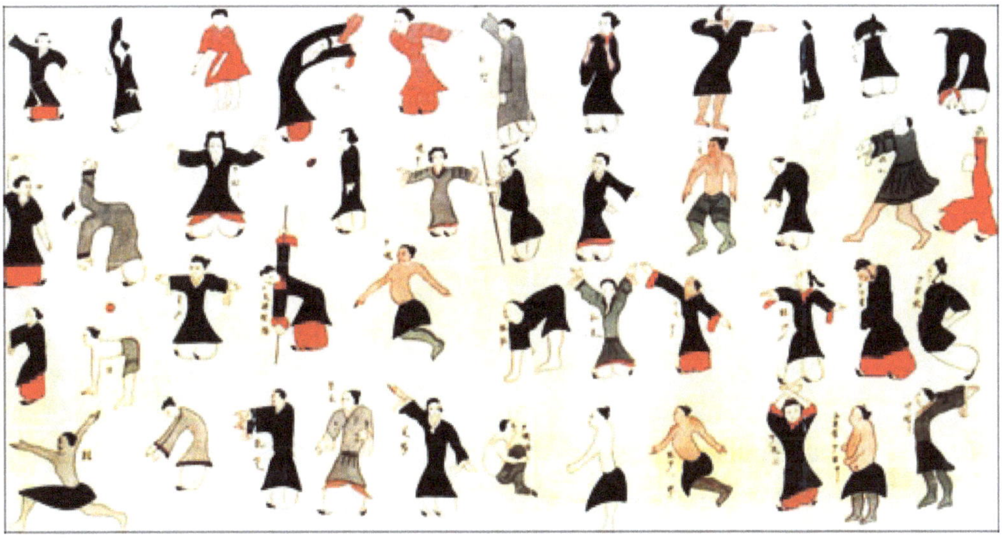

Fig. (3). Silkscreen Han dynasty (200 B.C. to 24 AD) in Mawangdui, Changsha, Capital of Hunan. The earliest forms of Qigong. (With special permission of Hegda).

The contents of adjusting body posture fall into two categories: external maneuver and internal maneuver, and the two affect and complement each other. The former focuses on the external posture and position; while the latter focuses on the maneuver of internal feelings and the relations of body parts.

I. External Maneuver

External maneuver includes operations on body posture and body movements, which are distinct but related to each other. Body movements are formed by connecting individual postures together, while body postures are the fixed constituents of body movement (Fig. **3**). The two transform interchangeably to each other.

a. Posture Maneuver

The most commonly used body postures in Qigong practice can be briefly classified into three forms: standing, sitting and lying postures. This type of posture maneuver is mainly applied in static Qigong.

1) Standing Posture

Standing posture is the basic body posture for standing pile Qigong. Depending on the post of different parts of limbs and body, standing posture can fall further into different types.

a) Holding-ball Style (抱球式 Three-circle Type, 三圆式)

Stand on both feet with shoulder width apart, turn the toes slightly inward, forming the image of Chinese character 'Eight' (some forms request the two feet to be either parallel or turned slightly outward, but not strictly). The five toes gently grasp the earth; the two knees bend slightly, but are not supposed to surpass the tip of the toes. Extend the waist; place the buttocks in a position as if they were seated on a high stool. Keep the upper body upright; draw in the chest to straighten the back; bend both arms in front of the body horizontally to form a semicircle, as if holding a round balloon. Relax the shoulder, droop the elbow and empty the armpits. Both hands are about one foot away from the body; keep the fingers of both hands opposite to each other at a distance of about 8~9 inches. The five fingers are separated, slightly curved, and are with the neighboring fingers approximately at a distance of one flat finger apart. Keep the head upright and both eyes slightly closed. Place the tongue naturally in the mouth rather than pressing it against the palate; draw the lower jaw slightly inward.

Relax the whole body after taking the postures. The so-called three-circle type refers to the three circles of the feet, arms, and hands, respectively.

b) Raising-ball, Pressing-ball and Lifting-ball Styles

These three postures are stemmed from the holding-ball type and can be transformed to each other in practicing, but one should avoid changing postures too often lest they exert a negative effect on the Qigong state.

Raising-ball Type: After taking the standing posture, lift both arms gently and extend them slightly to the front. Keep the hands at a distance of one foot from the body. Both palms face upward; the five fingers are separated slightly as if are raising a balloon. Other requirements of this standing type are basically the same as those of the holding-ball type. At the initial stage of practicing holding-ball type, if the arms are tired, change this posture by turning both hands upward, gently with two arms slightly extending to the front to alleviate fatigue.

Pressing-ball Type: Lift two arms and extend them forward, both palms facing downwards and five fingers being separated as if they are pressing on a table, the back of a chair or the water surface. Other requirements of the pressing-ball type are basically the same as those of the holding-ball type. At the initial stage of practicing the holding-ball type, one can also change this posture for taking rest when the two arms are tired.

Lifting-ball Type, is also known as Floating-lifting type. At the initial stage of practicing holding-ball type, when the shoulders and arms are fatigued, one may move both hands downwards below the navel with both palms facing upwards, fingers of one hand pointing at the other at a distance of about 8 to 9 inches. The hands are away approximately 5 or 6 inches from the body, as if holding and lifting a balloon. When practicing this type, be mindful to empty armpits, namely, keep the armpits hollow by keeping both arms slightly apart from the trunk.

c) Resting Type

The requirements of this posture are basically the same as that of the three-circle type, except that the both arms are required to hang alongside of the body. Turn both elbows outward so that the back of the hands gently touch the hipbone under the waist.

This posture requires fewer movements, helps relieve the fatigue of arms at the initial stage of practice, and is therefore, termed as the resting type.

2) Sitting Posture

The sitting posture is most commonly used in static Qigong and consists of three styles: plain sitting, cross-legged sitting, and leaning sitting.

a) Plain Sitting

This posture is most frequently employed at the beginning of practicing sitting. The practitioner should sit on a square stool or a hard chair. While sitting, it is imperative to sit only on one third of the chair area, instead of sitting on it completely. The height of the stool or chair legs should be the same as the length of the lower legs. After sitting down, the thighs should be parallel to the ground and vertical to the trunk with knees bent at a 90° degree, with legs shoulder-width apart, and the feet flat on the ground. The posture of the upper body, waist and head is the same as that in the standing form, while the buttocks are should protrude slightly backwards. The arms can take the posture of the holding-ball or raising-ball form. A second alternative posture is to spread the two elbows outwards with palms facing downwards and resting on the thighs joints. The third alternative is to have the arms hang naturally beside the body with the hands placed slightly touching the thighs.

b) Cross-legged Sitting

Cross-legged sitting is the most suitable posture for static Qigong practice. There are three styles: natural cross-legged sitting, single cross-legged sitting and double cross-legged sitting.

The seats for cross-legged sitting can be an ordinary bed, Kang [1], or a stool that is made especially for meditation and has a square and bigger size surface. A cushion is needed on the seat whenever one practices cross-legged sitting. If the practice takes place on the ground, the cushion should be extra thick.

Natural Cross-legged Sitting: Keep the head erect, mouth and eyes slightly closed. Relax the shoulder; droop the elbow; draw in the chest; straighten the back; straighten the waist naturally. Cross the two legs with either one folding over the other and place the feet on a cushion under the opposite knee. Lower the arms naturally; place the hands on the thighs or knees or over the lower elixir (Dan Tian, 丹田) with the hands slightly clasped. Cushion the buttocks approximately 1-2 inches higher depending on the individual preference.

Single Cross-legged Sitting: The postures of the head, trunk and arms are the same as those in natural cross-legged sitting only that one's calf is required to place over the other thigh, either the left over the right or the other way round, according to one's habit. In this sitting style, one's foot still remains on the cushion.

Double Cross-legged Sitting: The postures of the head, trunk and arms are the same as those in natural cross-legged sitting. Sit with the calves crossed by placing one foot on the opposite thigh, and then move the other foot on its opposite thigh, both soles facing upward without touching the cushion. It is the sitting form most Buddhists employ during meditation sitting.

Cross-legged sitting is also named Jia-fu sitting (跏趺坐) in Buddhist Qigong. 'Jia' means overlapping and 'Fu' refers to the dorsum of foot. Jia-fu sitting, therefore, refers to the sitting form with two legs crossing each other, including full Jia-fu (namely, double cross-legged sitting) and half Jia-fu (namely, single cross-legged sitting). Full Jia-fu sitting further falls into vanquishing devil sitting (Xiang Mo Zuo, 降魔座) and good fortune sitting (Ji Xiang Zuo, 吉祥座). In the former, the right foot is placed on the left thigh before laying the left foot on the right thigh. Consequently, the left hand is laid on the right foot. The vanquishing devil sitting, placing the left calf over the right calf, has been the major form adopted by Zen Buddhism. Good fortune sitting employs just the opposite posture with the right calf over the left calf, and is termed lotus position in Esoteric Buddhism.

c) Leaning Sitting

The postures of this form are the same as those in plain sitting, except that the upper back leans slightly on the chair or sofa. With the upper back leaning back, the feet can slightly extend forwards. It should be noted that the waist should be kept straight without touching the back of chair.

3) Lying Posture

Lying posture includes: supine position, lateral recumbent position, and semi-reclining position. The height of the pillow should be approximately 10 cm, or the same as the width of one's shoulder, so that the head can be kept in a horizontal position. The bed should not be too soft, and suitable bedding should be added on plank bed.

a) Supine Position

Supine position is the basic lying posture. Lie flat on the back in bed; keep the head straight, the face upwards, the mouth and eyes slightly closed. Stretch out the limbs naturally; keep both legs slightly apart or closed depending on the practitioner's habit. Tilt both feet naturally towards the side, or stretch the tip of toes forward. Place the arms on the side of the body naturally, with both palms facing inward and slightly touching the thigh. One can also bend the arms inward and put the hands on the lower Dan Tian (for male, right hand on top of the left; for female, left hand on top of the right).

b) Lateral Recumbent Position

Lie on either the right side or the left, but the former posture is more common. Retract the head slightly towards the chest, keep both eyes slightly closed. Place one leg on the other with both knees bent naturally and the leg on the top bent in a larger degree so that both feet are on the bed. Stretch the top arm naturally, with the palm facing downward to hip; bend the underneath arm to the head with the palm facing upward, the five fingers gently jointed together and placed near the ear.

Another posture of the lying form is to stretch the underneath leg naturally, raise and bend the upper leg to 90° before putting it on the bed. This way, one leg is placed in front of another with the sole of the front leg touching against the knee of the hind one. Extend the upper arm to the front with its palm placed on the knee of the front leg. Bend the lower arm upward with its palm rested on the elbow of the above arm. This posture is also called three-connecting form.

c) Semi-Reclining

On the basis of lateral recumbent position, raise the head and the upper body before leaning on the bed to form a semi-reclining posture. Stretch out both legs naturally, or raise the lower legs by putting a cushion under the knees. This posture is intended for bedridden patients.

4) Other Postures

In addition to the above mentioned commonly used postures such as standing, sitting, lying, the chapter of *Special Therapy* in this textbook also covers straight kneeling, squat sitting, *etc*. They are introduced briefly as follows:

a) Straight Kneeling (Hu Gui, 互跪):

Stand with both feet parallel to each other, body erect, and both hands naturally placed on the sides. After standing still for a moment, bend both knees slowly and kneel down on the bed mat or cushion. In the kneeling position, the paralleled feet are to be erected (the tip of the toe touching the ground with the heels raised). This being done, bend the body forward or lean back, depending on the requirements of the Qigong form.

b) Squat Sitting (Juz Zuo, 踞坐):

Sit in bed and rest the hips and feet on the bed with knees bent upright and legs paralleled to each other. Bend the upper body forward, with the hands clasping the top of the lower leg.

c) Sitting with Foot Extending (Shen Jiao Zuo, 伸脚坐):

Sit on bed with both legs stretched next to each other; keep the body erect and hands naturally dropped, or place fists on the mid-thigh. Eyes should be looking straight ahead with the tongue pressed against the upper palate. Relax the whole body.

5) Movement Maneuver

Movement maneuvers covers a set of movements with pre-set forms and spontaneous movements without any form. The former consists of a series of continuous and fixed movements, while the latter is made up of naturally occurring movements.

a) Set of Qigong Movement

Most dynamic Qigong consists of fixed routine movements which are conducted sequentially in Qigong practice. As dynamic Qigong forms differ in movements, one needs to be familiar with the specific requirements of each form in practice. For instance, Tendon Changing Classics (Yi Jin Jing, 易筋经) has twelve forms, Wild Goose Qigong (DaYan Qigong, 大雁氣功) consists of 64 forms in each of the two sections, and Five Elements Palm (Wu Xing Zhang, 五行掌) is based on five forms.

Routine dynamic Qigong can be divided into different types in light of their particular style in performance. The conventional ones are listed as follows:

1. Pliable type: Represented by Nourishing Qigong (Yang Qi Gong, 养气功) and Eight Pieces of Brocade (Ba Duan Jin, 八段锦), the movements of this type are gentle, slow and continuous.
2. Firm and strong type: Represented by Tendon Changing Classics and Five-Elements Palm, *etc.*, the movements of this type are vigorous and forceful. Static contraction method (contraction with the same length) is often applied for the purpose of achieving Qi sensations in this type of Qigong practice.
3. Massage type: Represented by Health Preserving Qigong (Bao Jian Gong, 保健功) and Relaxation Qigong (Fang Song Gong, 放松功), this type is characterized by manipulating Qi to the hands and then giving a massage (including patting) to certain parts of the body.
4. Life-simulating Qigong type: Represented by Five Animal Play (Wu Qin Xi, 五禽戏), Wild Goose Qigong, Soaring Crane Qigong (He Xiang Zhuang, 鹤翔桩), *etc.*, This type refers to forms that are created by imitating animals movements.
   a. Dancing type: Represented by some yoga forms, meditative dancing (Chan Ding Wu Dao, 禅定舞蹈), the movements of this type are derived from dancing, and are therefore elegant and beautiful.
5. Gymnastic type: Similar to gymnastics, this type is characterized by stretched and flexible movements, and is represented by eighteen Forms of Qigong Practice (Lian Gong Shi Ba Fa, 练功十八法).
6. Walking type: This type is characterized by specific steps and is represented by New Qigong Therapy (Xin Qigong Liao Fa, 新气功疗), Taiji steps (Tai Ji Bu, 太极步) and Plum Blossom Stake (Mei Hua Zhuang, 梅花桩).

The classified types may be mutually merging and overlapping as the classification is not clear-cut. One set of routine dynamic Qigong can cover the characteristics of several other types. Take Five Elements Palm for example: Its body movement belongs to the pliable type, but its hand movement is typical of static force, and therefore, belongs to the firm and strong type.

Moreover, there is a great difference in the maneuver between movements in general physical training and those in Qigong practice. The former mostly employs the strength of muscles, the latter, however, stresses movements induced by internal Qi to avoid stiff movements exerted by mechanic force. It follows that in dynamic Qigong practice, the muscles are supposed to be soft and relaxed rather than stiff and tight (except for the firm and strong type).

The force of dynamic Qigong comes from the energy created by the mind, which can suddenly explode, instead of that from muscle contraction. Stiffness, fatigue, aches and numbness in the limb muscles after dynamic Qigong practice are probably due to improper ways of exerting strength.

b) Spontaneous Qigong Movements

Spontaneous movements can either naturally occur during Qigong practice or be induced by 'spontaneous dynamic Qigong', which is intended to produce such results.

The movements in spontaneous dynamic Qigong are caused by the flow of internal Qi rather than pre-set or guided by the mind. A variety of movements may occur, ranging from slight movements to dramatic ones, soft movements to vigorous ones. It is crucial that spontaneous movements should be maneuvered under the control of the mind, and that the rhythm, pause and closing are to be directed by the mind as well. Otherwise, the practitioner is subject to Qigong deviation.

Spontaneous dynamic Qigong is, generally speaking, unsuitable for beginners since it is very hard to manage and liable to deviation.

c) Internal Maneuver

Internal maneuver, as mentioned previously, involves the exercise on the body parts' internal feelings and their relations during Qigong practice. Subtler than the external maneuver, the internal maneuver is of great importance, but easily neglected as it is often invisible on the exterior.

The internal maneuver and the external movement are closely linked and exert mutual influence. The practitioner has to adjust the external by regulating the internal feelings and their relations, as they cannot inspect their entire external movements.

The internal maneuver in static Qigong will be introduced in the order from head to toe in the following paragraph, some of which are also suitable for dynamic Qigong.

1) Head and Neck

The basic principle includes keeping the head erect and the neck relaxed, "withdrawing the sight and reversing listening", pressing the tongue against the palate, *etc*.

In some Qigong forms, keeping the head erect is often referred to as 'the head seems to be suspended' (Tou Ru Xuan, 头如悬) or 'suspending the head' (Xuan Ding, 悬顶). The feeling is obtained by imagining that there is a thread linked to the head which pulls it upward. In doing so, the pressure on the neck will be reduced. This helps relax the cervical vertebras and benefits the smooth Qi circulation of Governor Vessel (Du Mai, 督脉).

It should be noted that the head is kept relatively erect, and should, as a matter of fact, tilt slightly forward by drawing the lower jaw slightly inward. If the head is entirely upright, the cervical vertebras will be compressed, but if the head tilts slightly forward, the cervical vertebras can fully extend. Moreover, the maneuver of drawing the lower jaw back and tilting the head forward is closely related to the motion of drawing in the chest and straightening the back, which will be discussed later.

"Withdrawing the sight and reversing listening" (Shou Shi Fan Ting, 收視返聽) is a maneuver which reverses the outward-going attention in vision and hearing, resulting in looking without seeing anything, listening without hearing anything. *Clue to the Unseen* (Yin Fu Jing, 阴符经) put it 'The hidden wisdom lies in the eye'. *Spiritual Pivot On perplexity* (Lingshu Dahuo Lun 灵枢・大惑论) stated, 'The eye is the messenger of the heart, which houses the spirit'. The eye is the occult point in Qigong practice. Only when the eyes are not distracted the spirit can be stored. "Withdrawing the sight" helps get rid of hallucinations. It also helps the practitioner to concentrate on Qigong practice by blocking the impact of external light. The eyes should be slightly closed because complete closure may cause drowsiness due to darkness, and keeping eyes open diverts one's attention due to excess light. Consequently, a slight closure of eyes is required for static Qigong practice.

It is easy for beginners to get drowsy and distracted. When this happens, open the eye a bit to receive a glimpse, and look straight ahead or slightly downward at the tip of the nose. The requirement of line of sight is closely related to "keeping the mind on" (Yi Shou, 意守), but has little to do with the opening or closing of the eye. The exercise of focusing on the Dan Tian, for example, is similar to reflecting the elixir field. In general, the standing style requires looking slightly upward or horizontally, while the sitting style requires looking slightly downward or horizontally.

"Reversing listening" is the maneuver of listening inwardly, represented by the form of listening to one's own breath the so-called 'breath-listening'. As no sound is produced by breathing in Qigong practice, breath-listening suggests the idea of listening to silence instead of any other sound. Turning the sense of hearing back to oneself by listening to silence is a perfect state in Qigong practice and matches the saying 'silence is superior to any utterance'.

Keep the mouth gently closed and the tongue in its natural place. Raising the tongue to press against the palate, also known as tongue column (She Zhu, 舌柱) is pressing the tongue gently and naturally against the connecting area between the teeth and palate without exerting any force. This maneuver is required in many Qigong forms, Taoist Qigong in particular, for the purpose of linking the Conception (Ren Mai, 任脉) and Governor Vessels. When one attains certain level in Qigong practice, the pressure of the tongue against the palate will be increased gradually. Such phenomenon appears naturally and the practitioner should not intentionally pursue it.

Relaxing the brows and facial muscles is also required in the practice for both physical and emotional maneuvers. A smile is emphasized in many static Qigong forms, as it indicates a happy and relaxed emotional state, which in turn manifests in relaxed brows and a joyful face physically. It should be noted that smile is more emphasized with a sense of peace and joy than the facial expression of laughing that tends to tighten the corners of the mouth.

2) Upper Limb

Shoulder Relaxation and elbow drooping are the basic principles for upper limbs.

When practicing shoulder relaxation, one should avoid shrugging and keep them in a natural position. It is necessary because tightened muscles interfere with the downward flowing of Qi and hinder abdominal breathing. In the standing style, the shoulders are liable to shrug when lifting arms, especially when they are raised too high. Therefore, it is recommended that the arms stay at the height between Dan Zhong Point (膻中) and the Lower Dan Tian in either Holding-ball or Raising-ball form.

Relaxing the shoulder involves not only the relaxation of the shoulder, but that of the elbow as well. As an extension of the maneuver of the shoulder, drooping the elbows means exerting no force on them, which can be attained once the shoulder is properly relaxed. Since the elbow is considered a supporting and turning "point" for the dropping trend of the shoulder and the arm, the maneuver on the elbow is to make sure not to raise this point, while practicing either in standing or sitting position.

Moreover, one should leave a space between the arm and the body instead of pressing them against each other, while practicing in standing. An empty armpit can help relaxation and bring more comfort to the body, while the tightly squeezed one blocks the circulation of Qi and blood.

3) Chest and Back

Drawing in the chest and straightening the back are the essentials of maneuver on the chest and the back.

Drawing the chest slightly inward can relax the muscles on the triangle region of chest (formed by the lines drawn among Tian Tu Point (天突穴) and two nipples) for freer breathing, and helps the flowing of Qi move downward to induce abdominal breathing. Straightening the back can stretch the spine, and therefore, smooth the flow of Qi in the Governor Vessel.

Drawing the lower jaw inward is accompanied by a pulling-in of the chest, and therefore, the maneuver on the chest is directly related to that on the lower jaw and the shoulder. Drawing in the chest and straightening the back should be conducted simultaneously because the maneuver of the former, to a certain extent, determines that of the latter. Drawing in the chest excessively will result in a hunched back instead of a straightened back. The character 'straightening' stresses the idea of being straight and upright, but avoid bending. The proper maneuver on the chest and back naturally reduces the physiology curvature at the back and waist to bring about a more erect spinal column. In addition, the physiology curvature at the neck is also reduced by drawing the lower jaw inward. As a result, the spinal column can fully extend from top to end during Qigong practice.

4) Waist and Hips

The basic requirements for the waist and hips are briefed as extending the waist and lowering the hips. These two maneuvers are of great importance in both standing and sitting styles.

Extending the waist means stretching the spinal column to prevent it from lowering. Lowering the hips is a maneuver of sinking the hips by protruding them backward in the sitting form, and can be conducted in the way as if one is about to sit on a high stool in the standing form.

The two postures are not only helpful to extend the spine, but enable the practitioner to rest the center of gravity on the lower abdomen and help Qi to gather into the elixir field.

5) Lower Limbs

Keeping the lower limbs relaxed and steady is one of the basic principles in Qigong practice. One should stand up straight in the standing form with both feet as relaxed as possible and both knees slightly bent without surpassing the tip of toes. Keep the feet apart at shoulder width, toes slightly grasping the ground.

Both feet can show in three forms: inward splayfoot, outward splayfoot and parallel foot. Inward splayfoot is formed by turning the toes inward to enable firm footing. Outward splayfoot is formed by turning the toes outward to render flexible movements. The posture of standing with paralleled feet is also known as horse-riding stance, which is a posture conforming to the natural physiological condition with less intentional maneuver.

Moreover, when practicing the standing form, the lower limbs (including the entire body) should not be in a completely stiff and motionless condition. Under general circumstances, the body may be engaged in slight swaying, which can actually stabilize the standing posture rather than harming it. In addition, standing with slight swaying can save energy and keep the body relaxed. Generally, the lower limbs are more relaxed in the sitting form than in the standing form. In the standing form, the feet postures are similar to those in plain sitting. In cross-legged and kneeling sitting form, the lower limbs might suffer pressure. In this case, one should tap and massage them gently to help promote Qi flow and blood circulation.

ADDICTION THERAPY

Of particular importance was a pilot study in a residential addiction treatment center. The objective of this study was to explore the feasibility and efficacy of adding integrative Qigong meditation to residential treatment for substance abuse. The method was to introduce Qigong meditation, which blends relaxation, breathing, guided imagery, inward attention, and mindfulness to elicit a tranquil state, and to introduce a short-term residential treatment program. At first, clients chose to participate in Qigong meditation on a voluntary basis during their evening break. Later, they chose to participate in either meditation or Stress Management and Relaxation Training (SMART) twice a day as part of the scheduled treatment. Weekly questionnaires were completed by 248 participants for up to 4 weeks to assess their changes in treatment outcomes. Participants in the meditation group were also assessed for quality of meditation to evaluate the association between quality and treatment outcome. Results showed most clients were amenable to meditation as part of the treatment program, and two thirds chose to participate in daily meditation. While both groups reported significant improvements in the treatment outcome, the meditation group reported a significantly higher treatment completion rate (92% *versus* 78%, $p<01$) and more reduction in craving than did the SMART group. Participants whose meditation was of acceptable quality reported greater reductions in craving, anxiety, and withdrawal symptoms than those participants whose meditation was of low quality. Female meditation participants reported significantly more reduction in anxiety and withdrawal symptoms than any other group. The conclusions showed that Qigong meditation appears to contribute positively to addiction treatment outcomes, with results at least as good as those of an established stress management program. Results for those who meditate adequately are especially encouraging. Meditative therapy may be more effective or acceptable for female drug abusers than for males. Further study is needed to assess ways to improve substance abusers' engagement and proficiency in meditation [22].

REFERENCES

[1] Shinnick P. Qigong: where did it come from? Where does it fit in science? What are the advances? J Altern Complement Med 2006; 12(4): 351-3. [http://dx.doi.org/10.1089/acm.2006.12.351] [PMID: 16722782]

[2] Shinnick P. A twelve-year research report on the science of Qigong, disease, self care and recent discoveries. Proceedings of the Fourth World Academy of Medical Qigong. People's Republic of China. 2006.

[3] Shinnick P. Roy R. The Science of whole person healing: research data summary on Qigong and the differentiation of qi into body pathways, the physiology and properties of ind/body wholeness and its clinical application to disease and athletics. Science of Whole Person Healing: Proceeding of the First

Interdisciplinary International Conference.; New York: iUniverse, Inc.. 2004; pp. 87-126.

[4] Chen KW, Comerford A, Shinnick P, Ziedonis DM. Introducing Qigong meditation into residential addiction treatment: a pilot study where gender makes a difference. J Altern Complement Med 2010; 16(8): 875-82.
[http://dx.doi.org/10.1089/acm.2009.0443] [PMID: 20649456]

[5] Chen KW. An analytic review of studies on measuring effects of external QI in China. Altern Ther Health Med 2004; 10(4): 38-50.
[PMID: 15285273]

[6] Sancier KM. Search for medical application of Qigong with the Qigong Database. Townsend Letter for Doctors & Patients 2002; 222: 116-8.

[7] Sancier KM. Anti-aging benefits of Qigong. J IntI Soc Life Info Sci 1996; 14(2): 20.

[8] Sancier KM, Holman D. Commentary: Multifaceted health benefits of medical Qigong. J Altern Complement Med 2004; 10(1): 163-5.
[http://dx.doi.org/10.1089/107555304322849084] [PMID: 15025890]

[9] Sancier KM, Hu B. Medical application of Qigong and emitted qi on humans, animal, cell cultures & plants: review of selected scientific research. Am J Acupunct 1991; 19: 367-77.

[10] Sancier KM. Medical applications of Qigong. Altern Ther Health Med 1996; 2(1): 40-6.
[PMID: 8795871]

[11] Chen KW. An analytic review of studies on measuring effects of external QI in China. Altern Ther Health Med 2004; 10(4): 38-50.
[PMID: 15285273]

[12] Lin A, Li Y, Guo Z, Shen Z, Zhang H, Zhang T. Qigong: chinese medicine or pseudoscience?. New York: Prometheus Books 2000.

[13] Shao L, Zhang J, Chen L, Zhang X, Chen KW. Effects of external qi of Qigong with opposing intentions on proliferation of Escherichia coli. J Altern Complement Med 2009; 15(5): 567-71.
[http://dx.doi.org/10.1089/acm.2008.0408] [PMID: 19425820]

[14] Chen K, Yeung R. Exploratory studies of Qigong therapy for cancer in China. Integr Cancer Ther 2002; 1(4): 345-70.
[http://dx.doi.org/10.1177/1534735402238187] [PMID: 14664729]

[15] Chen K. Inhibitory effects of bio-energy therapies on cancer growth: an overview of recent laboratory studies in the US and it implications in cancer treatment World Sci and ech/modern of trad Chinese. Med and Mat Medica 2008; 10(4)

[16] Chen KW, Liu T, Zhang H, Lin Z. An analytical review of the Chinese literature on Qigong therapy for diabetes mellitus. Am J Chin Med 2009; 37(3): 439-57.
[http://dx.doi.org/10.1142/S0192415X09006965] [PMID: 19606506]

[17] Chen KW, Perlman A, Liao JG, Lam A, Staller J, Sigal LH. Effects of external Qigong therapy on osteoarthritis of the knee. A randomized controlled trial. Clin Rheumatol 2008; 27(12): 1497-505.
[http://dx.doi.org/10.1007/s10067-008-0955-4] [PMID: 18654733]

[18] Chen K, Liu TJ. Effects of Qigong therapy on arthritis: a review of report of a pilot trail. Med Poara 2004; 1(1): 36-48.

[19] Chen KW, Turner FD. A case study of simultaneous recovery from multiple physical symptoms with medical Qigong therapy. J Altern Complement Med 2004; 10(1): 159-62.
[http://dx.doi.org/10.1089/107555304322849075] [PMID: 15025889]

[20] Chen KW, Hassett AL, Hou F, Staller J, Lichtbroun AS. A pilot study of external Qigong therapy for patients with fibromyalgia. J Altern Complement Med 2006; 12(9): 851-6.

[21] Chen K, Berger C, Manheimer E. Meditative Therapies for reducing anxiety: a systematic review and meta-analysis of randomized controlled trials. Dep Anx 2012; 29: 45-562. [http://dx.doi.org/10.1089/acm.2006.12.851] [PMID: 17109575]

[22] Chen KW, Comerford A, Shinnick P, Ziedonis DM. Introducing Qigong meditation into residential addiction treatment: a pilot study where gender makes a difference. J Altern Complement Med 2010; 16(8): 875-82. [http://dx.doi.org/10.1089/acm.2009.0443] [PMID: 20649456]

CHAPTER 6

Organ Pulsed Electromagnetic Fields (PEMF): Critical Evaluation of Traditional Chinese Meridian Theory and O-Ring Contribution to Medicine

Abstract: The Omura O-ring non-invasive low cost test is a scientific way to gather data over time. The O-ring is able to image PEMF (Pulsed Electromagnetic Fields) organ pathways on the surface of the skin and compare these imaged pathways with the traditional Oriental Meridians. These pathways have only been theories and with the O-ring a deeper understanding can be realized. The biochemistry of these pathways is presented. A triple blind study shielding the O-ring process from two researchers and patient shown under toxic condition (holding tobacco and lung tissue in the hand as control reference) caused an aberration of the lung pathway. A two year - 400 patient-clinical study was initiated from this aberrant experiment to see pathways under various pain conditions. These pathways deviate in spinal herniations, infections, scars, breast implants, emotional stress and muscular spasms. This case study indicated that most myofascial pain comes from the dermatome of the spine (areas of innervations of each vertebra) and stimulation to that particular vertebrae resulted in pain reduction in 80% of the cases. About 30 cases were associated with organ dysfunction and manifest aberrant pathways or pathways not a part of Oriental medicine. Through O-ring imaging, infections can be located, usually inside localized muscle spasms and when given compatible antibiotics, the O-ring showed that the antibiotic did not penetrate these spasm areas. With stimulation *i.e.*, acupuncture, laser, manual stimulation or Qigong, the antibiotic penetrated the area and resolved the infection. The Hui theory, supported by this clinical study outlines the general phases and direction inside and outside the body, linear and nonlinear direction from the location of a Oriental meridian points or circles.

Keywords : Antidote, Asthma, Asymmetry, Diaphragm, Heart hypertension, Implants, Molecular identification, Mu points, Organ meridians, Organ PEMF, Organ representation, Pathological phases, Shu points.

INTRODUCTION TO THE O-RING TEST

My research into health care, while teaching at Rutgers University as an assistant

Phillip Shinnick & Laurence Porter

professor in the 1970's, found that the high cost of health care came from the new technological diagnosis instruments. A spontaneous gathering of surgeons at Robert Wood Johnson Medical Center, prompted by hearing of my interest in medicine thought I might help with difficult patients, even though my background was not in medicine. I treated patients at Robert Wood hospital who had been paralyzed from surgery gone wrong at Dr. Bernie Sandler's request. I just used my intuition, based upon my experiences as a frequently injured athlete due to my long career in sport, in treating these patients who did well. Clearly medicine needed new thinking and I was the New Jersey recruit. Dr. Bernie Sandler and Dr. Lee, at the Robert Wood Johnson Hospital in New Jersey, recommended I seek out. Yoshiaki Omura and electrical engineer, who practiced advanced Occidental medicine and understood Ancient Oriental medicine. Dr. Omura had developed a low cost form of diagnosis. Also Saul Heller, M.D., Chairman of the New York Medical Board, supported my inclusion into medicine as an equivalent since New York was looking for new ideas and approaches to medicine.

In the late 1970s Dr. Omura — physician, engineer, researcher and author, editor, healer — was testing arm strength using applied kinesiology when he felt that there must be a better and easier method than arm strength. Dr. Omura discovered the ORT (O-Ring Imaging Test) while he was testing brain laterality by the grasping strength of a hand of a subject who was being subjected to battery-generated positive and negative electromagnetic fields in close proximity. Both positive and negative fields were shown to have an effect on the grasping strength of the hand and finger, along with various sounds and whether the subject's eyes were open or closed [1]. He noticed that when applying pressure to create pain, the grip force decreased. He observed that (a) induced pain would decrease the grip force, and (b) even a light pressure on skin areas, very often related to "previous pain", also reproduced this phenomenon. However, pressure applied on "normal" areas did not cause the grip force to decrease. This also hinted at memory of an injury in previously injured areas of the body. This technique method has been published elsewhere as the references will show.

In the process he discovered testing fingers in an O-Ring was much more reliable than arm strength or hand grasping strength which could be valid but not reliable. The Bi-Digital-O-ring test, a sensitive, non-invasive diagnostic screening method can provide basic information about a variety of pathologies. The BDORT or ORT, is now taught at two schools in Japan but viewed with suspicion in the Western world because of its low cost and simplicity. It can be used in acupuncture, dentistry, and veterinary medicine. It is quick, safe and low-cost, and there is no expensive equipment to maintain — an important point in this era of ever-rising medical costs. Easily administered, it can discriminate between normal and abnormal tissue and, as a primary screening method, it can provide important information to health practitioners without exposing patients to more expensive and invasive procedures such as MRIs, CT scans, X-rays or exploratory surgery and the ancillary concerns about strong magnetic fields and radiation as well as surgical recovery [2, 3].

I worked with Dr. Omura as his associate editor of his journal, secretary of his college, co-author and as a trustee for 8 years. I scientifically exposed this test to real scrutiny, collecting data, drawing diagrams, and designed research methods. I was asked as a member to present to the New York Society for Physicians and Dentist for Acupuncture on my other clinical work. Members wanted to know about the O-Ring. I spontaneously demonstrated this method and the one of the board members afterwards thought this was improper, he was suspicion of this technique, which could reflect unfavorably on the society. I am now very careful with this information and do not speak about it very often because of this medical backlash for fear of compromising my own standing in the medical community. The information one gets from using the O-ring technique is informative and gives a very good new clinical understanding. In this way after years of use it is not necessary anymore to use it because of the sophistication it provides. I do not practice it except in extremely difficult situations for the reasons mentioned above. *All patients on whom I used this technique on for research signed informed consent form.*

An acupuncture point is really an area which has a diffuse pattern and is not two dimensional or linear but geometric with movement in and out and is an approximation of what a meditator roughly sees when being one pointed in space (Fig. **1**).

The ORT has many advantages. In 1984, Omura demonstrated, witnessed by me, that by touching a subject's organ representation point, like the stomach, Ren 12, the front-Mu or Alarm Point Zhongwan中脘) with a non-conducting probe while the subject was simultaneously holding a substance, an aspirin — known to be toxic to that organ — the O-ring test produces a weakening response. This confirmed the relationship between the Mu points and their respective organs as described in Traditional Chinese Medicine. In Traditional Chinese Medicine (TCM) qi has many forms. One differentiation of qi, there are pathways on the surface of the body called meridians, originating with PEMF of organs which have internal and external pathways, according to TCM.

In 1985 Omura showed that with the subject holding a microscopic slide (two layered pieces of glass with a substance inside) of a specific organ tissue as a *reference control substance*, a meridian-like pathway of that internal organ could be mapped or "imaged" on the surface of the skin [4, 5]. Later in this chapter we present pathways imaged in clinic and compared to Oriental Medicine. This technique was published in 1996 by Shinnick [6].

Circles represent toxic conditions to the lung and the other pathway is the normal imaged lung imaged using the lung tissue of a microscopic slide.

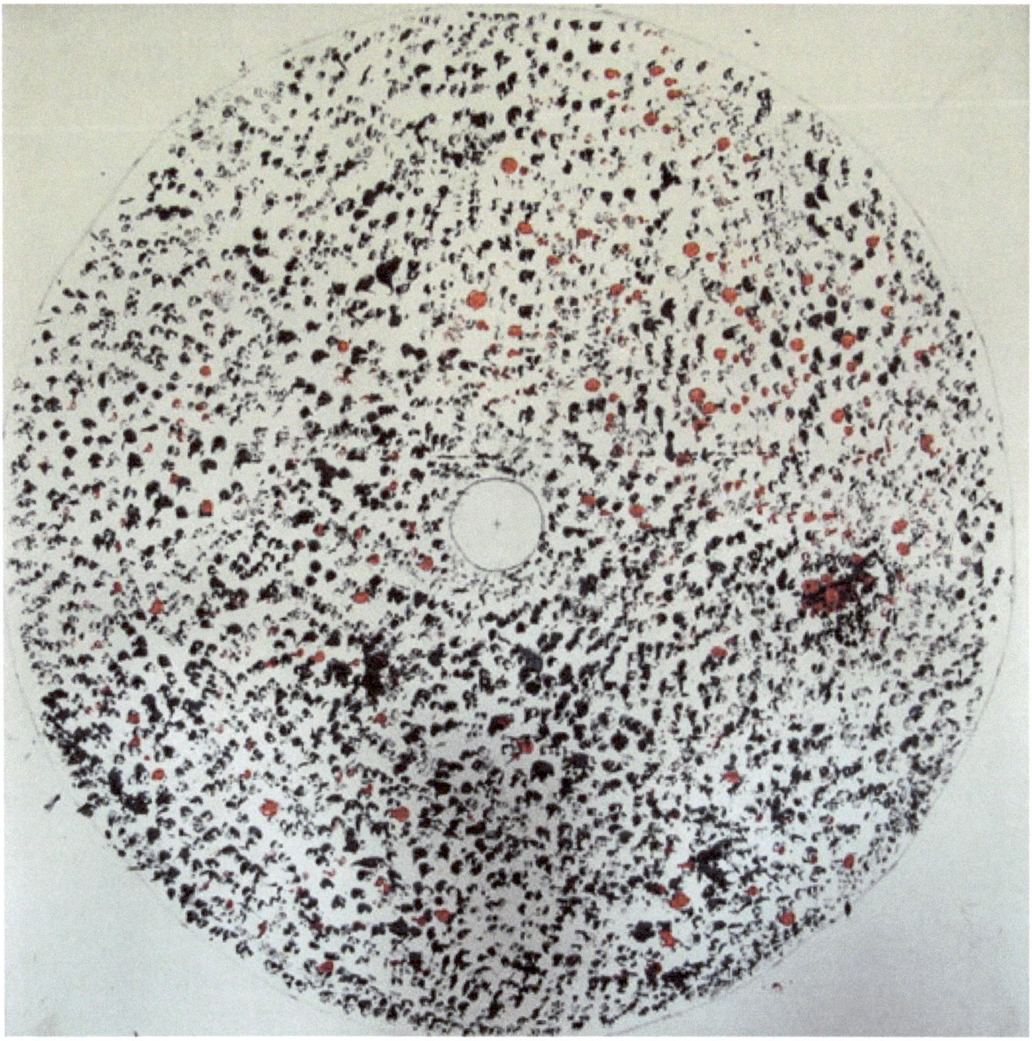

Fig. (1). Red and Black Dancing. (This painting is reproduced with special permission of Laurence Porter). Photo Herman Costa.

The idea that a known toxin reflected in a negative way to the meridian led to the idea to image toxin pathways. Shinnick and Celia Blumenthal, M.D. using a triple blind technique where the subject, tester and assistant did not view each other, imaged the lung pathway using the lung as a control reference but with more information, tobacco was held in the subject's hand [7 - 14] (Figs. **2, 3**). This pathway deviated from the classical meridian. With this new information, a differentiation or fragmentation appeared on the pathway. This was later confirmed by subsequent cases of patients with lung disease. Pathways change according to variables in the body such as a microorganism or a toxin to the organs, scars, breast implants and asymmetry to the spine creates organ pathway aberrations. Pathways are informational and the biochemistry of the pathway can be tested with various tested substances *i.e.*, holding a particular biochemical in the hand and to see if it matches the organ pathway tested.

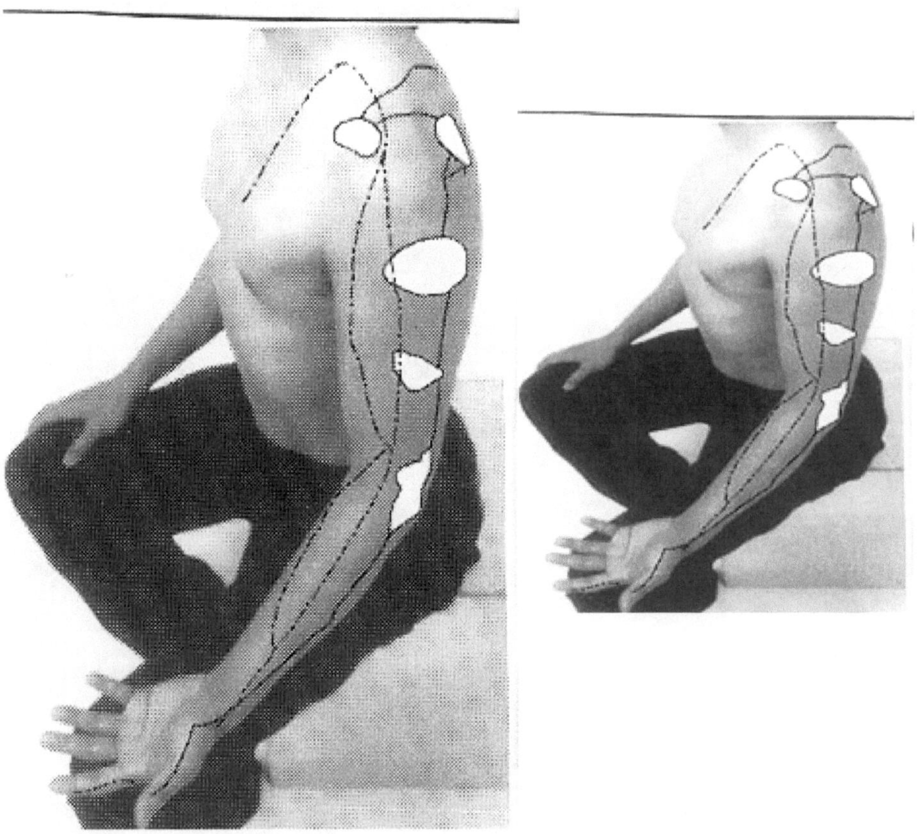

Fig. (2). Imaging of the lung pathway medial and the toxic lung posterior by Shinnick. (With special permission of Shinnick).

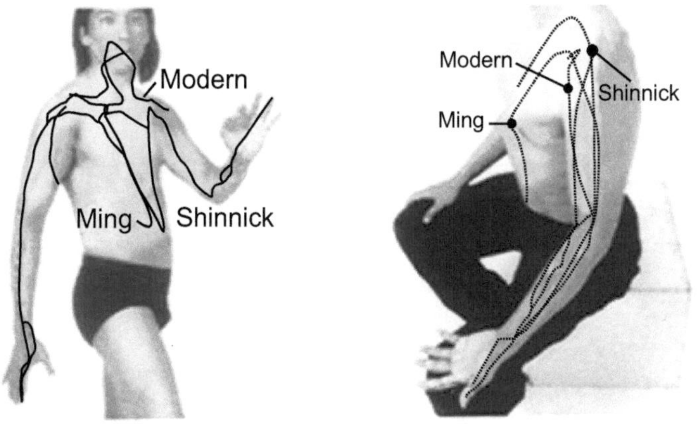

Fig. (3). To the left Shinnick, Modern and Ming Colon Pathways. On the right Shinnick, Modern and Ming Lung Pathways. (With special permission of Shinnick).

The modern is reflected in modern textbooks and the ancient appears in historical records. One can see that the Shinick imaged colon and lung pathway is closer to the ancient than modern abbreviated lung pathway. Multiple starting positions in the hand for the lung and colon were found and account for more variations due to either condition of the lung or colon, or dominant position of the hand throughout the day due to the reversible forearm. Oriental medicine shows just one starting point.

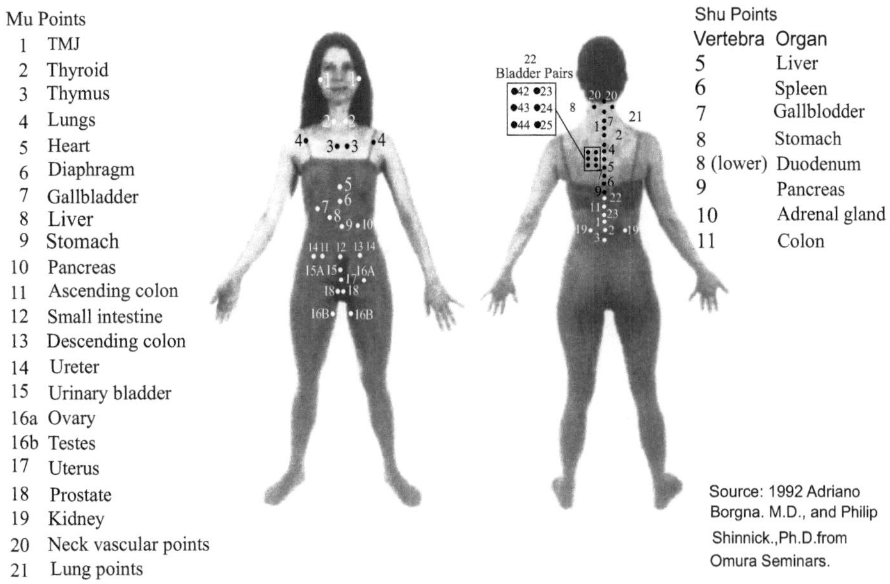

Fig. (4). The organ representation points on the (Mu) front and (Shu) back. (With special permission of Shinnick).

The above shows the organ representation points of the back (SHU) and front (MU) taken from Omura's lectures, our own research, put together by Adriano Borgna, M.D. and Shinnick from workshops and clinical cases [15 - 17] (Fig. **4**). The stomach meridian 胃经)weijing starts in the face, just below the center of the eye, and has multiple pathways going out from the stomach and across the abdomen. While only one pathway can be seen in the traditional charts.

O-Ring method showed multiple channels diverging and converging to the main pathway [18] (Fig. **5**).

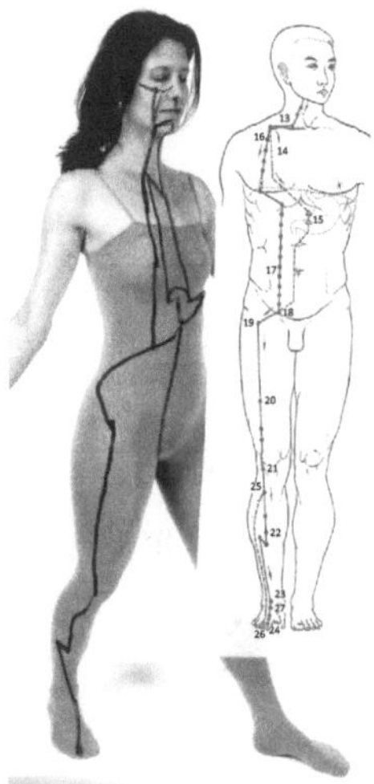

Fig. (5). Omura imaging of stomach meridian compared to traditional stomach pathway. The second dotted line on right of traditional stomach meridian is inside the body not outside. Omura shows multiple pathways.

Omura imaged the stomach pathway with stomach tissue which shows multiple pathways in comparison to the modern and ancient stomach meridian [16, 28]. This imaging of the Stomach pathway appears in the Shinnick Borgna book and generally a condensation of that book [16] (Figs. **5, 6**).

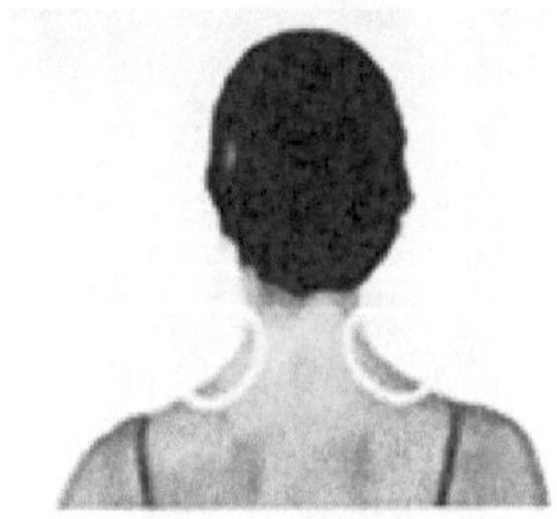

Fig. (6). Phase 1 Diaphragm. (With special permission of Shinnick).

Briefly, from 1985-1989 Shinnick looked at 400 cases and from those 30 cases could be matched to organs from clinical patients who complained of pain. The others were related to a dermatome field from the spinal cord. The protocol was simple, each organ representation point or alarm point, called Mu front points, was tested for abnormality then each spinal Shu vertebra points was tested. Acupuncture was given to abnormal Mu or Shu points; if patient did not get pain relief then we tested the abnormal points on the spine ignoring the textbooks understanding and instead tested with organ tissues, randomly (face down, not seeing what organ was being tested randomly), selected for comparison. Several interesting results came from this study [19-25].

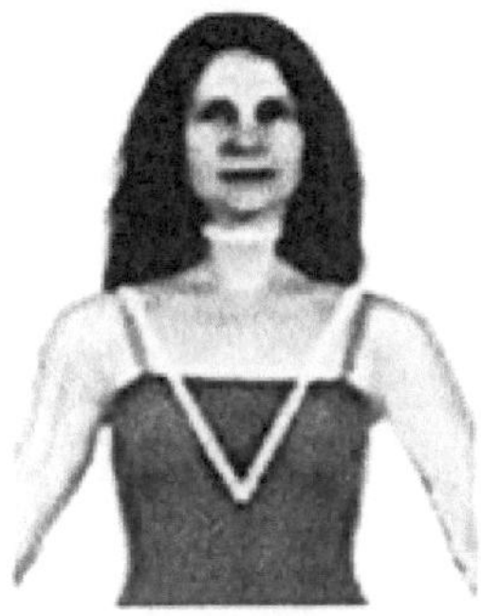

Fig. (7). Phases 1 Diaphragm. (With special permission of Shinnick).

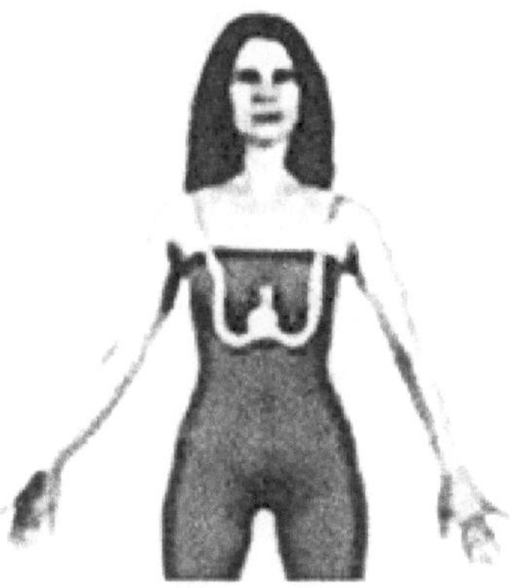

Fig. (8). Phase 2 after acupuncture. (With special permission of Shinnick).

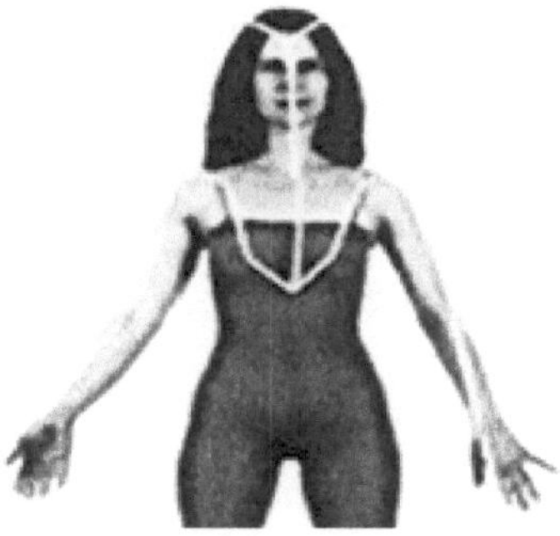

Fig. (9). Phase three after acupuncture Diaphragm. (With special permission of Shinnick).

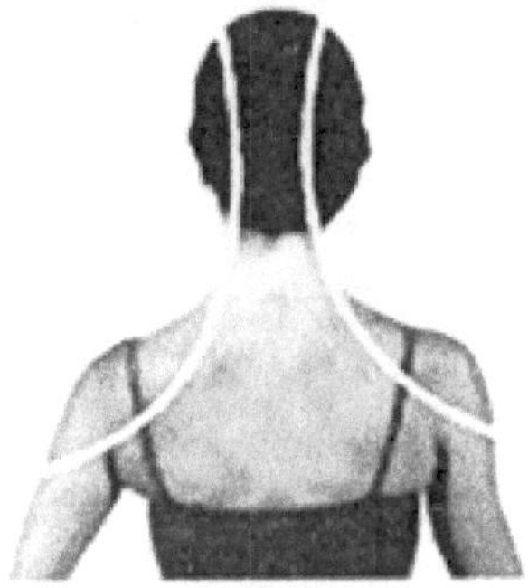

Fig. (10). Phase three after acupuncture Diaphragm. (With special permission of Shinnick).

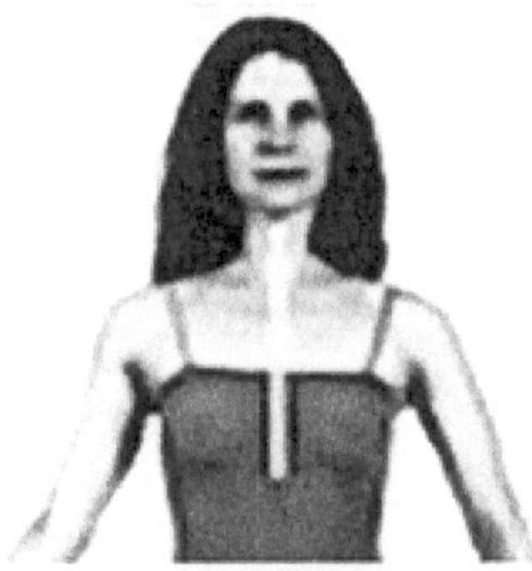

Fig. (11). Phase 4 after acupuncture. (With special permission of Shinnick).

The first was the four phases of the diaphragm. A woman complained of neck pain and this neck point was randomly matched to organs tissues and other non-organ tissue selected at random. A diaphragm tissue resonated to this point (Figs. **6 - 11**). After imaging the diaphragm pathway at random, acupuncture was administered to this point and the pathway changed. This was done three times until it stabilized. Subsequent clinical tests showed that people with asthma, allergies or respiratory problems get stuck in one of these phases. This particular patient had cervical neck problems. A diaphragm pathway was found in four phases.

This patient had a cervical herniation C6-7, imaging started from the xiphoid process randomly (Figs. **6 - 11**). In clinical tests, asthma patients tended to get struck in one phase as do smokers and individuals with pain along this pathway. Mechanical problems with the cervical vertebrae were associated with abnormal phases of the diaphragm as were pain in the neck, posterior deltoid or scapula. Constriction of the throat, chronic rhinitis, deviated nasal septum and stress were also associated with certain diaphragm phases. Pathways imaged with tissue after acupuncture usually resulted in the abnormal pathway disappearing or shifting more medial.

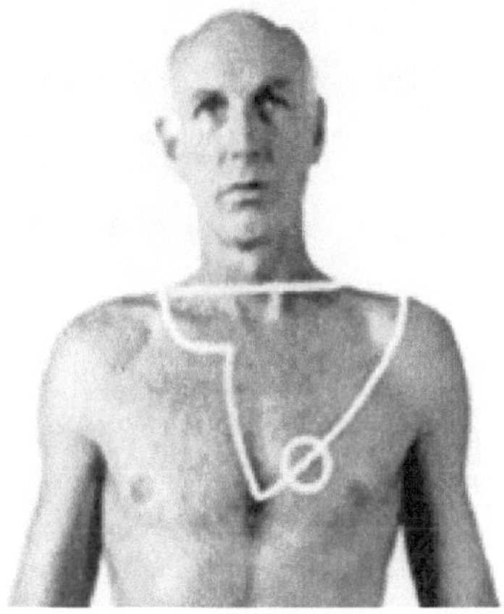

Fig. (12). Phase 1. Hypertension of the Heart (front). (With special permission of Shinnick).

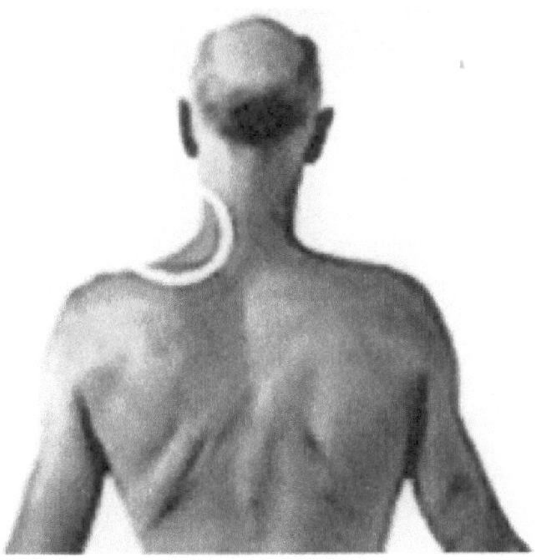

Fig. (13). (back pattern). (With special permission of Shinnick).

A patient with chest pains. The circle (Fig. **12**) was randomly matched to heart tissue which manifested in three phases after acupuncture (Figs. **12 - 16**). No laboratory test confirmed any heart abnormality. He suffered from emotional stress. This showed that stress and emotions can affect the qi pathways as well as microorganism or toxins.The heart pathway around the thoracic was associated with chronic costochondritis and hypertension and showed three phases.

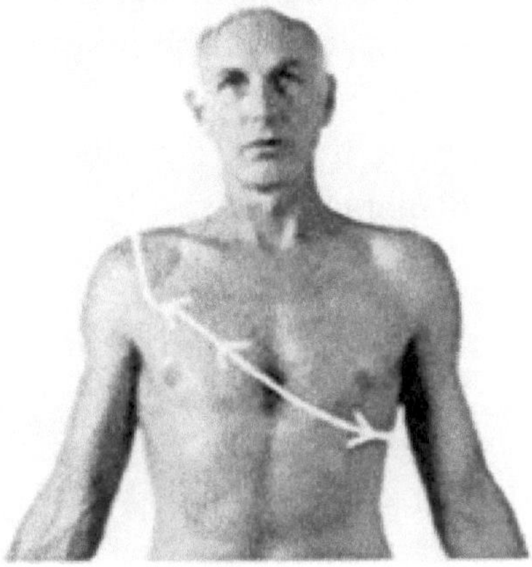

Fig. (14). Phase 2 Front Heart pathway after acupuncture. (With special permission of Shinnick).

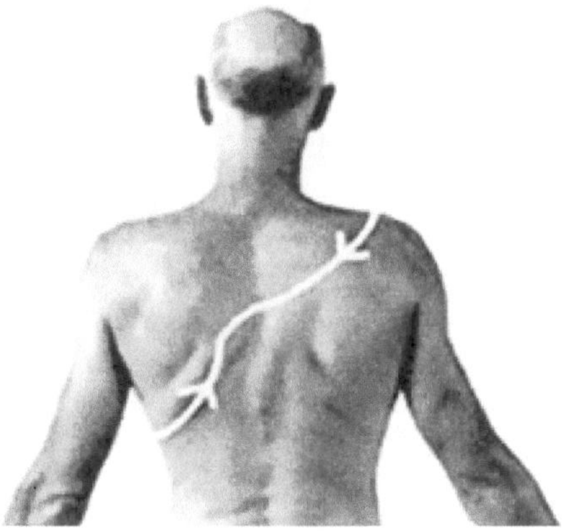

Fig. (15). Back. (With special permission of Shinnick).

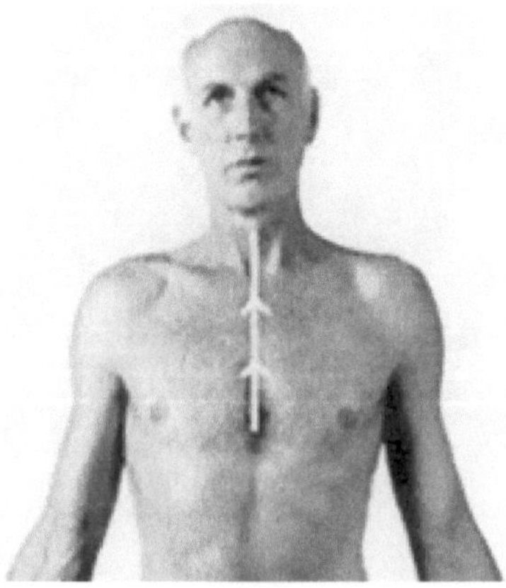

Fig. (16). Phase 3 after acupuncture. (With special permission of Shinnick).

One can see that due to emotional stress the thoracic rib cage tightens and causes back pressure to the heart through this constriction. One can see direction, after imaging this pattern with a unidirectional germanium diode. One can see on the front, the direction is away from the center and in the back the direction comes together in the mid upper back where the tension originates (Figs. **14, 15**).

Altogether, organ pathways deviate from the normal pathways under conditions of pain and injury to the body, disturbances of internal organs, or mental stress. The variable that connect various cases are asymmetry---scoliosis, short leg, rotated rib cage and the assortment of deviations from assumed symmetry. Also, scars on the pathway or plastic surgery cause deviations.

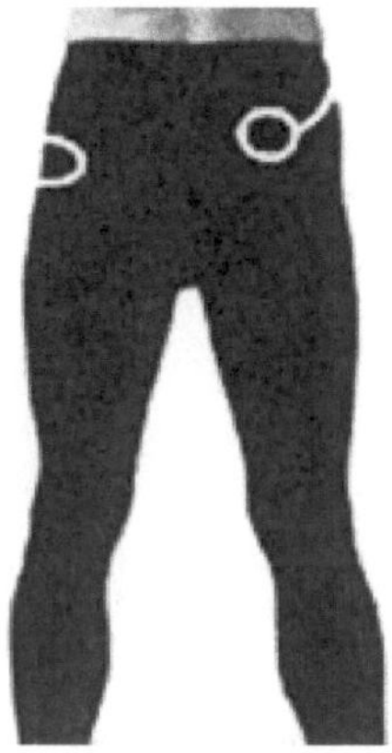

Fig. (17). Back gallbladder. (With special permission of Shinnick).

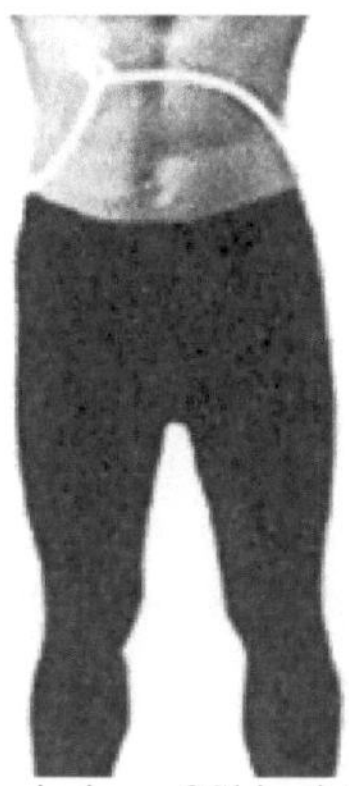

Fig. (18). Front gall bladder. (With special permission of Shinnick).

From this clinical study, the symptoms from the hip gallbladder aberration pathway were associated with scoliosis, infection, colitis, constipation, hip spurs, food allergies, parasites, gallstones, osteoporosis, mechanical problems with the vertebrae, emotional stress and spinal diseases of asymmetry (Figs. **17, 18**). See below. Oriental medicine does not reflect this understanding.

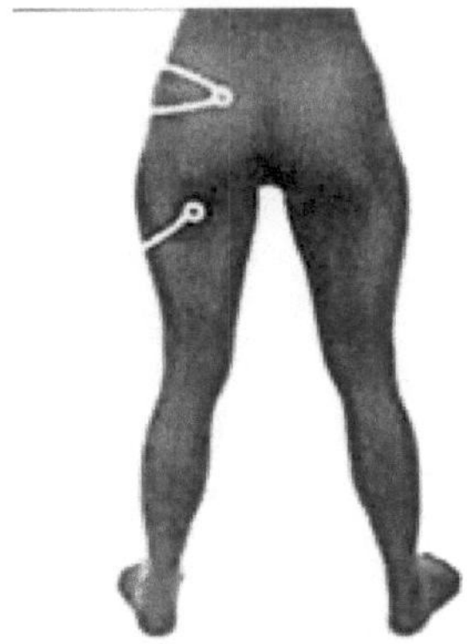

Fig. (19). left back ovary. (With special permission of Shinnick).

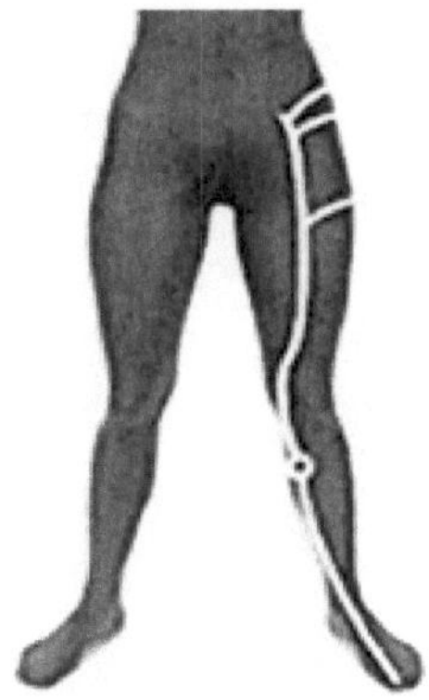

Fig. (20). front ovary. (With special permission of Shinnick).

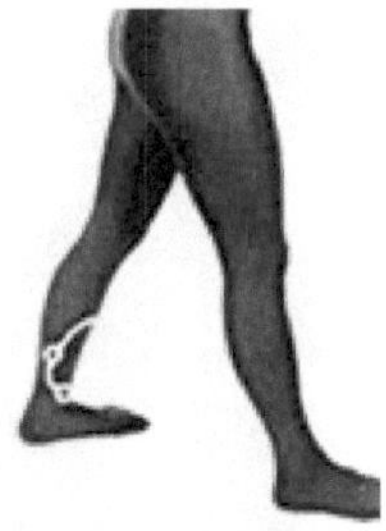

Fig. (21). Other case medial left calf. (With special permission of Shinnick).

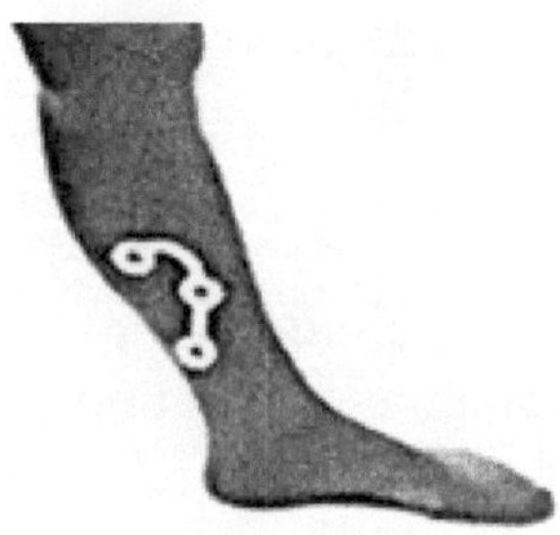

Fig. (22). Other case medial left calf. (With special permission of Shinnick).

In women, this same configuration was associated with the ovary rather than the gallbladder and went to a point directly over the ovary anatomically. See below The ovary aberrant pathway was associated with hip or sacral pain, medial calf pain, scoliosis, pronation of the feet, weakness of the calf muscles, cysts, herpes, infection to the ovary, lumbar radiculopathy, psoas insufficiency, obesity, depression, scoliosis, short leg, arthritis of the hip and postural imbalance (Figs. **19 - 22**).

The bladder prostate aberrant configuration crosses around the leg (Figs. **23,24**). Other bladder symptoms include scoliosis, weak abdominals, psoas insufficiency, and chronic immune deficiency. The colon hip pathway was associated with hip pain, constipation, herniation and bulging, scoliosis, pain to bottom of feet, and subtalar joint dysfunction.

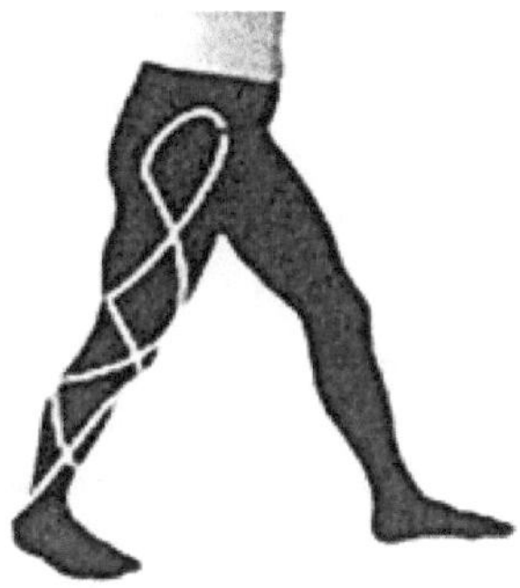

Fig. (23). Phase 1, Bladder and Prostate. (With special permission of Shinnick).

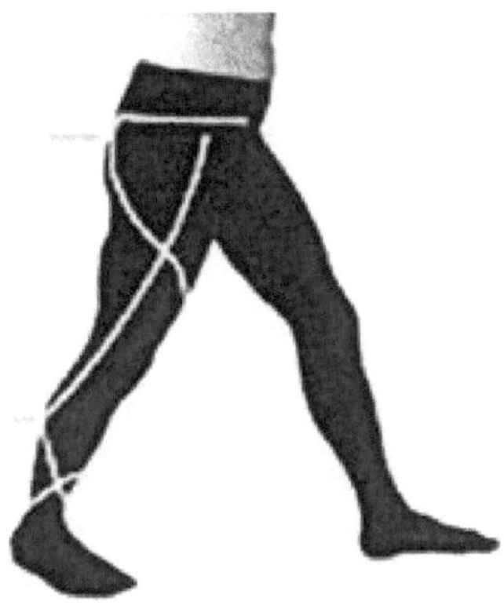

Fig. (24). Phase 2, Bladder Prostate after acupuncture. (With special permission of Shinnick).

From this study one can see PEMF organ qi pathways deviating under diseased conditions and go back to "normal" patterns after treatment with acupuncture or meditation. Qi is differentiated, to each internal organs but fragments due to disease or a variety of structural or skin abnormalities. If the organ is synchronized, then its pathway will be normal, if de-synchronized then it will be fragmented and deviate from that normal pathway. Aberrations were noted in the following organ pathways not reflected in Oriental Medicine, the gall bladder, ovary, bladder, prostate, colon, heart and lung.

In 1987, Omura's publications demonstrated that six of 12 traditional meridians could be detected not only by a reference control substance of its related organ (*e.g.* microscopic slide of stomach tissue for the stomach meridian), but also by the control substance of the preceding organ or pair organ. That is, the first of two organs that comprise a yin-yang "organ/pair system" (*e.g.* with the microscopic spleen slide you can detect the spleen and the stomach meridian). For example, lung precedes large intestine, spleen precedes stomach, heart precedes small intestine, *etc.* "The reverse does not work; with the microscopic stomach slide, the spleen meridian cannot be imaged, and so on" [26]. Along with these relationships Omura found that the pericardium meridian could be detected with the adrenal gland tissue sample and the triple warmer meridian by the ovaries and testes tissue samples. He also found that the SA node tissue sample can be used to detect the AV node. According to Omura, the starting point of the heart (1) 心 xin, Jiquan is not in the axilla but further up on the arm.

Omura used thymus tissue samples to detect its network. The internal network has long been charted by western science but not the external one. Later Omura re-evaluated his network and found a much more elaborated network on the mammary glands' thymus support system. In testing the homunculus in various parts of the body Omura experimented with the use of hormone samples produced by various organs as reference substances and found a correspondence with the weakening of the O-Ring, which represents a resonance between two substances. Examples are: natriuretic peptide could identify heart areas; gastrin the stomach; ovaries and testosterone estrone, estriol, progesterone; *etc*....correspond to the triple warmer organ system of TCM [27].

APPLICATION TO ORT TO CARDIOVASCULAR SYNDROME

Using a microscopic slide of a particular artery, Omura was able to accurately trace areas of brain circulation through certain arteries (posterior, anterior and medial). With the subject wearing a latex cap (like the one for swimming) he was able to draw the contours of the arteries on it and show areas of abnormality. Often acupuncture along the restricted artery could reestablish a good circulation and relieve the symptoms elsewhere (Fig. **25**).

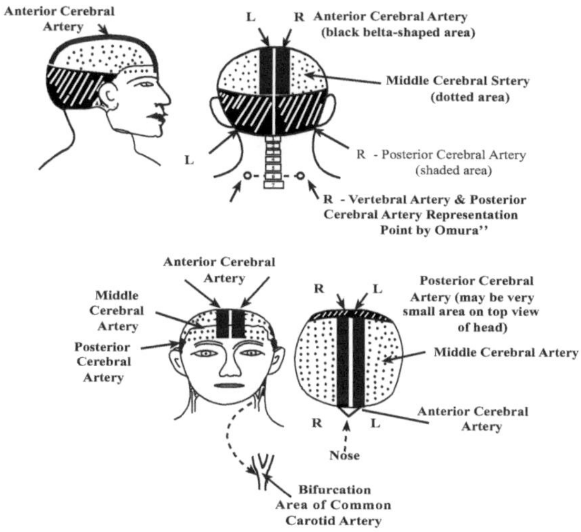

Fig. (25). Location map of blood circulation to the brain from the carotid and posterior cerebral artery. (This figure is reproduced with special permission of Omura).

Mapping of brain circulation on the surface of posterior cerebral arteries by Omura [16, 27] Fig. **25**).

Mapping of heart representation areas on the back of the neck over the medulla oblongata of separate individuals for changes in size according to normal and hypertension (Fig. **26**).

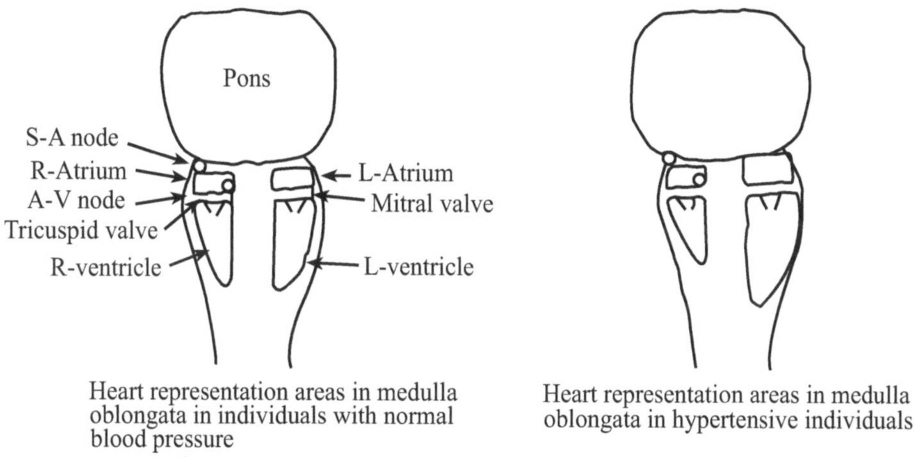

Fig. (26). Mapping of heart representation areas to the back of the neck. (This figure is reproduced with special permission Omura) [28].

Mapping of the right and left posterior spinal arteries and the anterior spinal artery (Fig. **27**). Seeing further up the basilar artery is where these arteries come together at the top of the Circle of Willis. Examining the picture above and below gives a good idea of how to treat heart hypertension the back of the neck and upper thoracic vertebrae (Fig. **25, 26, 27**). This understanding, of location in the brain of the source of arterial circulation and organ representation areas can lead to relieving many patients with arrhythmia and cervical pain with this simple technique. More blood flow to the brain eases the heart tension and systemically affects all organs as well as by stimulation to as the heart [28 - 30]. The AV nodes follow the rhythm of the SA node and disruption of this can lead to a heart attack. Release of the spasticity in the neck area results in heart functioning improvement. The spasticity in the neck is further complicated with asymmetry. In general, patients with asymmetric B/P readings, especially when the patterns were caused by asymmetrical posture, and asymmetry due to previous traumas or stress usually have pain and quickly responded to acupuncture (manual, electrical stimulation) given to the area where the narrowing of the artery had been detected by ORT.

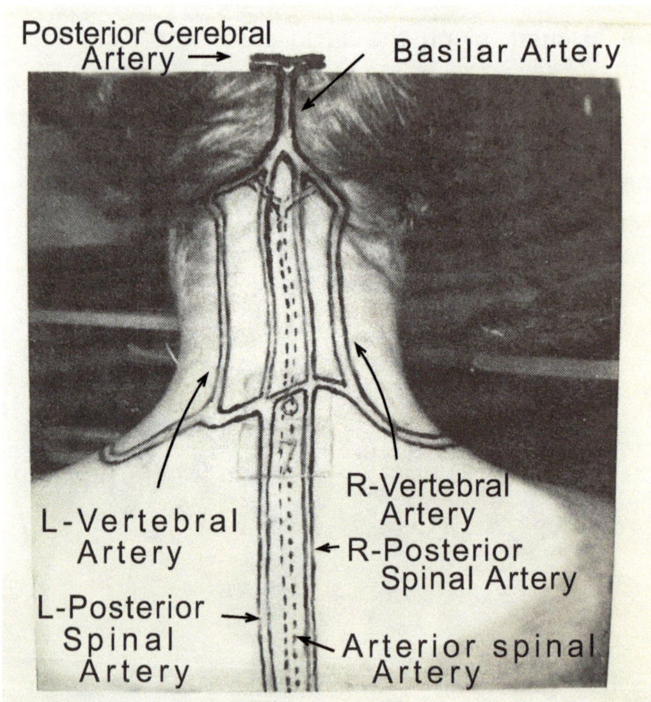

Fig. (27). Posterior arterial circulation to the circle of Willis. (This figure is reproduced with special permission of Omura) [16, 27].

In several cases of older patients who developed arrhythmia due to emotional stress, acupuncture to the heart organ representation points as shown in the Mu and Shu Points, and to the thoracic rib cage quickly resolved arrhythmia. This phenomenon was confirmed in other patients as well. Almost invariably ORT will show asymmetry and spasticity in the neck area and resulting asymmetrical circulation disturbances when clinical symptoms like pain are present.

FOOD AND DRUG COMPATIBILITY TO PATHOGENIC MICROORGANISM

A practical application of the O-ring in helping patients is to take the appropriate multi-vitamins or supplements. The procedure is simple. First the patient is tested for reliability by the normal procedure we described later for the direct ORT; then the control substance (vitamin or supplement) is placed in the hand of the patient that is free. If the ring formed with the most sensitive finger opens, the substance is not helpful for that individual. If the same ring becomes stronger the substance is helpful. The change in strength of the ring is also dose related, so you may observe no change in strength with one dosage but you may notice a change if the dosage is increased or decreased.

INFORMATION PROPAGATION WITH LASER

In the mid 80's, Omura, with the assistance of Shinnick, conducted an examination of a patient. But instead of using a non-conducting probe with direct O-ring application, or a conducting probe with indirect O-ring, a laser beam was used as a probe to stimulate the stomach representation point (Ren 12) 中脘 zhongwan. This was done from a distance of about eight meters. Placing an aspirin in the vicinity of the beam caused the O-ring of the subject holding the laser pointer to open when the beam was targeting the Mu point of the stomach. Dr. Omura deducted that an 8 mm watt monochromatic concentrated beam (laser) positioned in the proximity of the control substance carries the molecular information to the subject to be examined at a distance. It is obvious that the practical applications of this indirect method are innumerable: from difficult patients to dangerous animals, the laser beam method could help make a diagnosis without the need to touch the subject, all the while maintaining a safe distance [30].

Many things are now possible thanks to the ORT, like finding an infection on an X-ray, MRI or CT-scan and determining the proper agent for treatment; or even determining anomalies in tissue samples.

In one case in 1986 Omura found the migration of helicobacter pylori from the stomach to the heart. He had suggested the involvement of helicobacter pylori in stomach ulcers and cancer before the scientific community accepted the concept and rewarded Australian doctors with the Nobel Prize for that discovery.

CHANGES IN BIOCHEMISTRY DUE TO PAIN

Using the O-ring, Dr. Omura was able to localize neurotransmitters and other substances present in areas affected with changes in microcirculation and pain. When the area tested positive for a microorganism, taking a matched anti-microbial agent before acupuncture increased the relief of pain.

In most cases acupuncture can relieve pain, but when it was unsuccessful Dr. Omura almost invariably detected the presence of bacteria, virus or fungus. He also observed that even using the right antibiotic was often not enough to relieve the patient's symptoms. By testing the affected area he soon realized that abnormal areas are always affected by poor blood circulation, therefore the antibiotic could not reach its target.

Through the ORT, one can perform a compatibility test for microbial agents with the right anti-microbial agent, *i.e.* the right antibiotics for a particular bacterium. Once a match is found, giving acupuncture locally 20 to 30 minutes after taking the antibiotic yields a much better result. Acupuncture has a well-known effect of vasodilation at the level of the microcirculation, allowing the antibiotic to reach the affected area more quickly.

BIOCHEMICAL PRECURSORS TO CANCER AND CIRCULATION DISTURBANCES

Dr. Omura had an intuition early on about the importance of the blood flow in the area affected by pain, cancer or internal functional problems. He wrote in 1983:

"... And since any circulatory disturbance can (directly or indirectly) create pain, abnormal sensory function, muscle spasticity, muscle atrophy and many varieties of clinical symptoms, blood pressure and blood flow measurements at various parts of the body can be invaluable diagnostic tools, as well as a quantitative means of evaluating therapeutic effects. In fact, it is the author's belief that wherever there is an abnormality or a problem, there is also a corresponding circulatory disturbance" [31].

More recently he successfully used the ORT with Thromboxane-B2, a powerful vasoconstrictor, as the reference control substance to show that there is always a correlation with increased concentration of Thromboxane-B2 in a painful area, or an area affected with cancer or another functional problem. He also showed increased circulation from circulation disturbance by infusing paper with Qigong and placing the paper over the abnormal location [32, 33].

The research on the local sub-clinical infection prompted him to investigate the immune system and how infections of the thymus gland could affect its functioning and create an immune-deficiency syndrome. He then formulated the hypothesis that longstanding infection with the presence of heavy metal deposits and long exposure to PEMF is a formula for cancer. He was able to demonstrate that if you have the right cancer marker (oncogene C-*Fos),* a certain neuro-transmitter (acetylcholine), and a local hormone (*thromboxane B2*), you could reliably make a cancer diagnosis with the ORT. Because of his discovery there are now two schools of ORT for Physicians in Tokyo and his method has been adopted as an effective screening method in major Japanese hospitals.

When all four cofactors are present, then special attention for cancer is required.

Four cofactors:

1. Increase in Oncogene C-*fos* AB2,
2. Marked increase in Integrin a5b1,
3. Disappearance of acetylcholine (Ach)
4. Marked increase in mercury (Hg)

LONGEVITY

In the mid 90's Dr. Omura became fascinated with longevity and visited Mrs. Calumet in France, at 121 she was the oldest living human on record at the time. He asked her the secret ingredients of her long life. She mentioned three things: Olive oil, a small glass of Port wine every day, and... Cheerfulness! He also estimated her telomere. Telomere is the molecular structure located at the end of the chromosome that controls the programmed death of the cell, also called apoptosis. The amount of telomere decreases with age, therefore, infants have the highest amount and ultra-centenarians the lowest.

PEMF EFFECTS ON HUMANS BIOCHEMISTRY

Dr. Omura then started to look into environmental factors that could interfere with the therapies and discovered the effect of the PEMF (Pulsed Electromagnetic-Field) on the biological tissues and deposits of heavy metal as cofactors in the pathology he found.

Using the ORT he was able to detect the appearance of several well-known cancer markers after exposure to the PEMF generated by various common home appliances like TVs, computer screens, microwave ovens and cellphones. The presence of Thromboxane B2, Oncogene *C-fos* A 1 or 2, Integrin a-5 b1 in the areas exposed to EMF seemed to be related to the length of exposure and aggravated by the presence of deposits of heavy metals in the area. In the same article Dr. Omura reported changes in the stereoscopic structure of amino acids exposed to the microwave oven. He observed that most amino acids were converted from the normal L-form to a D-form and therefore could compromise the nutritional value of the food exposed to microwaves. This process could contribute to the development of cancer, Alzheimer's, and probably other diseases [34].

Other independent researchers, who found the ORT in 2001 at the University of Istanbul, showed the correlation for the grip force, measured with a standard dynamometer, and ORT results when a group of people were exposed to facial expressions indicating crying or smiling [35]. Exposure to a smiling expression increases the muscle strength while crying decreases it. Mrs. Calumet's ancient wisdom was confirmed!

In 2003 another independent researcher demonstrated the importance of ORT in managing a case with multiple hepatic abscesses. The patient had been treated unsuccessfully with three different antibiotics and the condition was deteriorating. With the use of ORT the pathogen was quickly identified and the drug compatibility test showed that two of the three antibiotics were ineffective, canceling the effect of the only effective one. Two different antibiotics were found to be compatible and effective, and the patient had an immediate clinical improvement [35].

In the same year independent researchers published another article about a case of MRSA (methicillin resistant *Staphylococcus Aureus*) infection treated successfully with the administration of antibiotics and cilantro according to the ORT results [36].

In 2003, using the ORT, L-Homocysteine was found to be the most sensitive and reliable control marker for the screening of cardiovascular diseases [37].

COMPARISONS OF ORIENTAL PATHWAYS TO CLINICAL TESTING WITH O-RING

In the International Chinese Medicine paradigm, organs have pathways on the surface of the body flowing in a linear fashion according to the time of day. In addition, the Triple Warmer is a pathway which regulates heat in the body throughout the upper, middle and lower aspects of the body. Omura showed the adrenal gland is the gland which images the pericardium while the ovaries and testes image the Triple Warmer. There are brother and sister pathways with one more dominant than the other. Evidence has been brought forth to generally prove such a system. The O-ring is a technique which makes it possible to image these organ pathways on the surface of the body, which Omura and I, working independently, have shown through publications during the last several decades through the O-ring. However, this evidence shows differences from the Traditional interpretation.

The confounding results showed an assortment of pathways and circles not typical of the Traditional Chinese Theory. Omura also produced results which in certain regards showed similarities. The acupuncture points were longer, changed shape and location after stimulation and, as Omura showed, had an assortment of organ bio-chemical substances on the pathways and circles. Inside the circle was different than outside in substances and polarity. Stimulation changed all of this.

Evidence also shows double circles through both my images and Omura's (Figs. **28, 29, 32 - 35**). After stimulation is an inversion so that the biochemistry inside goes outside and vice versa, and, shows lateral movement through the circle [27] (Figs. **28, 29**). *Pathways for both linear and nonlinear, not just linear as reflected in the main meridian system of Traditional Chinese Medicine.*

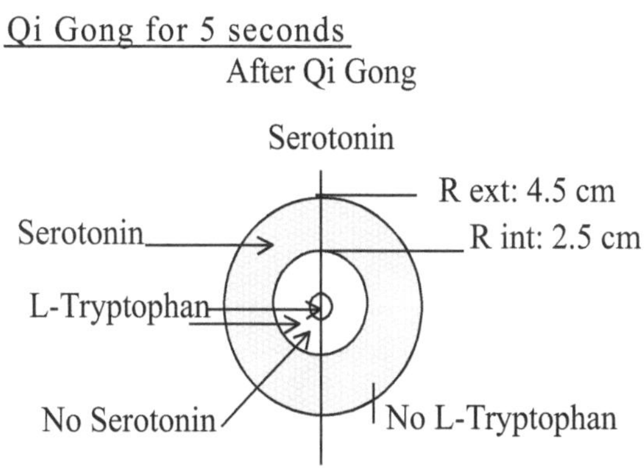

Fig. (28). Before acupuncture. (This figure is reproduced with special permission of Omura) [16, 26].

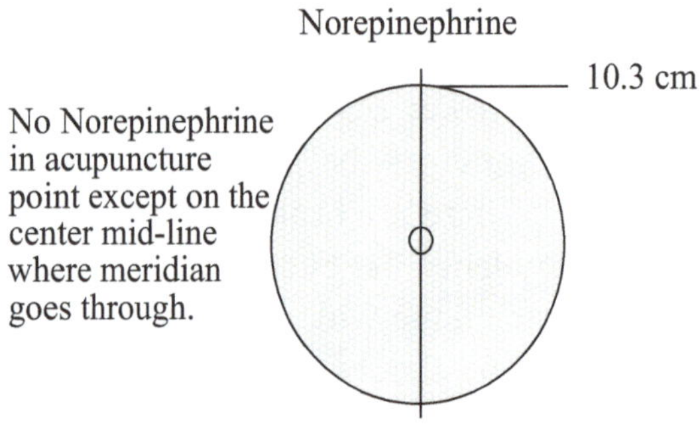

Fig. (29). After acupuncture. (With special permission of Omura).

In 1989 I presented the Hui Hypothesis to explain these confounding evidences. The essence of the Hui Hypothesis is that the non-linear circles are constantly changing by inverting, from inside to outside in four phases [38]. These circles are vibrating in constant flux in fields that differ from the outside to inside with diffuse boundaries. The O-ring test reflects a dominant phase of the circle. The phases move through changes constantly over the course of seconds but have dominant phases with distinctly different patterns. Images show an inclusive field inside the circle and outside, the boundary is different from the inside and outside (Figs. **28**, **29**) [39]. When this happens transverse linear movement can happen or be deviated from a direct route to the other side. Experiments proved this. This deviation can change angles or go up and out or down into the body, or simply concentrate to a point (Figs. **29, 36, 37, 38**).

The above shows what the Meridian point process looks like without the differentiation of the four phase spread apart but seen as a whole (Fig. **30**).

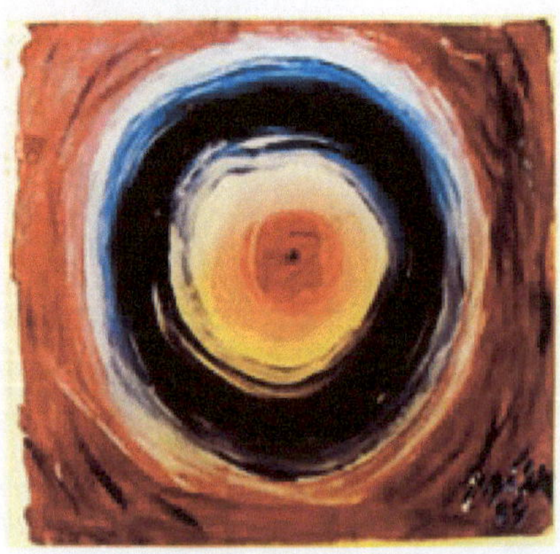

Fig. (30). One Pointedness. (By special permission of Phillip Shinnick).

Also, rather than the idea that there is a continuous flow (at certain hours the Hui hypothesis shows a distinct amount of energy emitted at times, presumably from the pulse generator of an organ or pathogen. Biochemical evidence supports this theory. Since external Qigong influences changes to the dimensions of the circle, internal Qigong presumably could also influence it as well through synchronization of the organism through various techniques of practice. In science Prigogine proposes similar diagrams supported by mathematical acceleration formulas in a nonequilibrium natural state. Traditional Chinese Medicine proposes a movement toward equilibrium or stability. In the Hui hypothesis there is very little equilibrium, in fact the basis is a non-equilibrium state, much like a biological organism experiences – changes in hot/cold, high/low atmospheric pressure, humidity/dryness, light/dark, invasion of pathogens, old age, growth, psychic disturbances, trauma, water balance in the body, cosmic bombardment, and modern electro-magnetic fluid fluctuation by electro-magnetic pulse generators (refrigerators, power tools, cell phones, *etc.*). See Chapter 2 [55].

A quantum amount of purple energy directed by a person's will can be directed outside the body for healing or inside.

Hui hypothesis is based upon the idea that the circle undergoes an inversion or reversal to the opposite; the inside of the circle goes to the outside and the outside of the circle goes inside. The first phase has a diffuse boundary between red on the inside and black on the outside with no distinct boundary. In the second phase the movement is inward, creating a circle within a circle. The inner circle still has red on the inside and, outside the two circles, black (with backgrounds of opposite colors). In the third phase, there is a return to the configuration of the second phases, but now it is black on the inside and red on the outside of the outer circle. The movement is outward. The space between the two circles is nondescript. This whole process is very fast. Phase 4 is like Phase 1 but opposite. This transformation takes about one second to go through its phases. Hui means circle in Chinese. The modern Chinese character for circle is a square line within a square line; not too long ago the character was a circle in a circle, and the ancient character for circle was a spiral in a circle, from a whirlpool.

Domonal changes are very quick, like a camera flash. This distinct quick movement (moving outward and inward) is illuminated with a gold ring of transformation (or an illuminated boundary) replacing the diffuse boundary of the red and black (Fig. **31**). When this happens, both inside and outside are nondescript and the opposite, hued with gold. Outside forces can transform this into circular spinning motion.

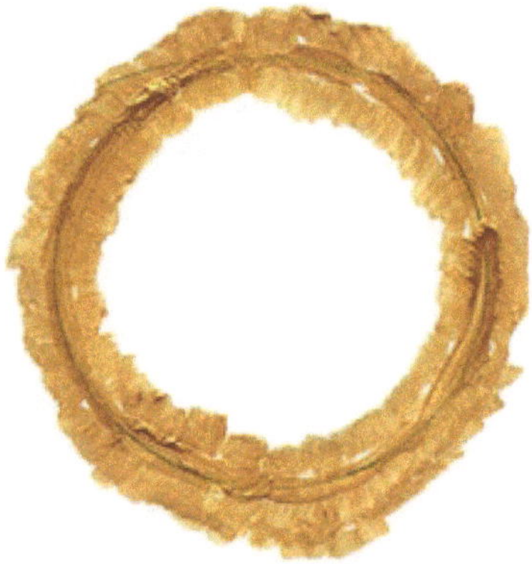

Fig. (31). Ring of transformation. (By special permission of Shinnick).

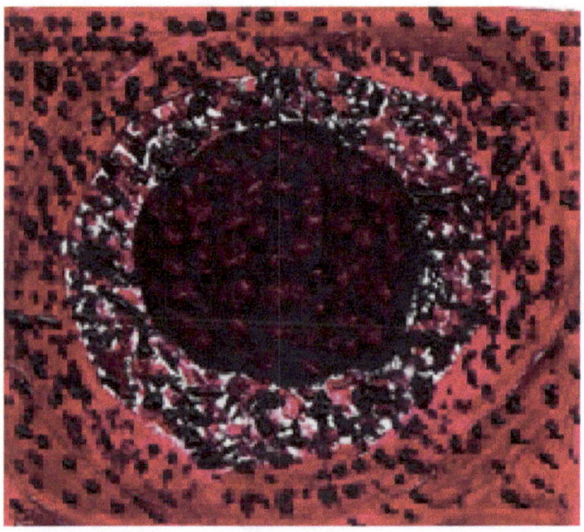

Fig. (32). Phase 1. (With special permission of Shinnick).

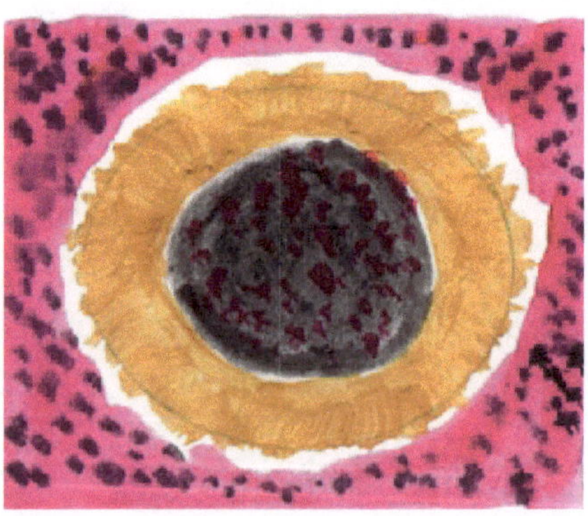

Fig. (33). Phase 2. (With special permission of Shinnick).

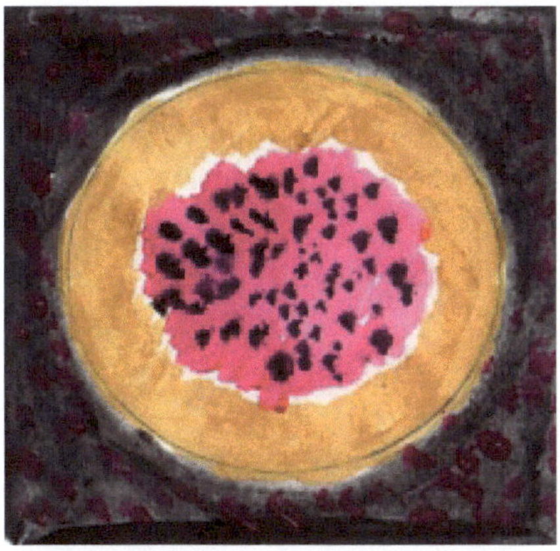

Fig. (34). Phase 3. (With special permission of Shinnick).

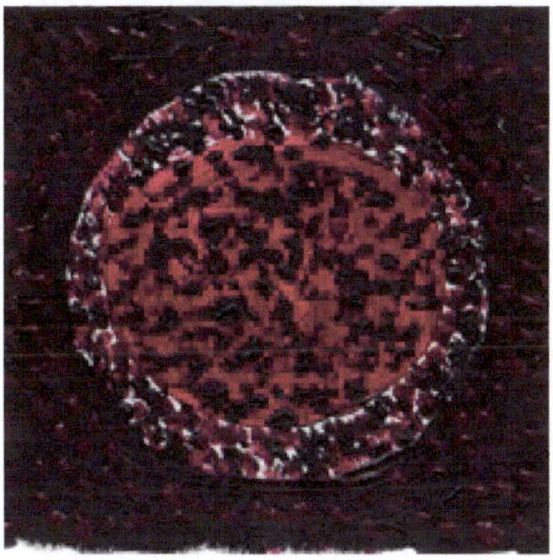

Fig. (35). Phase 4. (With special permission of Shinnick).

These are the distinct quantum energy entering the Domonal which can go in any direction, presumably initiated by the phases of the organs going through various cycles of functioning during the day or night or stimulation of some sort by internal changes to physiology through Self Help meditation (Figs. **36, 37, 38**).

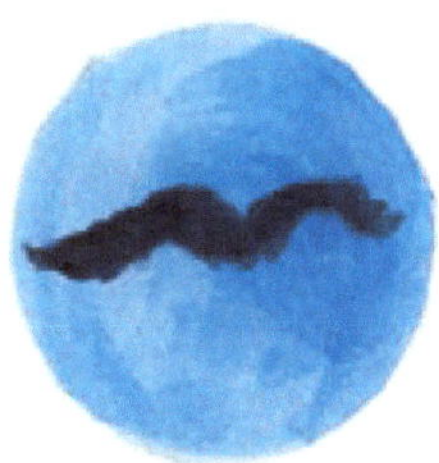

Fig. (36). Movement across. (With special permission of Shinnick).

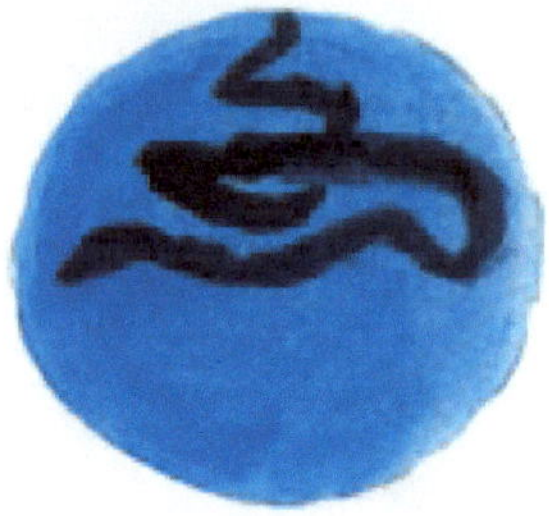

Fig. (37). Movement across and out to another direction. (With special permission of Shinnick).

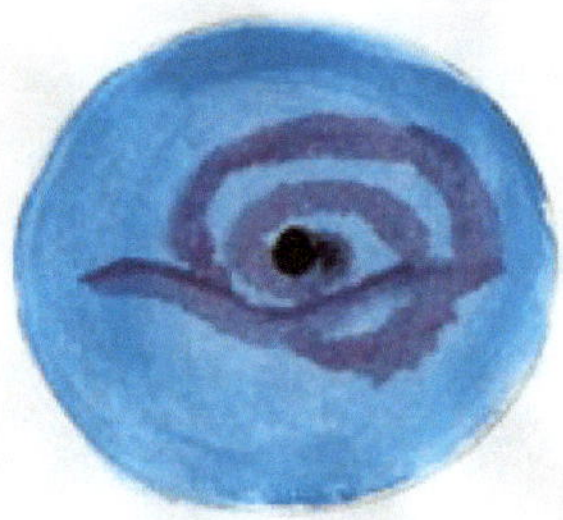

Fig. (38). This shows a movement through and to another dimension. (With special permission of Shinnick).

Tiller a material scientist who publishes on the structure of matter shows in his book the gold above as normal space time (D-space) and the background as reciprocal space time (R-space) [40] (Fig. **39**). The center diagram is similar to the reversal of the acupuncture points upon stimulation which changes direction shown (Fig. **37**). Upper left of Fig. **(39)** shows that the acupuncture point recedes to a point. The ring of transformation initiates (Fig. **31**). The acupuncture point reflects space time and reciprocal space time (symmetry) of another dimension upon stimulation.

At times there is a spinning of the linear movement around itself then to a point (proved by the O-ring after stimulation the domonal sometimes goes to a point) or disappears, or a flushing (in blue, yellow, green or red) as indicated and evidenced by Omura's bio-chemical reaction which spread over the whole body for a time. Patients also report a flushing feeling after acupuncture stimulation. Also Master Yogi report a flushing in colors during meditation. External Qigong influences this process in distinct ways, as Omura found. In Qigong, a Master can emanate energy from his hand to another, also a persons can direct Qigong emanation inward to their own.

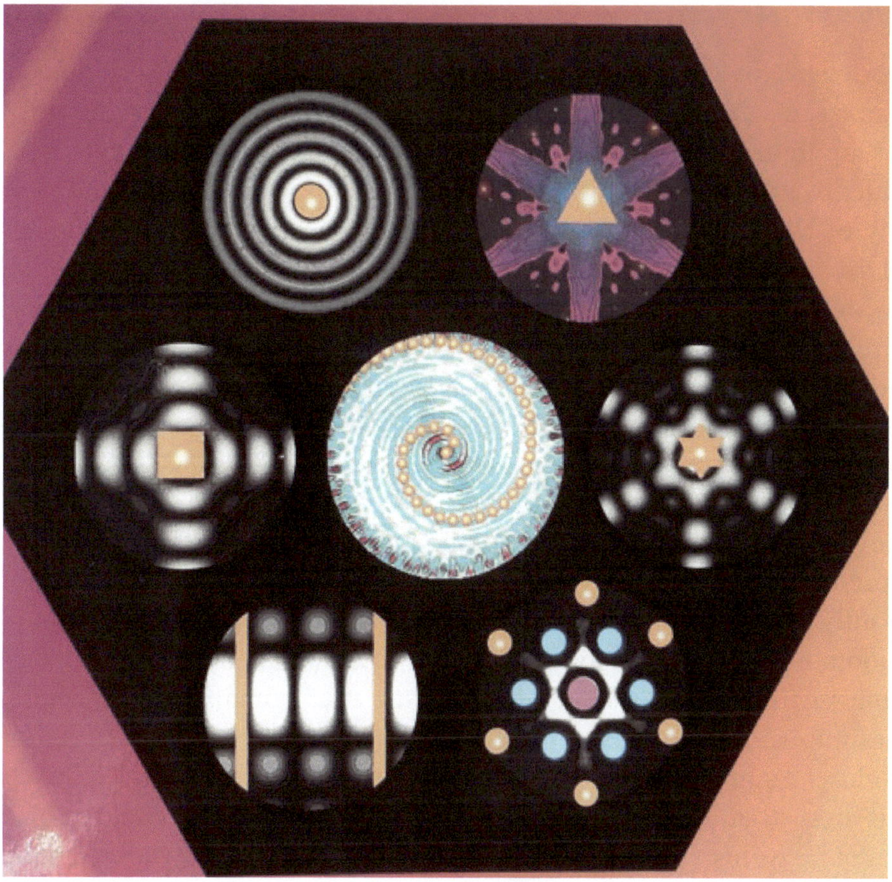

Fig. (39). Tiller illustrated different reciprocal structures of mater, normal space time (D-space) and background reciprocal space time (R-space). (Reproduced with permission, William A Tiller, Ph.D. www.tiller.org).

The third dimension of an acupuncture point (Fig. **40**).

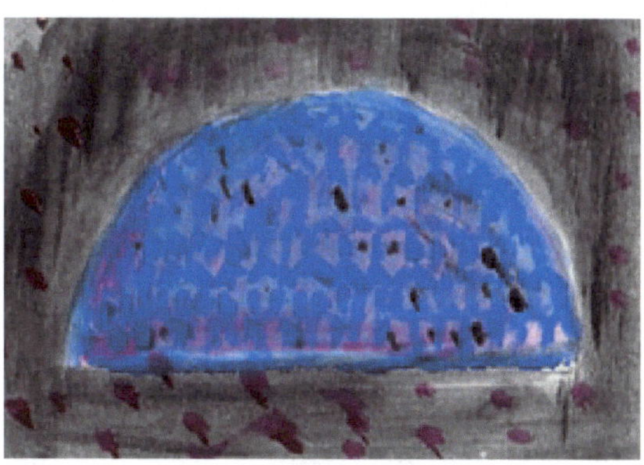

Fig. (40). Domanol 1987 (By special permission of Phillip Shinnick).

Summary

Supported by clinical cases where organ or other tissues were tested randomly on pain areas of the body resulted in the phases of the diaphragm and heart. Departing from Oriental understandings, circles appeared on the hips for bladder, prostate, ovary, gallbladder and colon with pathways downward to the legs in a variety of locations. Each of these research cases was done with a diode which could determine direction. Some of these circles with transverse pathways showed a flow only out, others only in, and others traversing in, then out the other side of the circle. Oriental understanding states these flow through an acupuncture points in one direction. Omura showed on a cadaver that acupuncture point ST. 36 on the stomach meridian 胃经 weijing dipped into the body several centimeters. Conversely this acupuncture point or circle raises above the skin by the same distance. This domonal or circular dome has the capability to go in any direction up, down, transverse in either direction coming in and going out. This domonal collapsed to a point verified by the O-ring after stimulation. Also the circle inverts constantly going into it opposite triggered by a golden ring called the ring of transition. Sometimes this point disappears after stimulation, or inside the circle become just one color and in certain cases after stimulation the whole body flushes into various singular colors depending upon the circumstance. However upon closer examination the blue color outside the circle is still a domonal but the blue is an shell of hexagonal lattice of blue with the underlying field of black and red. In other words, inside the domonal is a black background with red points and above the blue lattice is red background with black points like leopard spots.

As well, this domonal collapses to a point and also changes biochemical composition (inside to outside and *vice versa*) for pain relief from stimulation. At times a distinct or quantum of energy enters the domonal and can go in and out in any direction. At times the acupuncture domonal disappears after stimulation and a flushing of a clear color (blue, yellow, green or red) goes over the whole body, which is reported by patients as a sensation. The inside of the circle at times becomes a clear color as shown in Japanese paintings. However this is a delusion, the domonal has a hexagonal lattice like structure, the lattice is blue and illuminates seeming one color but on examination underneath is a pattern of red and black.

How is this known? Three years of imaging these circles and meditating on their meaning created an impetus to paint the figures being seen in meditation. This image at first was (Fig. **30**) then it became apparent in the meditation that the mind could be slowed down and then the phases Figs. (**32-35**) appeared very clearly. In reading scientific discoveries many scientists just meditated on their experimentation and the structure appears in their mind.

Microscopic Slides used for reference (Fig. **41**). These are held in the hand as a control reference and in the direct technique below part of the body is stimulated with a non conducting probe and if there is a resonance then the O-ring opens. For the indirect method the helper can hold the slide and stimulate the subject with a conducting probe, if there is a compatibility or resonance then the O-Ring opens. Without a substance in the hand, stimulating the Mu or Shu organ representation point on the front or back with a probe can tell if the organ is stressed by seeing if the O-Ring opens. Also stimulating a pain area can determine the boundary of the area which is usually a dermatome or neurological pathway of the particular vertebra and not an organ as indicated in Traditional Chinese Main Meridian understanding.

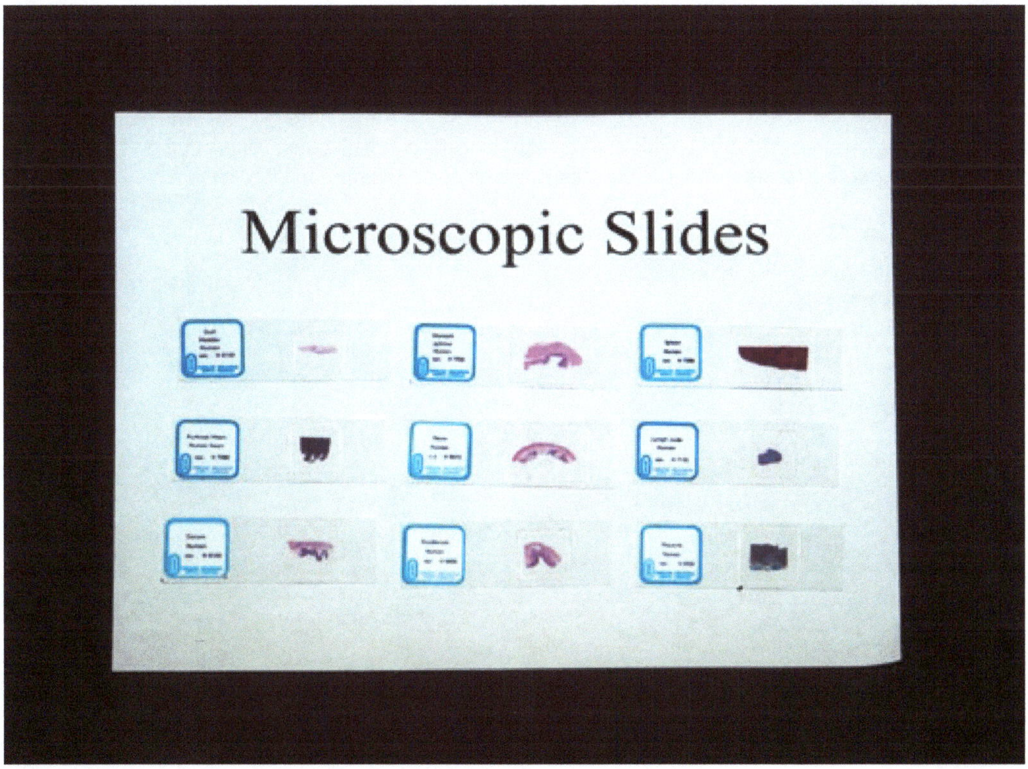

Fig. (41). Microscopic slides. (With special permission of Shinnick).

The technique of using the O-Ring can be found in Reference [6, 10, 16]. See Figs. (**42-45**) it was not the purpose of this book to explain the process of the O-Ring but to report the findings and contribution to medicine.

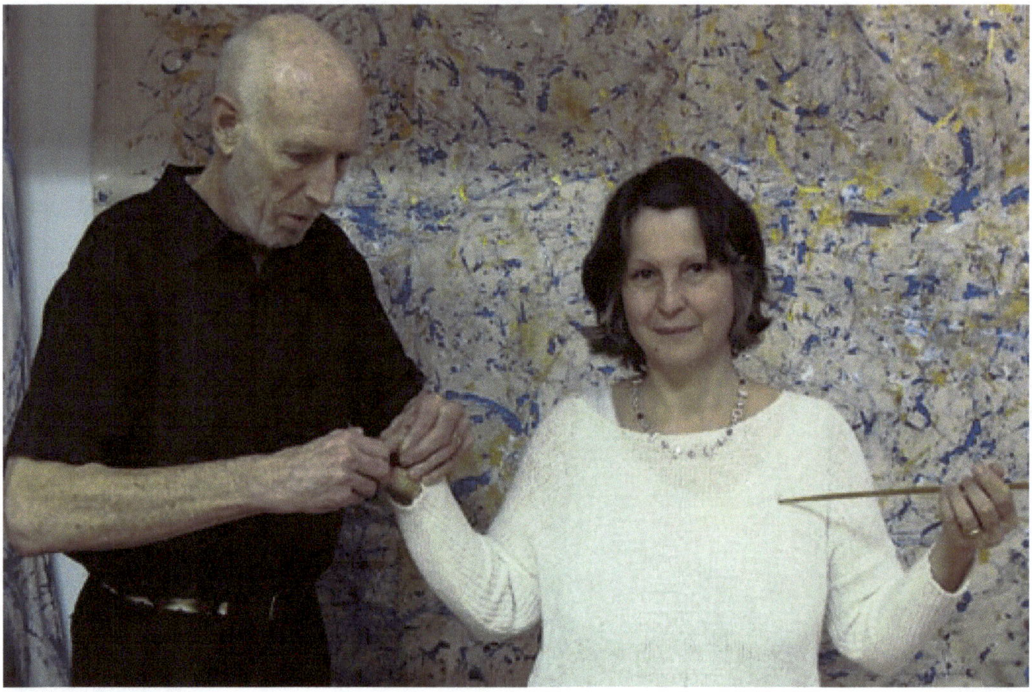

Fig. (42). Direct O-ring test: Subject holds control substance in hand with a non conducting probe pointed at the area testing. *Photo Herman Costa.* (With special permission of Shinnick and Porter).

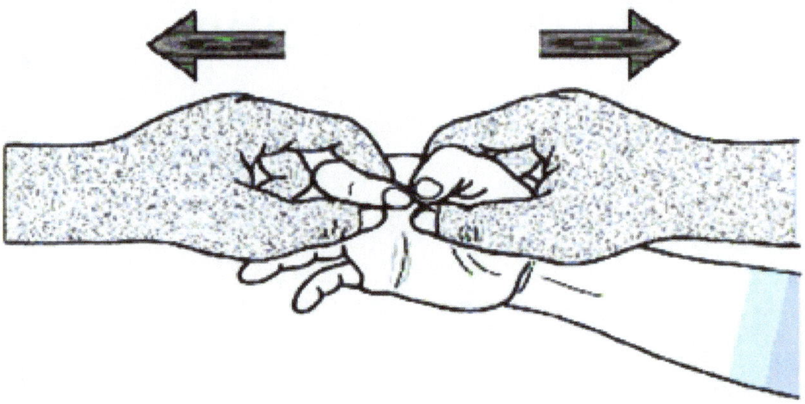

Fig. (43). O-Ring hand technique. (With special permission of Shinnick).

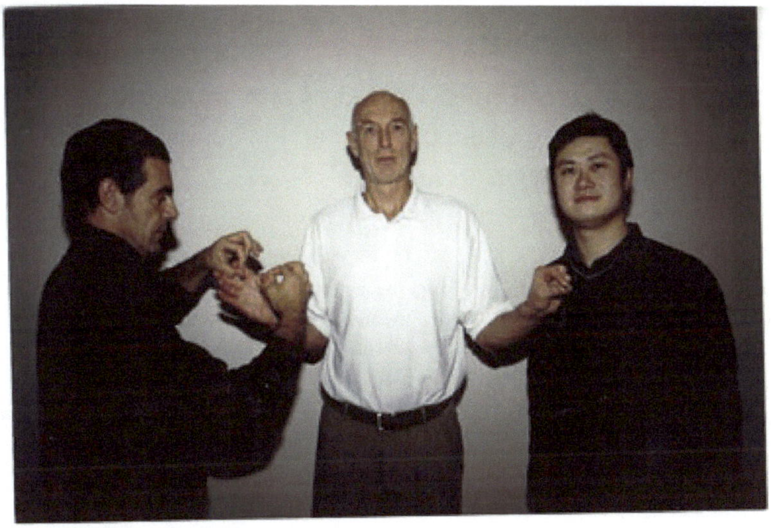

Fig. (44). Above Indirect O-ring using a third person who using a conducting probe and holds the control substance in hand while pointing to the area testing. Just above, another finger angle of the O-ring above. (With special permission of Shinnick).

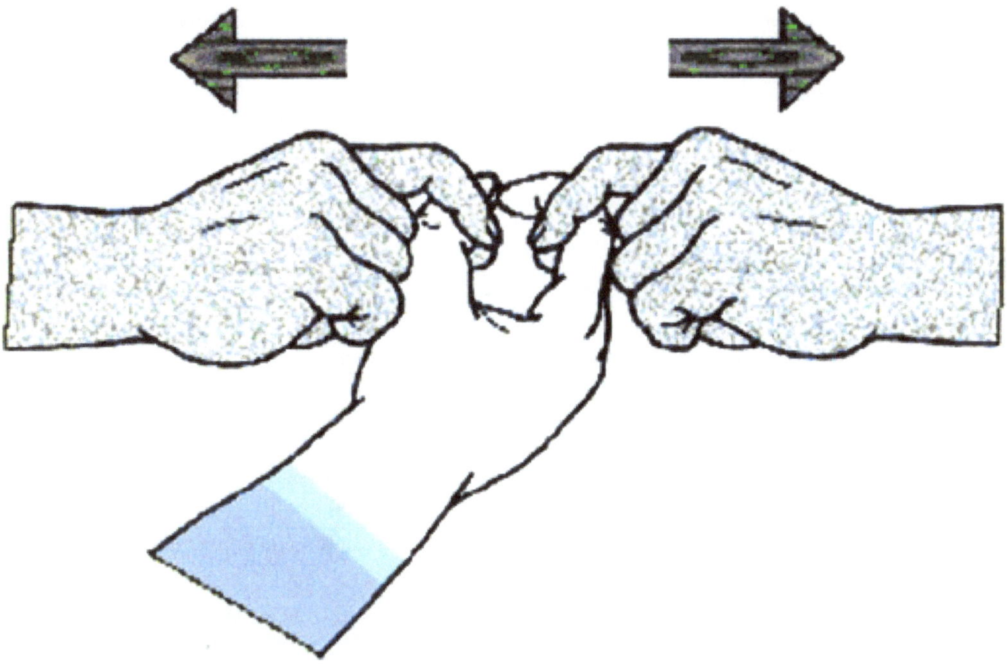

Fig. (45). Above is the direct and indirect O-ring finger technique using either a third person or using the subject with the same techniques. Hand position of O-ring. (With special permission of Shinnick).

ACKNOWLEDGEMENTS

All patients signed an Informed Consent Form from a Research Protocol of the International College of Acupuncture and Therapeutics, a New York State Permanent Charter College.

REFERENCES

[1] Omura Y. Applied kinesiology using the acupuncture meridian concept: critical evaluation of its potential as the simplest non-invasive means of diagnosis, and compatibility test of food and drugs-part 1. Acupunct Electrother Res 1979; 4: 165-83. [http://dx.doi.org/10.3727/036012979817552861]

[2] Omura Y. New simple early diagnostic methods using Omuras 'Bi-Digital O-Ring Dysfunction Localization method and acupuncture organ representation points, and their applications to the "drug & food compatibility test. Acupunct Electrother Res 1981; 6(4): 239-54. [http://dx.doi.org/10.3727/036012981816952199] [PMID: 6124084]

[3] Omura Y. Electro-magnetic resonance phenomenon as a possible mechanism related to the bi-digital o-ring test molecular identification and localization method. Acupunct Electrother Res 1986; 11(2): 127-45. [http://dx.doi.org/10.3727/036012986816359193] [PMID: 2879416]

[4] Omura Y. "Re-evaluation of the classical acupuncture concept of meridians in Oriental medicine by the method of detecting meridian-like network connected to internal organs using Bi-Digital O-Ring Test" Acupunct Electrother Res 1986; 11(3-4): 219-31.

[5] Omura Y. Meridian-like networks of internal organs, corresponding to traditional Chinese 12 main meridians and their acupuncture points as detected by the Bi-Digital O-Ring Test imaging method: search for the corresponding internal organ of Western medicine for each meridianPart I. Acupunct Electrother Res 1987; 12(1): 53-70. [http://dx.doi.org/10.3727/036012987816358968] [PMID: 2883838]

[6] Shinnick P. An introduction to the basic technique and theory of omura's bi-digital o-ring test. Am J Acupunct 1996; 24(2 & 3)

[7] Shinnick P, Blumenthal C. Application of the bi-digital O-ring test imaging method for acupuncture and electro-therapeutics in rehabilitation medicine. Acupunct Electrother Res 1988; 13(4): 248.

[8] Shinnick P, Blumenthal C. A study of the bi-digital o-ring test imaging method and organ pathways. Abstracts of Acupunct Electrother Res 1989; 14(4): 334.

[9] Shinnick P, Blumenthal C. Meridian-like pathway of the lung and large intestine as detected by the bi-digital o-ring test. Abstracts of International Symposium Acupunct Electrother Res 1989; 24(4): 334.

[10] Shinnick P. The application of the bi-Digital o-ring imaging test to toxic organ meridian and clinical medicine. Med Ac 2003; 14: 3.

[11] Shinnick P, Blumenthal C. Meridian-like pathway of the lung and large intestine as detected by the bi-digital o-ring test. Acupunct Electrother Res 1987; 12(3-4): 239.

[12] Shinnick P, Blumenthal C. Application of the bi-digital o-ring test imaging method for acupuncture and electro-therapeutics in rehabilitation medicine. Acupunct Electrother Res 1988; 13(4): 248.

[13] Shinnick P, Blumenthal C. A study of the Bi-Digital O-Ring Test Imaging Method and Organ Pathways. Acupunct Electrother Res 1989; 14(4): 334.

[14] Shinnick P, Borgna A. Electromagnetic Resonance Phenomenon: The Bi-digital O-ring Imaging Test; a Non-invasive, Inexpensive Diagnostic Method Applied to Medicine and Science. Proceedings of the

Society for Scientific Exploration 22nd Annual meeting. June 14th.; Kalispell, Montana. 2003.

[15] Shinnick P, Borgna A. Electromagnetic Resonance: the Origin and Discovery of the Omura O-ring Test (Bi-digital O-ring Test), Which is a Non-invasive, Inexpensive Diagnostic Tool for Medicine; Important Omura Discoveries for Medicine and Science. Proceedings of the Material Research and Living Systems. Boston. 2004.

[16] Shinnick P, Borgna A. Whole person healing the O-ring imaging technique influences to oriental and occidental medicine. Indiana: AuthorHouse 2009.

[17] Shinnick P, Borgna A. Electromagnetic Resonance: The Origin and Discovery of the Omura O-ring Test (Bi-Digital O-Ring Test), Which is a Non-invasive, Inexpensive Diagnostic Tool for Medicine; Important Omura Discoveries for Medicine and Science. Proceedings of the Material Research and Living Systems. Boston. 2004.

[18] Omura Y. Meridian-like networks of internal organs, corresponding to traditional Chinese 12 main meridians and their acupuncture points as detected by the Bi-Digital O-Ring Test imaging method: search for the corresponding internal organ of Western medicine for each meridianPart I. Acupunct Electrother Res 1987; 12(1): 53-70. [http://dx.doi.org/10.3727/036012987816358968] [PMID: 2883838]

[19] Shinnick P. Electromagnetic resonance: the discovery and use of the omura o-ring test (bi-digital o-ring test); implications for traditional chinese medicine and the meridian system, 400 clinical case study and important omura discoveries for medicine and science. Proceedings of the Second Hole Person Healing Summit and Second Qigong Summit. 2005, April 14-17th; Washington D.C.

[20] Shinnick P. Electromagnetic resonance: the discovery and use of the omura o-ring test (bi-digital o-ring test) implications for traditional chinese medicine and the meridian system, 400 clinical case study and important omura discoveries for medicine and science. Proceedings of the Second Whole Person Healing Summit and Second Qigong Summit. 2005, April 14-17th; Washington D.C.

[21] Shinnick P. The science of whole person healing: research data summary on qigong and the differentiation of qi into body pathways, the physiology and properties of mind/body wholeness and its clinical application to disease and athletics. Proceedings of the Science of Whole Person Healing Conference. Washington, D.C. 2003.

[22] Shinnick P. The science of whole Person Healing, The omura's bi-digital o-ring test: it's contribution to oriental and occidental medicine and science: an independent analysis Proceedings of the Second Interdisciplinary International Conference-2005.

[23] Shinnick P, Roy R. Research data from the bi-digital o-ring test, a low cost non-invasive diagnostic test for medicine and science J Sci Heal Outcomes 2011; 4: 13.

[24] Shinnick P. The science of whole person healing, The omura's bi-digital o-ring test: it's contribution to oriental and occidental medicine and science: An independent analysis. In: Proceedings of the Second Interdisciplinary International Conference.

[25] Shinnick P. The Science of whole person healing: research data summary on qigong and the differentiation of qi into body pathways, the physiology and properties of mind/body wholeness and its clinical application to disease and athletics. Proceedings of the Science of Whole Person Healing. 2004 March 14;

[26] Omura Y. Meridian-like networks of internal organs, corresponding to traditional Chinese 12 main meridians and their acupuncture points as detected by the Bi-Digital O-Ring Test imaging method: search for the corresponding internal organ of Western medicine for each meridianPart I. Acupunct Electrother Res 1987; 12(1): 53-70. [http://dx.doi.org/10.3727/036012987816358968] [PMID: 2883838]

[27] Omura Y. Connection found between each meridian (heart, stomach, triple burner, *etc.*) & organ representation area of corresponding internal neurotransmitters and hormones unique to each meridian

and corresponding acupuncture point & internal organ after acupuncture, electrical stimulation (including shiatsu) soft laser stimulation or Qiong. Acupunct Electrother Res 1989; 1(2): 155-86.

[28] Omura Y. Simple and quick non-invasive evaluation of circulation of cerebral arteries by clinical application of the "Bi-Digital O-Ring Test". Acupunct Electrother Res 1985; 10: 146. [http://dx.doi.org/10.3727/036012985816714469]

[29] Omura Y. The Bi-Digital O-Ring Test: critical evaluation of its abnormal responses with laboratory tests including blood pressure & blood flow method, blood chemistry, *etc.*, and neutrological method. Acupunct Electrother Res 1983; 8(1): 37-43. [http://dx.doi.org/10.3727/036012983816715037] [PMID: 6135302]

[30] Omura Y, Losco M, Omura AK, *et al.* Bi-directional transmission of molecular information by photon or electron beams passing in the close vicinity of specific molecules, and its clinical and basic research applications: 1) Diagnosis of humans or animal patients without any direct contact; 2) Light microscopic and electron microscopic localization of neuro-transmitters, heavy metals, Oncogen C-fos (AB2), *etc.* of intracellular fine structures of normal and abnormal single cells using light or electro-microscopic indirect Bi-Digital O-Ring Test. Acupunct Electrother Res 1992; 17(1): 29-46. [http://dx.doi.org/10.3727/036012992816357855] [PMID: 1351338]

[31] Omura Y. The Bi-Digital O-Ring Test: critical evaluation of its abnormal responses with laboratory tests including blood pressure & blood flow method, blood chemistry, *etc.*, and neutrological method. Acupunct Electrother Res 1983; 8(1): 37-43. [http://dx.doi.org/10.3727/036012983816715037] [PMID: 6135302]

[32] Omura Y. Storing of qi gong energy in various materials and drugs (qi gongnization): its clinical application for treatment of pain, circulatory disturbance, bacterial or viral infections, heavy metal deposits, and related intractable medical problems by selectively enhancing circulation and drug uptake. Acupunct Electrother Res 1990; 15(2): 137-57. [http://dx.doi.org/10.3727/036012990816358270] [PMID: 1978504]

[33] Omura Y. Unique changes found on the Qigong (chi gong) Masters and patient's body during qi gong treatment: their relation to certain meridians & acupuncture points and the recreation of the therapeutic qi gong states by children and adults. Acupunct Electrother Res 1989; 14: 61-89. Omura Y, Interrelationship between the heart and central nervous system: localization of Neurotransmitter sand imaging of their associated nuclei, including raphe nuclei & the locus coeruleus, as well as the imaging of the heart and its representation areas in slices or the human central nervous system using the Bi-Digital O-Ring Test. imaging method. Acupunct Electrother Res 1987; 12(½): 139-164.

[34] Omura Y, Losco M. Losco M, Electromagnetic fields in the home environment (color TV, computer monitors, microwave oven, cellular phone, *etc.*) as potential contributing factors for the induction of onogene C-fosAb 1, onogen C-fosAb2, Integrin alfa5 b1 and the development of cancer, as well as effects of microsave on amino acid composition of food and living brain. Acupunct Electrother Res 1993; 18: 33-73.

[35] Alwasa S, Neves LB, Lopes AC. The importance of bi-digital o-ring test in the treatment of multiple hepatic abscesses-a case study. Acupunct Electrother Res 2003; 28: 201-6.

[36] Asou T, Hayashe T, Jitsuik I, *et al.* A patient with MRSA infection to prosthesis of femoral head diagnosed noninvasively using the bi-digital o-ring test: a clinical case report. Acupunct Electrother Res 2003; 28: 69-72.

[37] Omura Y, Shimotsuura Y. Ohki. 2 minutes non-invasive screening for cardiovascular diseases: relative limitation of C-reactive protein compared with more sensitive L-homocysteine as cardiovascular risk factor; safe and effective treatment using selective drug uptake enhancement method. Acupunct Electrother Res 2003; 28: 35-68.

[38] Shinnick P. The hui hypothesis with clinical evidence from a 400 person study. Proceedings of the Third Science of Whole Person Healing Conference. October 12.

[39] Omura Y, Shimotsuura Y. Ohki. Interrelationship between the heart and central nervous system: localization of neuro-transmitters and imaging of their associated nuclei, including the raphe nuclei & the locus coeruleus, as well as the imaging of the heart and its representation areas in slices of the human central nervous system using the "Bi-Digital O-Ring Test" imaging method. Acupunct Electrother Res 1987; 12(½): 156.

[40] Tiller WA. Psychoenergetic science: a second copernican-scale revolution. California: Pavior Pu 2007.

CHAPTER 7

Self Healing in Chronic Heart Disease: A Clinical Study Using Heart Medication

Abstract: In Chronic Heart Disease, exertion, overstrain or cold wind and temperature can create symptoms of tiredness, fluid in the lung, coldness symptoms, sputum production, cough, rapid breathing, nausea and abdominal spasm, no appetite, mental disturbances, insomnia and restless sleep, and fear. These were our questions: What techniques of meditation, Qigong and acupuncture can alleviate the symptoms of Chronic Heart Disease? Which complementary treatments and techniques can help alleviate heart medication side effects such as a drop in blood pressure? How effective is Traditional Chinese Medicine acupuncture techniques for symptoms of Chronic Heart Disease? What new techniques can be learned from this study in acupuncture, meditation and Qigong for particular symptoms? From these question came the desire to test and measure these states of Chronic Heart Disease in an acute state (with traditional heart medication) using meditation, acupuncture and Qigong. These transcendent states could help theoretically in the terminal phases of life *i.e.*, escaping from conditioned thinking associated with fear. We wanted to test this general understanding with a particular case.

Keywords: Acupuncture, Albumin, Blood lactate, Breath count, Chronic heart disease, Diaphragm, Digitalis, Disturbed sleep, Dyspnea, Fluid retention, Kidney deficiency, Lasix, Meditation, Moxibustion, Oxygen consumption, Phlegm, Qigong, Synchronization, Vasotec, Zazen.

INTRODUCTION

This article was a joint project between Dr. Shinnick and Dr. Freed as they explored scientific approaches to body, mind and spirit healing during a life threatening illness of Simon Freed, (SF). Their discussions about appropriate therapy, including acupuncture, meditation, Qigong, massage, and Western medicine were an outgrowth of their interest in developing a scientific understanding of the mind/body connection in health and healing. This present study incorporates several complementary therapies used in treatment over a 6-week period during an acute period of Chronic Heart Disease. This began midway in the course of a terminal illness due to cancer of the esophagus (Appendix **A** & **B**).

Death resulted ultimately from a weakened nutritional condition due to restriction of the esophagus from the cancer. SF chose not to have a shunt in his stomach.

Besides thermal changes brought about through acupuncture and meditation, Qigong studies led us also to believe that this therapy might be important in a terminal illness when cold and lack of heat aggravates the condition. For a year in the late 1980's, every six weeks, at the International College of Acupuncture and Electro-Therapeutics, Qigong was studied by inviting various Masters in Qigong to treat patients and discuss their technique. The Qigong state and effect on the patient and the person doing the external Qigong was measured. "External" refers to a person giving Qigong to another either to demonstrate or to help the healing process in pathology. "Internal" refers to a person doing Qigong for his or her own health and directs the Qigong energy inward. Slowly through observation and practice we developed some skills in internal and external Qigong developed. It is the internal Qigong technique, which SF developed and used during the terminal illness to raise his body temperature.

My friend Simon Freed did a Ph.D. in magneto chemistry at UC Berkeley under GN Lewis who said Freed was the brightest of the nine Nobel Prize winners he taught during his time. He and I experimented around ideas of mind/body connections for eight years. It appears from our experiments, that brain incoherence, differentiations of heart rhythms and not being at ease, results in higher amount of lactic acid (stress), oxygen consumption (low when at rest) and consequently disease.

Dr. Freed's meditation for 30 years was to focus on the upper lip, watching the breath go in and out. This is like sitting in a tower, watching people come in and out of the gate below, seeing them without following them with curiosity. This way, the mind can stay empty, not following thoughts or outside stimulus.

Dr. Freed (SF) did his meditation every day for thirty years. At ninety-six, he suffered from chronic heart disease, with periodic water in his lungs, a panting breath, nightmares and weakness. He did Qigong meditation to balance heat in his body and continued his Zazen meditation, watching the breath on his upper lip. He descended into the abyss, the great vacuity where subtle vast vibrations are underneath a vast expanse of emptiness and space. One hears celestial sounds in meditation especially when chanting mantra. In this meditative state one can see many unusual images (Fig. **1**).

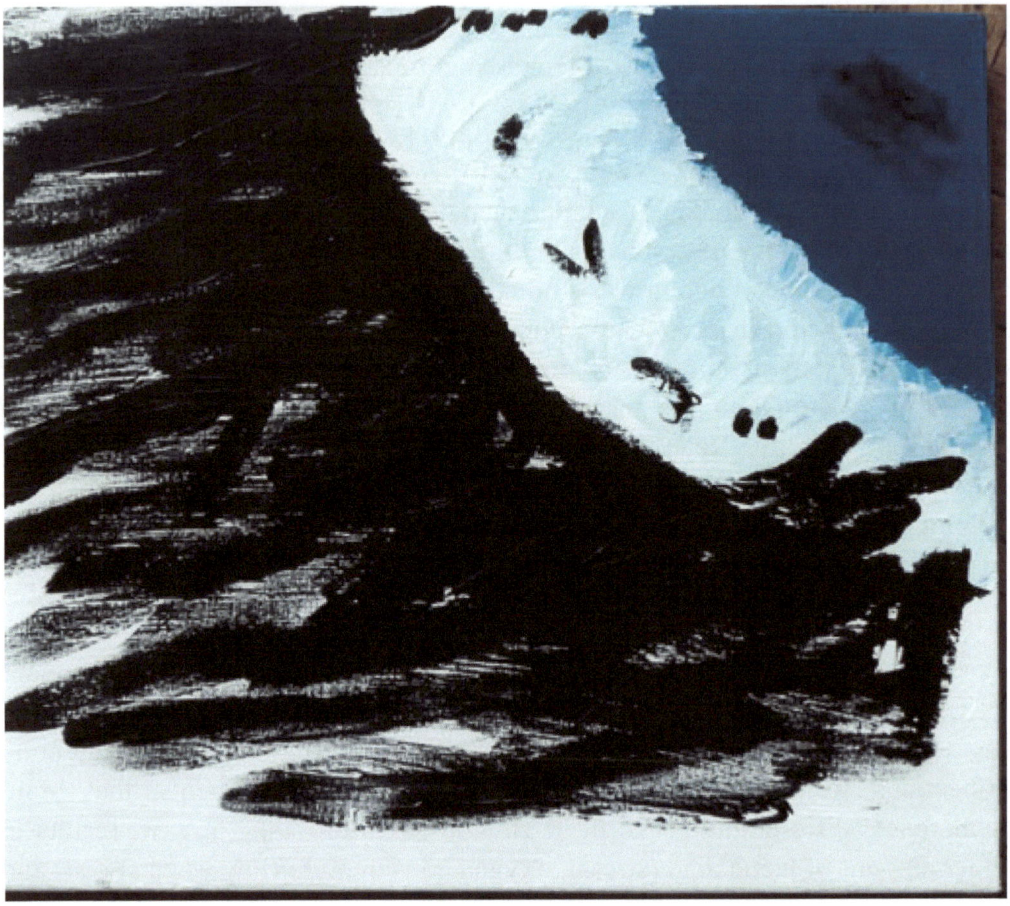

Fig. (1). Blue and Black Dancing 2009. (This painting is reproduced with special permission of Shinnick).

SF, with a recent pacemaker, overextended himself the winter of 1994 by delivering a technical paper in Israel and consulting in Czechoslovakia. SF had a pacemaker inserted the previous Fall but no clinical records of EEG recordings could be found in the hospital records to determine if it was operational or an on demand pacemaker. Therefore, the effect it had on this study cannot be determined. X-rays showed the pacemaker was not connected to the heart and presumably disconnected in the fall. In Israel, when his foot got caught in a bus as the driver pulled away and was dragged extending his thoracic rib cage and was hospitalized for water in lung from the trauma. Upon returning to New York during a severe winter storm, he experienced a quick (twenty minute) drop in external temperature (25°F to 5°F) with a 12-mile an hour wind during a long walk. This exposure left him weak and full of phlegm, which required hospitalization in March. At first, he was treated with an intravenous antibiotic for ten days but later X-rays showed water in his lungs rather than pneumonia. In

Traditional Chinese Medicine cold and wind are two of the six excesses along with heat, dampness, dryness and summer heat. "When environmental forces become excessive [*e.g.*, a particular cold spell in winter]...they may cause disease" [1].

Previous to this six-week study, the authors worked together weekly for eight years around the theme of global physiological states. The term "global" in our studies means a state that requires the whole organism to be synchronized as in Chapter 2, of the EEG patterns of meditators compared against a more "normal" state. Shown are two brain fields: a) one meditator's brain field in a homogenous or synchronized state of a resting electroencephalogram at 10/sec, alpha rhythm "relaxed wakefulness"; and b) the other a non-meditator's brain field in a differentiated state of desynchronized alpha waves. These would be examples of global measurement with the first state being more "global" and synchronized and the second differentiated and de-synchronized.

Besides SF the author had been a meditators for over twenty years and understood the various forms of meditation, researched the physiology of meditation on global characteristics and studied the heart [2 - 6]. In this study, our techniques were derived from a variety of sources but ultimately were our own techniques. In meditators, other global physiological characteristics are apparent as we show in previous chapters which show that over time oxygen consumption in meditators drops relatively quickly as compared with sleepers.

BEFORE, DURING AND AFTER THE "QUIET"

This case of Chronic Heart Disease, through its symptoms, represents a de-synchronized, differentiated state which includes an agitated mental and emotional state while facing death, respiration rhythm difficulties of all deadly sorts and the side effect of modern medication (Appendix **A**). As indicated above, meditation helps bring a quiet state to the brain field and a decrease in oxygen consumption and blood lactate. Moving toward a more synchronized and more global physiology is possible through meditation. This study reflects sitting meditation such as Zen and Qigong but there are other sorts of meditations, which will be discussed later such as watching the breath for length of inhalation and exhalation. Our techniques changed as symptoms changed.

Acupuncture also shares some of these same global characteristics as meditation. A before and after picture of a Single Photon Emission Computed Tomography (S.P.E.C.T.) to the brain shows an asymmetry inside the brain before acupuncture in a normal or pain state and an increased symmetry inside the brain after acupuncture [7]. This can be seen in Chapter 2, (Fig. **6**). Other global measurements such as infrared imaging show thermal changes after acupuncture [8]. Acupuncture can also help in affective disorders and psychosomatic illnesses [9, 10].

This method will be discussed in more depth later. Briefly, however, he assumed a position, in his case bent legs, arms in a circle with fingertips a centimeter apart, breathed naturally and looked through the space between the fingers onto the floor about a meter ahead. After an undefined period, depending upon practice and the day, when tingling in the fingertips was experienced or the space between the fingers changed color then he would think of a part of the body. Once this Qi was experienced through sight or sensation then we relied upon the axiom- wherever the mind goes, energy follows. SF had been doing inner Qigong for about five years [11]. He had a rash on his back from swimming in a river in Central America about fifty years ago, which never went away which he wanted to treat with this method. SF concentrated on this rash on his back after experiencing the Qi and then with some concentration felt his back become warm. After doing the meditation for about five to ten minutes each day over a period of five years; the area improved by 90% and returned only 20% more during his illness.

In addition to our studies on the synchronization and symmetry of the brain field, oxygen consumption and blood lactate, and thermal changes, we also studied the characteristics of fragmentation. We studied a fragmented state of confusion, dualism, ill health and emotional turmoil and the relation between the mind and body [12 - 14].

Appendix **B** is an attempt to look at what happened on a timeline and a measurement of quantity from a particular date such as the start of enalapril (Vasotec) and fluid volume in parts of the body. We needed to differentiate medically induced fragmentation from symptoms of Chronic Heart Disease. These relationships can be seen in this context.

DESIGN AND METHOD

The overall method of treatment was a joint effort of the two authors, the experimenter (PS) and the subject (SF). SF died two months after this six-week study period. Each day physical symptoms, acupuncture points, the form of daily meditation, and Qigong were recorded in a journal. (See Appendix **A**) SF's private and attending physician at Beth Israel Hospital in New York City coordinated and consulted on the progress of this study.

SF's heart condition stabilized, relatively, after four months of combining medication, meditation and acupuncture. A rough-sounding breath pattern late in our study triggered another X-ray, which revealed a mass protrusion at the level of the 7th cervical vertebra, diagnosed as cancer. He also had an anterior osteophyte fusion at the same level. He refused a shunt into his stomach or cancer treatment. In the end, six weeks later, he died due to narrowing of the esophagus and a restriction of food intake. Lack of albumin in converting nourishment to blood resulted in water accumulation throughout his body. He remained quite comfortable with the continuation of meditation. In the last days, he suffered from constipation due to weakness. Two needles on the superior and inferior descending colon (St-21, 28) were connected with electrical stimulation at a heart beat frequency for 15 minutes then needling opposite the eleventh thoracic vertebra on the bladder point which resulted in a complete elimination, being the last before his death several days later.

This single case study is based upon observation of the relationship between breath rate (or anxiety), frequent urination, bad dreams, and abdominal spasms and sputum production (our dependent variables) and acupuncture, meditation, Qigong and meditation (our independent variables). In order to create a timeline, a daily diary or log was kept which quantified the signs and symptom. The breath was observed in three ways: (1) the ratio of seconds of inhalation to seconds of exhalation, (2) breaths per minute, and (3) smoothness of the process ---pressure or absence of hesitations or jerkiness in the inhalation, exhalation and conversions. Sputum production came from observation of the number of expectorations per day and estimated volume of each expectoration (10 cc per day at peak). SF wrote down daily such things as nightly dreams, sleep quality, as well as any other observations. Blood pressure measurements were taken the same time each day and later in the day if required. The initial fluid in the lung measurement came from an X-ray and subsequent decrease or increase measurement came from daily listening to voice quality and fullness of the lungs from back thumping. Amount of swelling was determined by observing the malleolus and degree of bone obliteration and over the pedal bridge obliteration. Urination volume first came from an average normal volume per day 900cc and variations from that determined by frequency per day and volume of each urination were recorded as large, medium, below average and poor volume.

This journal was transcribed by PS and proofread by SF. After the subject died, PS constructed charts (See Appendix **B**) for urine volume, fluid in lungs, amount of drug, fluid in ankles, breaths per minute, phlegm, and blood pressure. In order to create a timeline, each variable was quantified at particular points in time. The journal included measurements of cough, ratio of inhalation to exhalation, the expansion and contraction of the abdomen while breathing, acupuncture, amount and type of meditation, meditative thoughts and Qigong practices.

MEDICATION

Digitalis (Digoxin) at 0.125 mg a day and furosemide (Lasix) at 20-10 mg a day were used throughout the crisis for the heart. After four weeks, enalapril (Vasotec) at 2.5 mg a day was introduced. During the subject's hospital stay and after the study, other medications were used.

Prescriptions from Traditional Chinese Medicine were given for the first month and in the last two weeks acupuncture was used in larger areas to improve respiratory and physiological functioning and to release spasms *e.g.*, from points to circular acupuncture to the lower diaphragm dome (Appendix **A**).

Acupuncture treatment method went from (1) treating specific symptoms such as decreasing phlegm, stopping rapid breathing, expelling fluid from the lungs, stopping the cough, and lowering edema, to (2) treatment of the psychosomatic aspects of the terminal disease: feeling of terror due to fear of imminent death.

Moxibustion was used because of low body temperature (95.7°F, see Appendix A, 5/5/94) once to twice a week for a month. As the body temperature increased and stabilized and it became warmer, Moxibustion was discontinued. This occurred after a month on 6/1/94 when body temperature reached 98 °F. moxibustion is putting an herb on the needle and lighting it which creates heat inside the body.

MEDITATION: VOLUNTARY

This technique used volition to move or hold voluntary muscles, as in breath control (coordination of abdominal muscles with the breath) or in Qigong, by assuming certain physical position while coordinating breathing. In SF's case of internal Qigong, he held the Qigong pose without moving, as done in other forms of Tai Chi Chuan and Qigong.

BREATH CONTROL

These breathing techniques were used to calm a cough, expel phlegm, break the short breath cycle, harmonize the fragmented breath, and relax abdominal spasms [15]. During the time of fluid in the lung, it created a more efficient breath and calmed panic. We developed these techniques from previous experiences and by observing the results through changes in symptoms. We had no particular guide as to what to do at a point in time so we thought through the process and consulted the journal and came up with the following principles, which seemed to take into account cause and effect. The principle for rapid breathing and fluid in the lungs was to extend exhalation and inhalation, and after a large inhalation relax the exhalation and let the air out slowly. In this regard, the exhalation is twice as long as the inhalation until the breath is brought under control. For cough and phlegm with an uncoordinated breath (which may have good volume) and abdominal spasms, the breath was harmonized. This means watching the cycle to see hesitations, contractions, and the sequence of the abdomen to the breath. Ideally the abdomen extended out upon inhalation. During a crisis it was important to first extend the length of time of the inhalation and exhalation and then coordinate and harmonize the cycle with the abdomen. For rapid breathing, we attempted to extend and slow the exhalation by relaxing at the top of the cycle after inhalation. For spastic breath, we focused each breath on the obstacle or hitch in the exhalation or inhalation cycle, and tried to create smoothness. For abdominal spasm, we used the internal force of the breath to extend the abdomen on inhalation and lower the abdomen on exhalation. This method stabilized the subject's emotional state and left him in comfort although he was slowly becoming weakened.

SF was in a deficient state and small disturbances such as the start of a bath or shower, or overdoing something would ignite a rapid breath episode. This out-o--control physiology seemed all consuming; it felt like an invasion from somewhere else, totally unfamiliar, consuming, and frightening. The emotional reaction was fear; this fear compounded any condition resulting in a rigidity of the body, and an uncoordinated state of the breath and stomach. A crisis could occur spontaneously if this state persisted. When the breath came under control (body) then dreams came (mind) not in themselves frightening, just vivid, in clear color of past events. Dream events of seemingly no meaning, then another, and another, in a fragmented sequence or order. Each dream seemed to reflect an actual time. This was very unsettling for SF. This is reflected in Appendix A 5/27/94. This state called for another meditation, getting out of the mind (see Involuntary Meditation) and this is where SF's previous discipline with Zen meditation became important and very stabilizing. SF stayed in this meditative state for up to four hours. Once after two hours in a Zen state SF opened his eyes. When questioned as to where he had been, he said. "In the great vacuity". Previous chapter shows a rapid drop in oxygen consumption, blood lactate and a synchronization of brain waves under deep meditation.

QIGONG

Generally speaking there are two types of Qigong: internal and external. Internal Qigong strengthens one's own Qi or warmth and external Qigong can benefit others. Before his winter crisis the subject regularly did five to ten minute of daily internal Qigong meditation as follows.

Generally, volition or will is used to recruit the voluntary muscles. The subject would stand with knees slightly bent and arms in a circle as if holding a ball. His fingers were about an inch apart and he gazed at the ground through fingers, focusing on the floor about one meter ahead. When his fingers started to tingle then his mind focused on a particular part of the body, and the sensation of warmth to that part followed. Sometimes after assuming the correct position he would swing his arms to each side. The arm in the direction of movement would swing further out to the side as if holding a bow and the other hand would remain as if there was an arrow in the other hand.

INVOLUNTARY USE OF THE WILL OR VOLITION

Zen meditation was introduced briefly with breath control, to stabilize the mind. SF especially liked and practiced Zen meditation in good health for many years. Zen meditation is involuntary meditation or not using volition or will to move voluntary muscles [16, 17]. The technique seems relatively simple -- sit or lie still, not moving any muscle, and watch the breath but don't try to do anything. One can focus one's consciousness on the upper lip and feel the breath coming in and out. With experience, eventually the breath quiets, thinking becomes minimal, and a quiescence or equipoise (harmonious balance) appears. This is not always possible but even with an active mind this state creates a time when dualism and contradictions can flourish without ill health from the normal physiological fragmentation it brings. In other words Zazen meditation may not quiet the mind but with the spine erect non psychosomatic transfer happens from this agitation, without it the body fragments become desynchronized. In heart disease, with this capability one can experience a disordered physiology and still maintain the meditation and improve. This sitting state was SF's daily meditation for years. For a beginner, against heart disease, in a fearful state, this is difficult to impossible. Zen meditation is not possible in a crisis situation such as panting or dream disturbed sleep or intense fear. After SF's near death crisis when he was able to use this meditative technique, a calm physiology resulted. SF felt a profound thankfulness for this quiet and ability to meditate in the Zen state.

RESULTS AND DISCUSSION

Appendix **B** are graphs (A-G) in an attempt to measure quantity over time.

Before May 15th, one can see a steady improvement and even stable periods even though he would later not be stable in two weeks (Appendix **A**). In Graph A Appendix **B** (lung fluid volume). This created the condition for SF to practice more meditation reflected in Graph B (breaths per minute). This stability and period of mental clarity from meditation created a general peace of mind, up to the 18th of May. Then the subject started dreaming in vivid color of past events, at random, without order or central understanding, *i.e.*, unrelated scenes all night. One can see this reflected in Graph I by a slight increase of fluid in the lung, drop in urination volume Graph D, abrupt changes in breaths per minute (Graph C-May 18th) and increase in phlegm volume Graph E. SF felt terrorized yet he saw no reason from any particular dream scene to say that he had anything but good luck all his life. Then he realized through his physiological response to the dreams that it was a psychosomatic response to the illness itself, and the thought, "Will this be my death?" In fear, the jaw, back of neck, and mid-thoracic tighten and in the subject's case, the Kidneys, the organ associated with the emotion fear was deficient in yang Qi.

When the symptoms became frightening, the treatment was to calm the terror by taking away the physical manifestations through acupuncture. The strategy was to release the diaphragm, relax the spastic abdomen, and change the ability to breathe and increase blood to the brain. The acupuncture method changed from points to areas of the body -- the diaphragm (circular acupuncture), the spine (each vertebra from cervical to the lumbar,) the hips (piriformis, quadratus lumborum and external oblique) and abdomen (rectus abdominis), supplemented by master points.

In Graph D one can see blood pressure lowering and becoming unstable in the ratio of systolic to diastolic during the time of enalapril or Vasotec shown in Appendix **B** Graph H from May 28th to June 26th. The relationship between Vasotec Graph H and swelling of the ankles Graph F seems clear- it decreased. The medication Graph H tended to drive blood pressure down and acupuncture was able to counter this side effect by bringing it up. Blood pressure Graph G instability can be misleading because acupuncture to raise blood pressure increased blood pressure values by 20-30% for 3 to 7 hours.

Acupuncture combined with Vasotec can be seen in Graph F Appendix **ii** ankle-swelling decrease, Graph D urination volume increases, Graph B lung fluid decrease and Graph E sputum or phlegm volume decreases.

Again area acupuncture was used to decrease fluid volume in the body, see Appendix **B** (6/12/94). This acupuncture departed from the point location to areas of the body *i.e.*, the lower abdomen around the Bladder Mu Point or Alarm Point. Concomitant to this was the traditional heart acupuncture to raise blood pressure.

Qigong is a good art against deficient yang Qi of the kidneys and heart which results in a lack of warmth. With daily practice of Qigong the subject was able to bring warmth to any part of the body on which he focused his mind. One morning after the six-week research had ended; SF was still in bed when PS arrived. He said, jokingly, "I've got one foot in the grave. It's time for Qigong". PS examined SF and felt cold on his forehead and entire body. With great effort he slowly sat up and then stood. He did the usual standing Qigong meditation but nothing happened. He then made upward arm motions (rotating the ulnar aspects of his wrists toward his body and up), and within a half dozen movements he said he felt some warmth. After laying down, a small area of warmth in his abdomen was noted below the umbilicus. When PS returned six hours later SF was working in his study, I could see only his foot with a slipper hanging off his toe twirling it, so I knew that his energy was back. He was editing the article.

CONCLUSION AND SUMMARY

Acupuncture, meditation and Qigong are most effective in treating the changeable symptoms of Chronic Heart Disease. Even when conditions become stable and general energy is good, a psychosomatic response to such symptoms can trigger a crisis. In this case the psychosomatic aspects of the illness became apparent -- feelings of hopelessness, bad dreams, and a general weakening even though objectively the subject had stabilized. No improvement over sleep or appetite could be induced up to that time, and then the fluid in the lungs got worse.

To ameliorate these symptoms and to complement other treatment, the acupuncture regime shifted from particularized local point-needling to extensive needling in general areas around the solar plexus and stomach, lower abdomen, across the back of neck, shoulders and down the paravertebral muscles to the lumbar so that a complete release of the body could be obtained.

If the system is not calmed down digestion and breathing will not work. This release reversed the pattern of insomnia and loss of appetite and made it possible for the subject to sleep and eat. Slowly there was a general improvement and his bad dreams disappeared. The subject's appetite and strength came back as well as a feeling of hopefulness. The breathing was constantly watched and monitored.

Along with this was a certain peace, absence from fear, lucidity, and a feel for life that included creating a rhythm for the process by controlling the breath and being aware of what would happen when the breath got out of control. More time was spent in Zen (involuntary) meditation (a form of Qigong) in a certain void and peace of mind. Qigong (voluntary) helped in a most critical time when the subject became extremely cold and through artful practice of Qigong changed his own body temperature. The unified use of the several complementary therapies stated above observably produced better results in this subject than would have occurred with routine administration of usual medications [18].

APPENDIX A

Chronic Heart Disease and Treatment Strategies

The particular method of acupuncture, (or meditation and Qigong) varied according to the changing conditions of the disease and can be seen under Results and Discussion.

The strategy for our study on Chronic Heart Failure came from Acupuncture a Comprehensive Text by the Shanghai College of Traditional Medicine (See Reference 1. p. 595). This disease is considered Deficient Yang Qi of the Heart and Kidneys because the yang functions of the heart are weak and blood congeals in the blood vessels. Consequently because Kidney Qi is deficient, it "lacks the strength to take in the Lung Qi". Normal Qi flows is disrupted and "water and dampness overflow". The principle is to aid and secure the source, the Kidneys, and to strengthen the Heart and spirit.

Treatment Strategies

General needling points: 1st P-6 (Neiguan), P-5 (Jianshi),

H-8 (Shaofu) 2nd P-6 (Neiguan), P-4 (Ximen), P-3 (Quze)

Supplemental: Gastrointestinal; Ren-12 (Zhongwan), S-25

(Tianshu), REN-6 (Qihai), S-36 (Zusanli) Strengthen

Source: REN-4 (Guanyuan), S-29 (Guilai), REN-6 (Qihua)

Facilitate urination and eliminate edema; REN-9 (Shuifen),

S-28 (Shuidao), K-7 (Fuliu), K-5 (Shuiguan), Bl-58

(Feiyang), Sp-9 (Yinlingquan), REN-3 (Zhongji), REN-2

(Qugu)

Distention of the Liver: Li-3 (Taichong), Li-13 (Zhangmen) and Bl-18 (Ganshu)

Relieve panting suppress coughing and eliminate phlegm Bl-13 (Feishu),

REN-22 (Tiantu), K-27 (Shufu), REN-17 (Shanzhong), H-8 (Shaofu), and LI-4

(Hegu)

In order: Symptom, Treatment Strategy, Acupoints, Progress

5/5/94

S. Panting, cough, phlegm, weak 95.4°F:

T. Aid and secure source (Kidney)

and strengthen Heart and Kidney:

A. REN-4关元,17膻中,22天突 K-7复溜. S-36

三里. LI-4合谷,11, Bi-13肺俞, H-8少府, K-27俞府.

Moxibustion.

5/18/94

S. More phlegm and adhering to side of throat, noisy lung

like growling, no urination, fluid in lung, tinnitus after

walk,dizzy.

T. Concentrate on breathing pattern.

A. REN-9水分. S-28水道.K-7复溜 ,5水泉. Bl-58飞扬 . Sp-9阴陵泉 .

REN-2曲骨,3中极 ,4关元 ,6气海. Bl-13 肺俞 . REN-22天 突. K-27俞府 .

REN-17 膻中. H-8 少府 . LI-4 合谷 . Moxibustion

5/21/94

S. Phlegm, panting, dizzy when lay down, stomach knotted, bad appetite and taste in mouth, edema in ankles.Pulse strong and stringy Uncoordinated breath--- exhalation jerky in three parts.

T. Elementary breathing exercises.

A.REN-13上脘,15巨阙. DU-22囟会. S-36 足三里. Liv-3太冲. Electrical stimulation (WQ-C2) Watching the breath for one hour

P. Less phlegm, breath brought to quiet and zero intensity after exercise

5/23/94

S. Diffuse Headache. Edema in right foot, left better. Breath opposite.

T. Watching breath with stomach going up. A. REN-12中脘,13上脘,14巨阙,22天突.K-9筑宾, REN-12中脘. Electrotherapy电疗 S-36 足三里 to Liv-3 太冲 (Bilateral).

P. Less phlegm, better sleep and breathing. Qi obtained at St-36.

5/25/94

S. 97° Sleeplessness, mouth and gums dry, strange taste, headache, fatigue, legs swollen.

T. Massage legs. S. Less phlegm, more warmth in abdomen,

swelling in legs down after massage.

5/26/94

S. Panting, legs swollen, phlegm with blood, inner mouth dry, Shen disturbances. Breath 1:2

T. Calm Shen

A. K-27 俞府. H-8 少府. LI-4 合谷. S-36 足三里

Moxibustion

P. Breathing better ratio of inhalation to exhalation 1:3 ½ after Acupuncture

5/27/94

S. Bedeviled sleep, one hour sleep

T. Calm Shen

A. S-36 足三里. H-8 少府 .

REN-13 上脘,14 巨阙,3 中极,4 关元. K-27 俞府,5 水泉,9 筑宾. Area acupuncture around xyphoid process

P. Phlegm less, abundant urination, nose clear, breathing good.

5/29/94

S. 95.8° Good sleep, looks good

P. Urination moderate until late afternoon.

T. Deep breathing for 20 minutes induced 20 of deep sleep.

A. S-36 足三里. Bl-20 脾俞,23 肾俞. Area acupuncture on left side-trapezius, scapula and paravertebral muscles from vertebrae C-3 to L-5 with gluteus minimus and piriformis

Bilateral.

P. No phlegm, good sleep and urination, more heat in body, slept deep one hour.

6/8/94

S. Hear water in lungs rattle, urinating at night, tongue reddish pitted in middle, constipation, and blood in sputum.

T. Qigong, standing knees bent and arms in

circle looking at floor through fingers one meter ahead. Arms move to side with alternating breath like shooting an arrow from a bow.

A. S-36足三里. Bl-11大杼, 12风门,13肺俞,14厥阴俞,41隔关. SI-9肩贞, 11天宗,13曲垣.

P. Taste in mouth better. Drank more water, phlegm less, no dizziness, eyes open and bright, good nourishment.

6/12/94

S. Weak.

A. S-36足三里,25天枢. K-9筑宾. REN-3中极,6气海. Area acupuncture to around Bladder alarm point.

P. Good appetite, good color, good sleep, breathing good, less fluid in lungs. Slept during treatment.

6/14/94

S. Pitted red tongue, wider than on 3/15. Ugly taste.

T. Zen meditation for long periods

A. S-36足三里,25天枢. K-9筑宾. REN-3中极,4关元,5.

LI-4合谷,11曲池.

P. Good color and fair appetite, no AM phlegm, good

sleep.Editing journal and writing.

6/19/94

S. 97.4° Stable

T. More Qigong

P. Napping. Calm breath, legs not swollen.

APPENDIX B

Summation of Variables

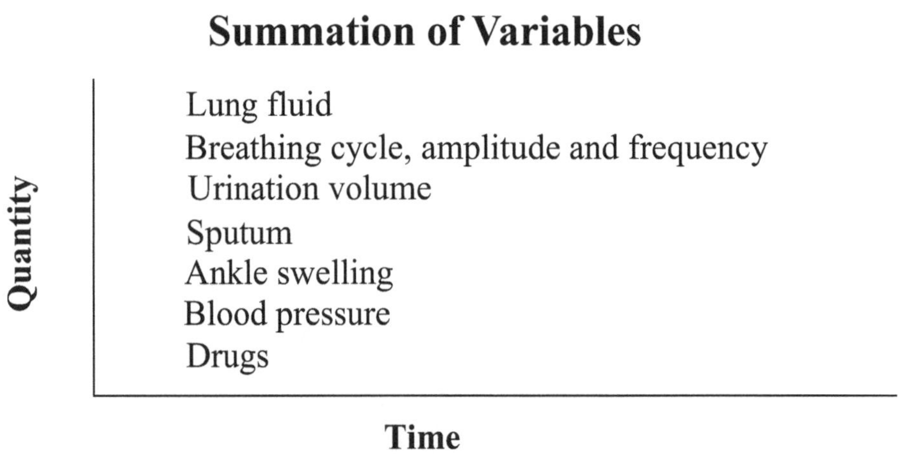

Graph A

Appendix B contd.....

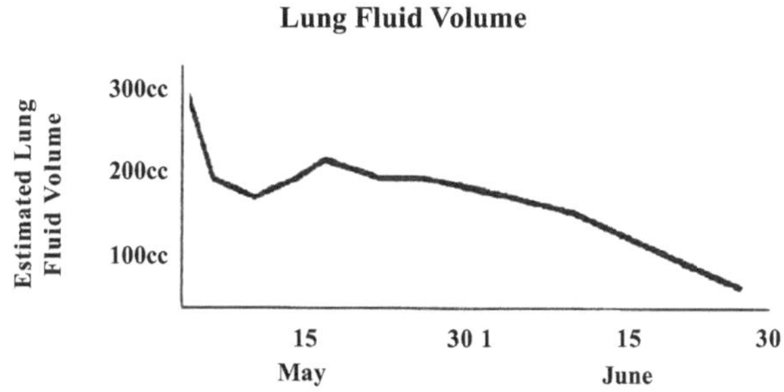

Graph B

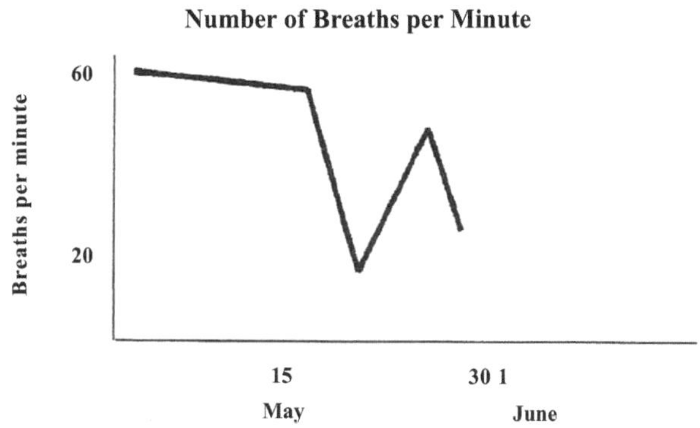

Graph C

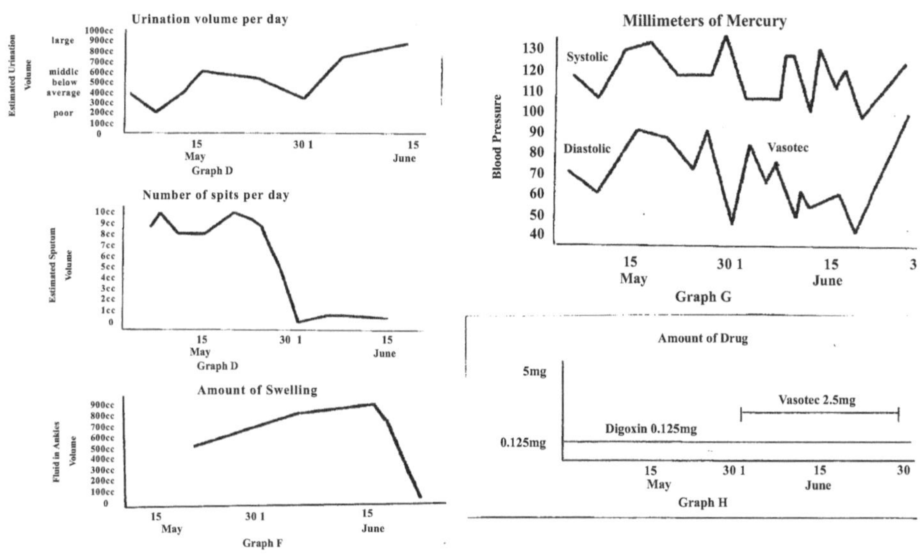

REFERENCES

[1] O'Connor J, Bensky D. Shanghai College of Traditional Medicine D, Acupuncture a Comprehensive Text. Seattle, Washington: Eastland Press 1987; p. 17.

[2] Shinnick P, Freed S, Blumenthal C, Omura Y. The heart. Brooklyn: The Heart Disease Research Foundation 1990.

[3] Shinnick P, Freed S. Organic life energy in physiologic states of chan (or zen) buddhism and ino analogous state of superfluid helium quantum liquid. J Sci Healing Outcomes 1995; 3(12): 4-10.

[4] Freed S. Induced specific immunological unresponsiveness & conditioned behavioral reflexes, in functional isomorphism-meditation and conditioned specific unresponsiveness. Int J Neurosci 1989; 44(3-4): 275-81.
[http://dx.doi.org/10.3109/00207458908986207] [PMID: 2656566]

[5] Anand BK, Chhina GS, Singh B. Some aspects of Electroencephalographic studies in yogis. Electroencephalograph Clin Neurophysiology 1961; 13: 451-6. Studies on Sri Rahahand yogi during his stay in an air-tight box. Ind Jour Med Res 1961; 49(1).
[http://dx.doi.org/10.1016/0013-4694(61)90015-3]

[6] Kasamatsu A, Hirai T. An electroencephalographic study on the zen meditation (Zazen). Folia Psychiatr Neurol Jpn 1966; 20(4): 315-36.
[PMID: 6013341]

[7] Alavi A, LaRiccia P, Sadek A, *et al.* Neuroimaging of acupuncture in patients with chronic pain. J Altern Complement Med 1997; 3: 47-53.
[http://dx.doi.org/10.1089/acm.1997.3.s-47]

[8] Lee MH, Ernst M. The sympatholytic effect of acupuncture as evidenced by thermography. A preliminary report. Orth Rev 1983; 12: 67-72.

[9] Freed S. Acupuncture as therapy of traumatic affective disorders and of phantom limb pain syndrome. Acupunct Electrother Res 1989; 14(2): 121-9.
[http://dx.doi.org/10.3727/036012989816358452] [PMID: 2575343]

[10] Freed S. Implications of physiological and behavioral states of extremely low noise-levels for acupuncture. Acupunct Electrother Res 1985; 10(4): 297-303.
[http://dx.doi.org/10.3727/036012985816714333] [PMID: 2871700]

[11] Omura Y, Lin TL, Debreceni L, *et al.* Unique changes found on the Qi Gong (Chi Gong) Masters and patients body during Qi Gong treatment; their relationships to certain meridians & acupuncture points and the re-creation of therapeutic Qi Gong states by children & adults. Acupunct Electrother Res 1989; 14(1): 61-89.
[http://dx.doi.org/10.3727/036012989816358506] [PMID: 2568074]

[12] Bykov K, Gant WH. The cerebral cortex and the internal organs. New York: Chemical Pub. Co 1957.

[13] Freed S. A possible physiological basis for effectiveness of acupuncture against psychosomatic disorders. Acupunct Electrother Res 1987; 12(2): 113-23.
[http://dx.doi.org/10.3727/036012987816358850] [PMID: 2890273]

[14] Anokhim P. Characteristic of the afferent apparatus of a conditioned reflex and its importance for psychology. Prob of Psych 1955; 6(15)

[15] Dyczkowski MS. The vibration of power, the aphorisms of siva. New York: State University of New York 1992.

[16] Hirai T. Zen meditation and psychotherapy. New York: Japan Pub 1989.

[17] Kapleau P. The three pillars of zen teaching, practice, and enlightenment. New York: Anchor 1980.

[18] Shinnick P, Freed S. Acupuncture, meditation and qigong as complementary treatment in chronic heart disease. Proceedings of the Seventh Symposium for the Society for Acupuncture Research. University of Maryland. 2000.

CHAPTER 8

Whole Person Family Healing: How a Daughter Heals Her Mother

Abstract: This is the case study of an elderly woman who underwent dangerous surgery that was not even needed because she felt too intimidated to question her doctor. This study shows that when we are tuned into our Self and our Nature, we can heal anyone who might be in a compromised state of health, including ourselves. We will also explore Wholeness, or the lack of it, and how it relates to disease.

Keywords: Afraid to upset the doctor, Anemic, Blood flow, Collateral damage, Creativity, Directions to the body, Education, Fragmentation, Greed, Healing, Healing work, Herbalist, Heroic medicine, Infection, Internal bleeding, Laparoscopic surgery, Life, Machine mechanization, Mental map, Negative entropy, Oath of Hippocrates, Organism, Palpation, Polyp, Power to heal, Quantum Physics, Reason, Relationship to the body, Responsibility, Societal injustice, Specialization in medicine, Teacher, Technology, Thought, Violence, Wholeness.

THE OATH OF HIPPOCRATES

In its original version, the Oath of Hippocrates is sworn to Apollo. It states: "With regard to healing the sick, I will advise and order for them the best diet, according to my best judgment and means; and I will take care that they suffer no hurt or damage. Furthermore, I will comport myself and use my knowledge in a godly manner".

Repeating, in mantra, the Medicine Buddha Sadhana one can get interesting images (Fig. **1**). The Medicine Buddha is the deep space of healing. A blue light shines its healing vibration. As we direct our attention toward Nature, subtle manifestations appear to guide us along our path.

Phillip Shinnick & Laurence Porter

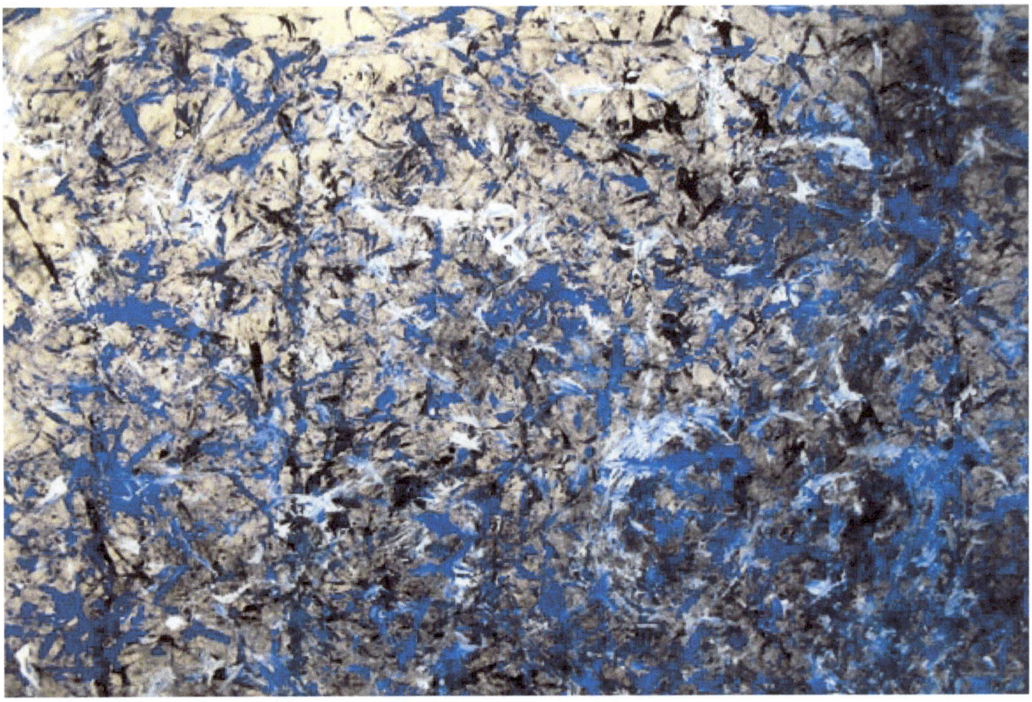

Fig. (1). Medicine Buddha. LP. 2010 (With permission of Porter).

INTRODUCTION

Every day thousands of people are subjected to costly, often unnecessary, medical tests. Patients are not being examined by their doctors. Instead, they are treated like machines that are all identical. Pharmaceutical companies have designed a pill for every possible symptom, and then some. Routine surgeries are performed on all kinds of problems that could be resolved more appropriately by other means.

The case presented here is quite a common one. This is the story of how my mother allowed herself to be subjected to a major surgical procedure she did not need. Because she was intimidated by "the aura of the white coat" and afraid to question a medical professional, she almost lost her life.

Maybe the Oath of Hippocrates has been compromised, but we can still restore it when we honor our natural connections.

Applying my skills as a healer, I did a few simple things that helped my mother get herself out of a dangerous state. Learning about our experience can help everyone see that we are not powerless in the face of illness. I will tell you about my background as a healer, and I will describe the impact Quantum Physics had on my quest for Wholeness.

TWO SIDES OF THE SAME COIN

In 1992, I was living in Washington, D.C. with my husband and son. A few years earlier, I had moved to the United States from France, where I was a dancer. Since childhood, dancing was my passion. It was cathartic for me to move to a different country. I began to question everything I had previously learned without understanding what was happening to me or why, but trusting in the process. Opening to a new language -- speaking and thinking in English for the first time -- offered me the freedom to explore myself anew.

“How can I be substantial if I do not cast a shadow? I must have a dark side also if I am to be whole”.~C.G. Jung (Fig. **2**).

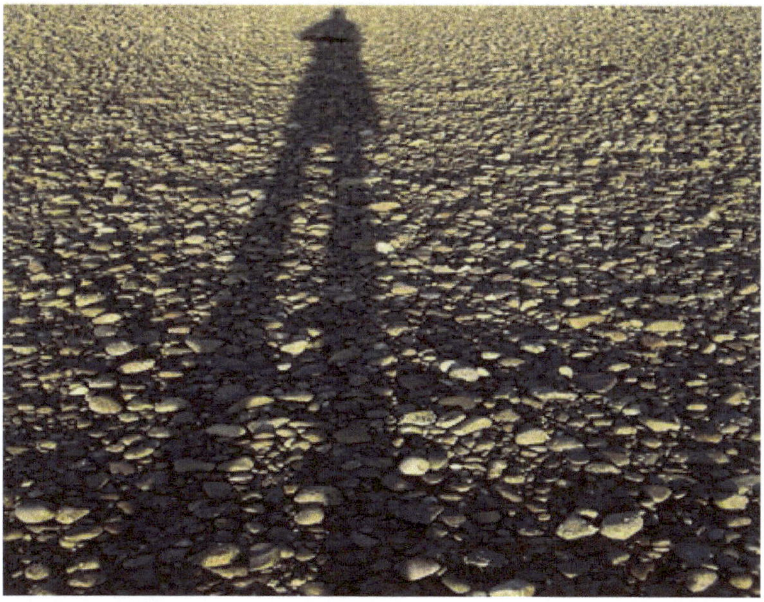

Fig. (2). Shadows. (With special permission of porter).

I was diagnosed with pneumonia during the winter of 1992, and I decided not to take antibiotics. Without understanding why, I knew it was the right choice for me at that time. I suffered intensely for a month. I retreated into myself, allowing my body to do what was necessary to heal itself. I ate very little, sometimes nothing. I did not speak. It allowed my body and mind to cleanse and regenerate. I just kept following my intuition. I plunged into the darkness and brought what I found back to the light. The process continued to unfold for many years, allowing me to face difficult events from my past. The light and the dark were inseparable, two sides of the same coin.

WHOLENESS

As I emerged from my deep retreat at the end of that month, I spontaneously wrote about dancers that were holograms. Each character in the elaborate story I wrote represented a different aspect of me. As soon as I saw the word "hologram" written on the page, I felt an urgency to learn more about holograms. I rushed right out to the nearest bookstore. There I bought The Holographic Universe by Michael Talbot and immediately devoured it. That book led me straight to David Bohm, a prominent physicist, who spoke to me directly. I soon read most of his books and discovered a whole new world, the world of Quantum Physics, a world of wholeness.

Though I had no prior knowledge of physics, I deeply understood what he was saying about the reality in which we live. He was describing the wholeness I had experienced when I danced. Quantum Physics revolutionized physics at the beginning of the 20th century. Observing the microscopic world and seeing the behavior of atoms revealed that the physics of Sir Isaac Newton no longer applied at that level of reality. Until then, the world was believed to work like a giant clock. It followed a predetermined path, and the lives of human beings were equally predetermined. In the 15th century, there was Copernicus's belief-shattering discovery that the Sun, not the Earth, was at the center of our solar system. It forever changed man's perspective of himself and his place in the universe. Now Man, no longer the center of the universe, slowly began to separate from Nature. At an atomic level, the reality of Nature looked different. Nature is not a machine made up of different parts. Instead, there are networks of interrelationships in which the observer plays a fundamental role.

The circle has always been a representation of wholeness (Fig. **3**). This is our natural state.

When physicist, Werner Heisenberg, said: "The common division of the world into subject and object, inner and outer world, body and soul is no longer adequate", his new paradigm once again changed our position in the universe. No longer merely observers, we had now become co-creators of our universe, our lives and our health. Through our thoughts, we create and define the world and the society in which we live. What happens outside of us, happens inside of us. There really is no separation between the inside and the outside. Thoughts, emotions and the body are deeply interconnected. When our personal, political or other systems are out of balance, division and illness are created. What we can create we can also un-create. Therefore, we can heal illness. Disease is merely another form of creation.

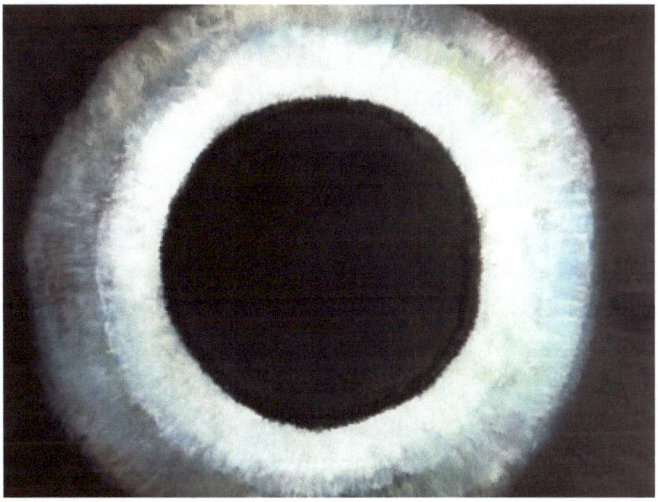

Fig. (3). Inner Space. (With special permission of Porter).

David Bohm's view of Wholeness included us; it was not just theoretical. Still, we mainly live our lives from mechanistic understandings. Bohm felt no one would need approval from scientists to explore the implications the concept of Wholeness can have on collective humanity or individual humans. All of us would be helped if we could only understand the significance of fragmentation and see the limitations we impose on ourselves by accepting a mechanistic model of reality.

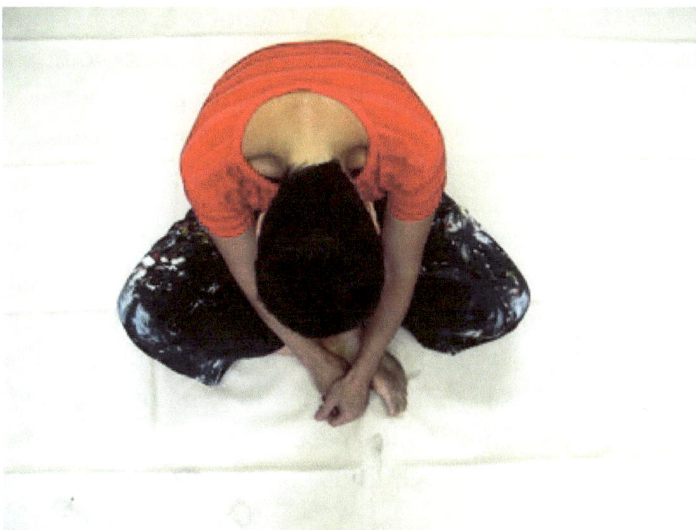

Fig. (4). Veneration. (With special permission of Porter. Photo by Herman Costa).

Before Creation . . . here, before starting a new painting, one has to bow in humility to the Infinite Potential at hand. Healing oneself requires the same recognition. One must go beyond the limitations imposed by thoughts and the fragmentation they cause (Fig. **4**).

HEALING MEDICINE IS AN ART

After healing by giving myself over to a process that liberated me from past conditioning, I looked at dance and life as one and the same. Life itself was now the art that captured my full attention. In the words of David Bohm, "The unbroken wholeness of the totality of existence as an undivided flowing movement without borders". This ongoing process led me to Dr. Phillip Shinnick, as things continued to unfold when I injured my leg while dancing. I knew the injury was an intrinsic part of my overall healing. Treatments I received from Dr. Shinnick helped me see my own ability to heal others as well as myself, and I began to develop as an intuitive healer. From Dr. Shinnick, I received a transmission of knowledge that was, and remains, of the highest nature.

Dr. Shinnick and I share the same vision of medicine. Medicine directly addresses the processes of Life. Therefore, it is naturally creative. Treating patients is informing patients. It is helping them to see what processes brought them to their sickness or injury. It is teaching them to breathe and to take care of themselves by becoming aware of their old habits and patterns, conscious of the dynamics in their relationships. It is showing them how they can take responsibility for the cause and effect of their thoughts and actions. Each person is unique and should be treated as such. Diseases and injuries are not our enemies; they are our teachers. Watching them, knowing them, accepting them is real work. Since they are not static, they can be reversed. Though it might seem scary at first, if we trust the process, there will be Light.

Disease can be the dark side of us we do not want to see, but repressing our dark side removes us from Nature, which has light and dark, day and night, life and death. By separating that which cannot be separated we create fragmentation and ever more darkness. When we see the oneness of the movement of life, we reside beyond duality. We see that we are the flowing of light and dark, life and death, health and illness. This is the space where we can heal as we learn that our demons are constructs of the mind, products of the past, mental agitation.

Looking at different levels of reality, we see that we reside here and there and that the space between things is alive. We feel the vibration of space (Fig. **5**).

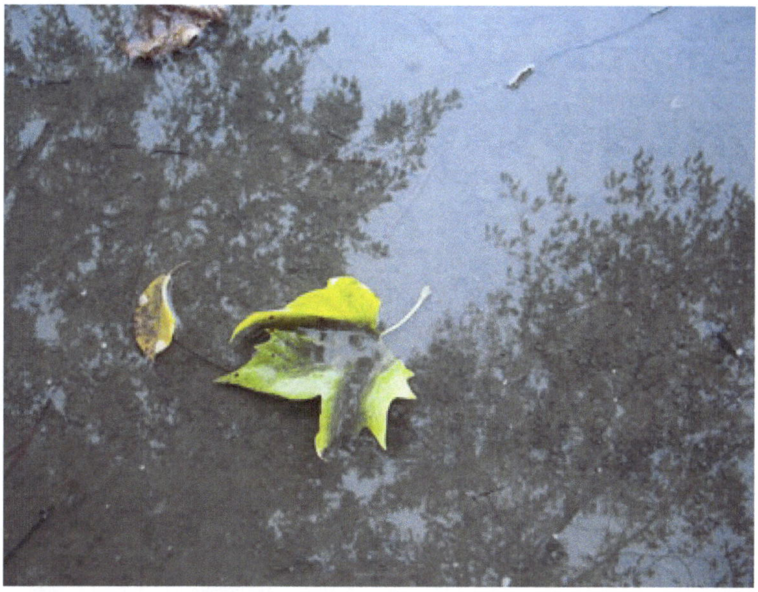

Fig. (5). Dimensions LP 2014. (With special permission of Porter).

MY ELDERLY MOTHER'S UNNECESSARY SURGERY

When my mother was 84, she was a widow with an active, creative life in France. She did ceramics and quilting, she knitted, loved to cook and to bake, and she had a busy social life with many friends, who ranged in age from quite young to elderly. My mother had a mild heart condition, a pronounced kyphosis, that could sometimes be painful, and she suffered from various other minor ailments. Most of her health problems were managed with medication. In November of 2014, she told me she had a malignant polyp, which needed to be removed from her colon. A couple of years previously -- on the anniversary of the death of her second husband -- she suffered from stones in her gallbladder that spilled into her pancreas causing severe pancreatitis. She was hospitalized, and her gallbladder was removed. She also suffered from a urinary tract infection for years. I understand that all of those manifestations were related to the emotional difficulty my mother had in resolving traumatic events from her past.

After hearing the news that she had a polyp, my mother came to New York for a month to spend the Christmas holidays. I suggested that she could benefit from Dr. Shinnick's treatment in addition to my own. Among his many accomplishments, Dr. Shinnick is an acupuncturist who responds in an intuitive, creative way to his patients and their problems . I work hands on , feeling my way toward unlocking whatever needs to be released from the body.

Like Dr. Shinnick, I work with the whole person at many different levels. I have learned from the work I have done with myself for many years. From being a dancer and observing Nature, I have experienced how all aspects of the human being are connected, that the emotional, the physical, the mental, the spiritual are various expressions of the same movement.

Being receptive to the idea, my mother was treated four times by Dr. Shinnick for about two hours per session. She received acupuncture and electrostimulation treatments for the purpose of releasing tension from her hips, back, shoulders and neck so that more blood could flow into her abdomen and create a terrain that might change the nature of the polyp. It was apparent to me that my mother, who was very present during the treatments, went to a different state of consciousness. Dr. Shinnick did Taoist meditation on her as well. After the first session, the difference in her abdomen was remarkable. What had felt contracted, congested and dead before Dr. Shinnick's treatment, now felt warm, relaxed and flowing. The blood flow in her legs improved immediately. As each treatment went deeper, my mother released more and more tension.

Manifestations of nature appear and disappear -- sometimes very quickly. If we are present to the moment we see them. This rainbow is a moment of perception that involves different levels of reality. The rainbow doesn't really exist, but its colors bring us a deep feeling of beauty and awe, affecting us in a real way (Fig. **6**). Even if we do not understand what the rainbow is, we feel happy anyway. Something happens that is from a different order than the thought process.

Fig. (6). Dragon Rainbow LP 2012. (With special permission of Porter).

During a successful treatment, the body and the mind grow quieter. They slip away from the agitations life presents, and the body becomes cooler. The same way that nature regenerates during winter time, the body regenerates and synchronizes when it gets into an empty state. This emptiness allows the space for life to unfold despite all its challenges. Stillness and movement are one. One does not exist without the other. Often oblivious to stillness, we identify with movement. But without stillness, movement can very quickly become agitation. Dancers and martial artists know that movement comes from stillness and dissolves back into it.

After each session there were discernible transformations. She was able to feel the changes. Between her sessions with Dr. Shinnick, I worked on her as well. During this time she and I also discussed her past and how it impacted on her in the present. She suffered family hardship. Her French father was assassinated in Algeria when he was an administrator there. Her husband, suffering from war trauma after his experience as an underground intelligence guerilla in the French Vietnam war, abandoned her and her two little children. She was responsive to our talks. She began to show signs of evolving in her understanding of the importance of releasing old memories which blocked her mind and body. On Cape Cod we visited an herbalist who made a special formula for her colon and polyp and another one to boost her immune system.

Observing how beautifully it was all unfolding, I suggested one morning while the two of us were having a lovely breakfast that she might consider waiting a few more weeks before deciding whether to have the surgery or not. After a short period of rest, she could have another colonoscopy to determine the status of the polyp and then decide. I reassured my mother that I would completely support whatever decision she made. The next day she told me she was afraid to upset the doctors. She believed she would look foolish if she declined the surgery, then the problem became serious. She felt unable to fight the system alone. If Dr. Shinnick or I could have been with her in France, things might have been different. She and I continued to talk about it. I even offered to speak with her doctor, but she asked me not to.

Each person is different and yet the same. We need to recognize what we share as human beings and see that our differences are part of the glorious diversity of creation. We are Whole, and on a deeper level we are all the same, but the circumstances of life, like our parents, place of birth, *etc.*, make each of us unique and different (Fig. **7**). These two poles must be reconciled to achieve individual and global healing.

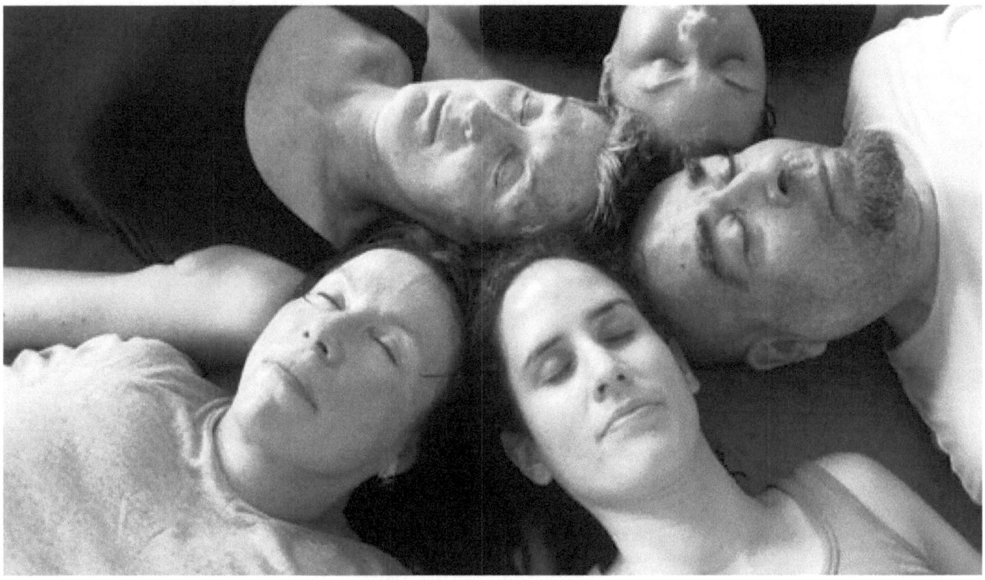

Fig. (7). Heads Together 2013 LP. (With special permission of Porter).

When my mother returned to France, she met with the surgeon and asked him what would happen if she did not have surgery. He replied that she could end up with an obstruction and need emergency surgery. My mother was examined only once, and that was by Dr. Shinnick who palpated every inch of her body to get an accurate landscape of what her patterns were. Touch is fundamental to the human experience. Palpation is essential in the practice of medicine. The hands have the ability to connect, to understand things at subtle levels, to transmit energy and love. To rely entirely upon technology for a diagnosis may yield higher profits, but it is unhealthy, even dangerous. The batteries of tests that are run whenever a person visits a doctor or a hospital have completely changed the relationship between the doctor and the patient. I remember when I was a little girl that our family doctor used to examine us thoroughly and from the examination was able to make a diagnosis. From depending more on technology than ever, our society has developed unprecedented communication networks, but actual communication is breaking down. Technology is not the problem. The real problem is the mechanization of the human being. None of the doctors my mother saw connected to any understanding of what was happening to *her*. She was one number among many numbers, just another number with a routine condition that just needed another routine procedure.

No two human beings are alike. Even when cases seem similar there are subtle differences that need to be considered. The body is a creation. It is Whole. It conceals the Divine within it. "He who penetrates the body's nature is liberated", says Abhinavagupta, the great 10th century tantric philosopher from Kashmir. The body is a marvel of relationships and processes that allow us to experience our passage on Earth in a connected way, not in isolation. It might be a temporary suit, but it is perfectly suited to our needs. In my healing work, I see how much we abuse the body. It is often treated as a commodity that we use to assert ourselves from what we believe to be a limited, restricted place. Since we are creation, it is only natural that medicine could be creative. The body is in constant flux. Its cells can morph into any function as required. The body has the ability to regenerate, reverse the direction of disease and heal itself when given the chance to do what it does naturally. To honor such a marvel of intelligence, medicine and the practitioners of medicine might better assist in the process of healing the body if they would be more alive to their own creativity, and not merely act as mechanized technicians. It is too often forgotten today that the Practice of Medicine is an Art. If we keep on using technology in our currently fragmented way, we will continue to generate ever greater chaos. But if we can integrate the benefits technology offers with a whole human being, who is living a healthy life, we will prosper.

Since her surgery was already scheduled for a couple of weeks later, I flew to France to be with her during that time. Surgery that involves the digestive system is generally heavy duty. The surgeon had warned her of bad consequences if the procedure did not go forward. Yet the problem was gone, undetected by the doctors who did not physically examine her, but had continued to rely upon an image that was taken six weeks before. The surgeon performed a laparoscopic procedure. He removed a segment of her colon. When I asked the surgeon what he had found, he replied that it was not much . . . and there was no reason to worry about the results! For a few days after her surgery, my mother remained in intensive care. She began to feel very weak. She became anemic. She was given a transfusion, but her blood work still showed that something was wrong. There was probably bleeding in her abdomen. On the fourth day after the initial surgery, she was taken back to the operating room. She was opened up for a second time. It was discovered that she was, in fact, bleeding. They suspected that she might be bleeding because her blood was so thin it was leaking out of her veins. She was given five kilos of blood and two kilos of plasma. We later found out that they put her back on anticoagulant medication too soon because they were concerned she might have a heart seizure.

When I saw my mother's condition, I feared for her life. I felt angry when I saw the state she had been brought to. On the spot, I recognized the anger, realized it would not be productive and let it go. All my energy was needed to help get her out of this dangerous state. Her heartbeat was very fast. Her blood pressure was too high. She had a fever and was incoherent. All of her systems had lost their sense of direction. They were in shock. I put my hand on her chest and told her, "Rally all of your energy . . . right now". I said it from my heart with all the power I had in me at that moment. The intention was clear. Her body responded with a jolt, and I knew it had heard me.

My mother was able to follow directions. She brought order back to the chaos in her body. Order and chaos are two sides of the same coin. I kept telling her to rally her energy. Her kidneys were not working well. I placed my right hand on her left kidney. I spontaneously focused on the energy of my kidney and let that energy flow into her kidney. A few hours later, the nurse told me that her kidneys were working normally. I did the same thing with her bowel to help restore activity. I kept reinforcing that she had to give her body directions. I basically guided my mother toward saving her own life, but her ordeal still was not over. She suffered an infection. The doctors could not localize her infection so they put her on five different kinds of antibiotics. The one she responded to indicated that the infection was in her abdomen. She also had water in her lungs due to her heart problem. I was able to help her with that through releasing her left side, under her armpit, her neck, shoulder and jaw. From my association with Dr. Shinnick, I knew the cardiovascular points for the heart. Exhausted, my mother slept a lot during the day, but she was too agitated to sleep well at night.

This purple ray feels like the power of intention. It is direct. Again we need to be present to know clearly what to ask for and to see the healing manifestations of nature and the constant exchange of energy between all living organisms (Fig. **8**).

Little by little my mother actively rallied her energy. With the good care she received from my sister and from me, with the loving energy she received from family and friends, and with the help of the calming influence of meditation she began to get more stable. She was released from intensive care. She started to eat and drink after not being allowed to drink anything -- not even a drop of water -- for at least ten days. She went home after spending a month in the hospital. The recovery process was slow. She took herbs and supplements to help her body return to a more balanced state. Depression was lurking, which was not surprising given the shocks her body went through. A nurse who saw the result of the polyp biopsy told my mother that all she went through had been for nothing. She did not even need the surgery. The obstruction was gone.

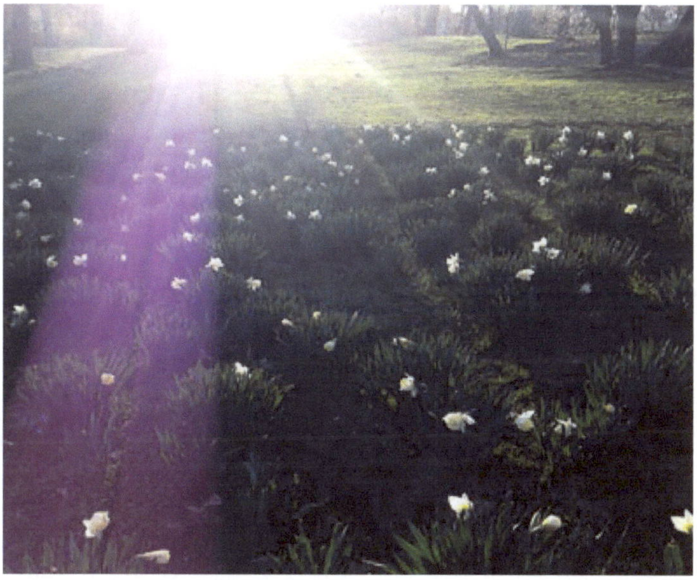

Fig. (8). Purple Beam LP 2012. (With special permission of Porter).

The spiral of life reminding us that we are beings of light (Fig. **9**).

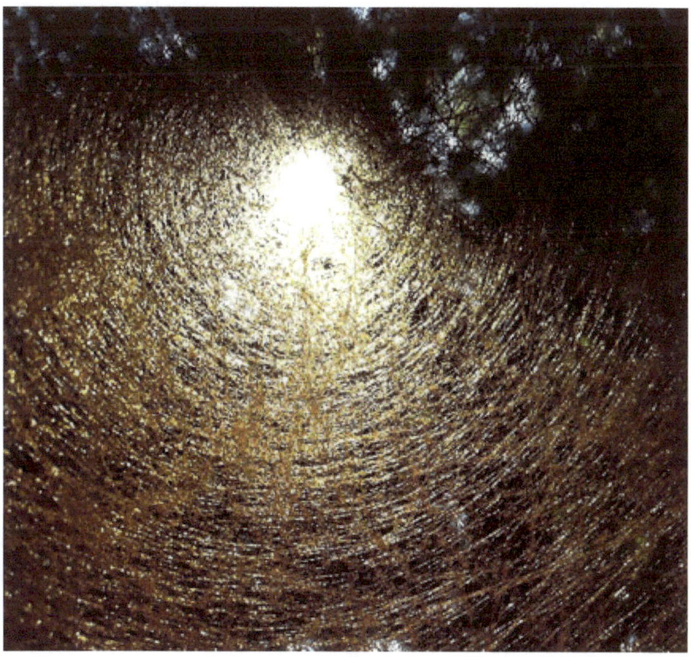

Fig. (9). Healing LP 2009. (With special permission of Porter).

Henry Miller said "Our own physical body possesses a wisdom which we who inhabit the body lack. We give it orders which make no sense". I agree. It makes no sense at all for so many people to subject themselves to procedures and drugs that are not necessary. Their choice is costly to society but lucrative only to a small, select group. Everything was done to save my mother at the age of 84 from a polyp that had become nothing, no threat at all, after being treated by acupuncture, herbs, meditation, deep emotional change, love and compassion. Even if the polyp had been stronger or more aggressive, there still would have been more viable choices than surgery.

I would like to share some important things that can be learned from this story. If we are in touch with ourselves, we all have natural powers we can use when faced with difficult situations no matter what the difficulties are. In this case, my mother's vital systems were in chaos, but order was restored when I gave commands to her body. Directions have to be clear and direct. They must come from the heart. The person giving directions can transmit energy, with the intent of the mind, directly from his or her own body. This brings order to chaotic situations. When faced with challenges, we are being called upon to show up, which means we must be present in the moment. We must listen and focus without tension and simply allow the information to flow. Each situation will require something different, but if we show up we will always know what is needed. This is done from the heart with no attachment to, nor expectations of how the process might unfold or what the outcome will be. This is not a thought-centered process. Therefore, it is necessary neither to analyze what happens nor to understand how it happens. To break this process down into knowable parts means losing it. As simply and quietly as possible, we need to open the heart, show up, listen, trust, and expect nothing. That is all.

Science has tried to break life down, to come up with an elegant formula on the origins of life, but the closer we look, the more we examine, analyze and think about it, the farther we find ourselves from life or its meaning.

In The Ending of Time, David Bohm and Krishnamurti engage in a dialogue on thought and consciousness, the nature of existence [1]. David Bohm: *" But I think that the main point, which could communicate it, is to see that knowledge, in all its forms, subtle and obvious, cannot solve the psychological problem; it can only make it worse. But then there is another energy which is involved".*

Nature is not divided. Knowledge can divide, and the more division there is, the more the Wholeness of Nature is lost. Knowledge is necessary, like maps are necessary, as tools to orient ourselves. But we must be aware they are abstractions that cannot be confused with the Whole. Life can never be less than the totality from which it is extracted. Knowledge does not grasp everything. Something beyond words is required.

Shakti energy, the creative force shooting straight up through matter to join Shiva, destroying all illusions and revealing the Oneness of all things (Fig. **10**). Opposites are binding forces that belong together. They dance until they realize that they are One. We have a certain independence but it is only relative to the whole and the union of opposites.

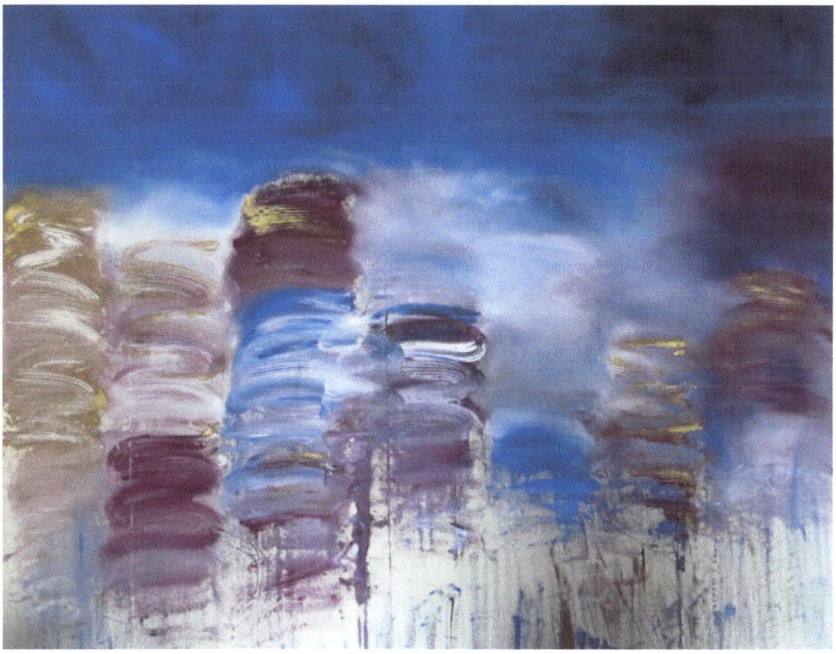

Fig. (10). Pure Energy LP 2007. (With special permission of Porter).

PROGRESS REPORT

The next time I returned to France for a visit with my mother, I offered her whatever help she might need. She was still very pale and tired. When I examined her, I found that her digestive system was still not functioning well, particularly the liver. She also had a lot of gas. Her right side was still painful from residue of water in the right lung. I treated her hands with needles. The liver responded well. The gas diminished. I guided her through a lot of deep breathing every day. I cooked mostly vegetables for her. That also had a good effect on her digestive system. It was Spring then, so we took advantage of its life-giving energy force and sat in the sun, nourishing ourselves from it. She was having physical therapy to help her back get better. Proper treatment, appropriate food, communion with

Nature, walking, some exercise, breathing, love and affection all go a long way. After spending a week with my mother, she felt stronger and had more color in her cheeks. She was on her own for the first time since the surgery. Although my mother had many good friends looking after her, it was still a big challenge.

CONCLUSION

Yes, in my mother's case, the Oath of Hippocrates was greatly compromised, but we are here to learn from each experience and to keep evolving no matter what the circumstance might be. Suffering, which is part of our human experience, can enlighten us. Suffering can be transformed into awareness, and it can provide us with information we can share with others. This is how we move consciousness. Perhaps my mother was ready at that time to accept that she did have choices.

Sometimes trees grow right through cement. With a tiny amount of soil and enough sunshine, life will sprout anywhere. Because we are Whole, we can heal ourselves. This is free medicine for all, like the limitless energy we can access through breathing and exchanging energy with our environment. Like all living organisms, we evolve creating order. As we exchange energy with our environment (the sun, the earth's magnetic field, food, water, *etc.*), we can change our physiology and our thoughts by creating more order within and without. By being conscious and appreciative of these life sustaining energies, we acknowledge the healing energy of life.

We have the same kind of faith in science that we have in religion. Forgetting our own natural powers, we give ourselves over to those belief systems, and we lose ourselves. We become dependent and weaken ourselves. Science and Medicine should benefit Mankind, guiding and assisting us to live in greater harmony with Nature. We are all healers because we are Nature and Life. The very nature of everything is to endlessly transform itself. Order transitions into chaos, then it turns back into order once again.

That is what happened during the treatments my mother received. When we tamper with and try to control Nature, we pay a high price, but when the head, the heart and the body are integrated, the cosmic flow makes itself heard. It is the most beautiful song of all. The earth and sky align creating tremendous power. In that space, everything is in balance. When we soften, we are able to love, and we have compassion for everyone, including ourselves. Then we are no longer separated by the artificial boundaries we have created. Consciousness is like clay, and we are all sculptors. We must each decide how we will shape our own world, but we all live by the same breath in the end.

"If [man] thinks of the totality as constituted of independent fragments, then that is how his mind will tend to operate, but if he can include everything coherently and harmoniously in an overall whole that is undivided, unbroken, and without a border, then his mind will tend to move in a similar way, and from this will flow an orderly action within the whole".

~David Bohm, Wholeness and the Implicate Order

This is the power of transformation from one thing to another in endless loops. We do have the ability to regenerate, to evolve (Fig. **11**).

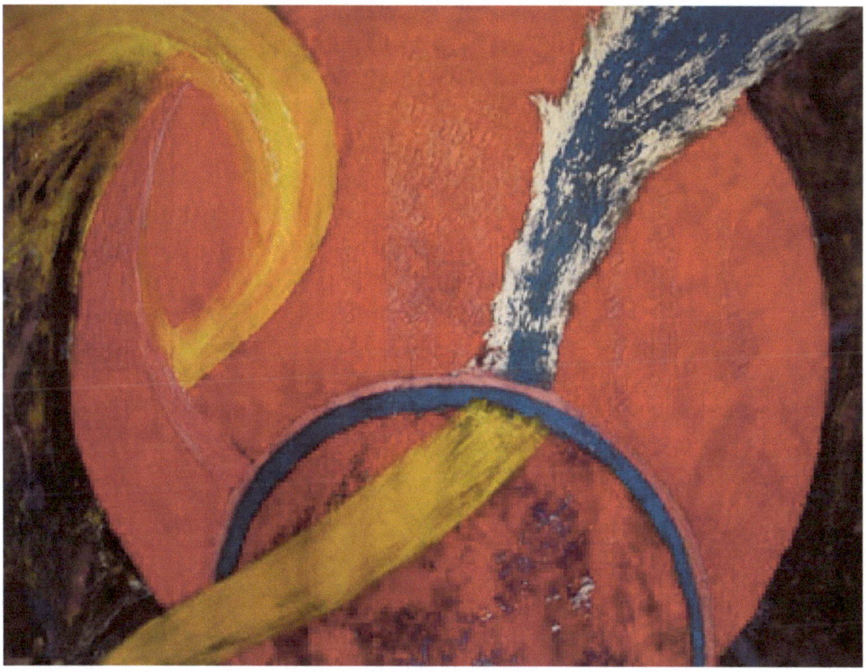

Fig. (11). Swooping Energy LP 2009. (With permission of Porter).

REFERENCES

[1] Krishnamurti J, Bohm D. The Ending of Time. San Francisco: Hall 1985.

CHAPTER 9

Multi Cultural Self Healing For A Spinal Injury

Abstract: This is a two and one half year report of a compressed and fractured vertebrae from a traumatic spinal injury subsequent to a one and one half year report previously published. The purpose of this study is to provide a non-manufactured drug, non-surgical, Oriental, Occidental, Indian/Tibetan and Native American approach to rehabilitation for a serious spinal injury. Besides stainless steel acupuncture needles used as emergency pain relief, the only material used was the mind, breath, body movement and posture positions. The method was based upon a variety of traditional cultural techniques as well as modern physical exercises for rehabilitation and a scientific case based pattern of reactivity from a Post Traumatic Shock Disorder (PTSD). Daily progress notes over a year and one half, and an understanding of Oriental, Occidental, Euro-American, Native American and Indian/Tibetan treatment provided the framework for recovery. This chapter explores using the Native American Indian practice of calling upon the animal spirit for healing, this is also a tradition in ShaoLin Gung Fu five animal forms as a Qigong practice. These technique are discussed here. The multiplicity of symptoms, changed constantly, arrhythmia, visceral dysfunction, concussion, herniated disks, dislocated ribs, whiplash, cervical and lumbar spine pain symptoms and emotional agitation.A quick recovery was followed by constant regression based upon reactions to posture, weather, noise in environment, travel and stress. It appeared that the effects of Post Traumatic Shock of anxiety, apprehension, fear and agitation became the most difficult to treat and continued after two years and one half year but at a more moderated occurrence

Keywords: Acupuncture needle, Animal spirit, Anxiety, Arrhythmia, Brain circulation, Clinical notes, Cold weather, Compression fracture, Computerized axiomatic scan, Fear, Herniated disk, Hot weather, Involuntary mediation, Magnetic resonance instrument, Non-drug treatment, Non-surgical treatment, Opiates, PTSD (post traumatic stress disorder), Spondylolisthesis, Visceral dysfunction, Voluntary meditation, Whiplash, ZeZen.

Phillip Shinnick & Laurence Porter

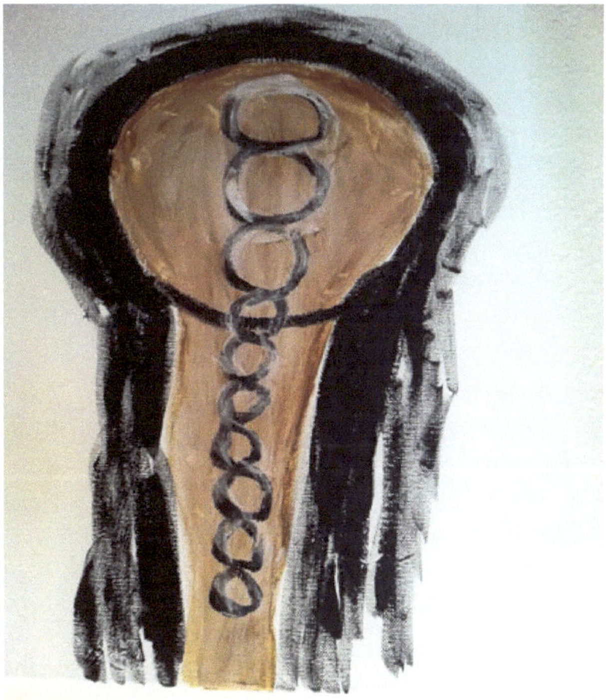

Fig. (1). Within PKS 2009. (With special permission of Shinnick).

The original Hippocratic oath. " I swear by Apollo the Physician and by Asclepius.". In honor of Asclepius, a particular type of non-venomous snake was often used in healing rituals, and these snakes — the Aesculapian Snakes — slithered around freely on the floor in dormitories where the sick and injured slept. These snakes were introduced at the founding of each new temple of Asclepius throughout the classical world. From about 300 BC onwards, the cult of Asclepius grew very popular and pilgrims flocked to his healing temples (Asclepieia) to be cured of their ills. It is said that in return for some kindness rendered by Asclepius, a snake, licked Asclepius' ears clean and taught him secret knowledge (to the Greeks snakes were sacred beings of wisdom, healing, and resurrection) (Fig. **2**).

Many strange visions appear in deep healing meditation, strange, which never appeared again and seemed very unusual (Fig. **1**).

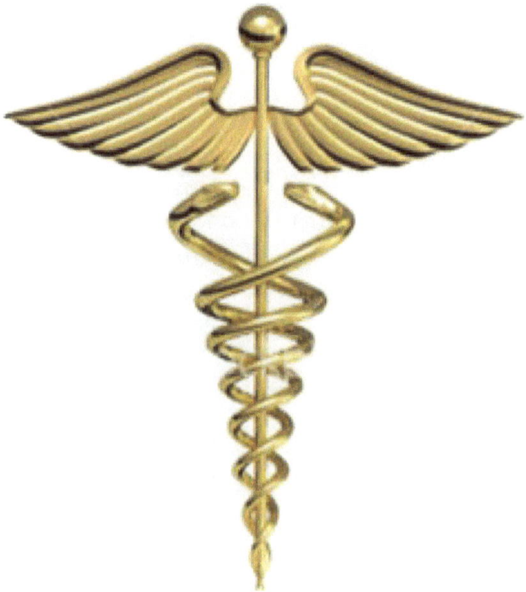

Fig. (2). The Rod of Asclepius. The God of Healing and Medicine.

INTRODUCTION, REPORTS, TECHNIQUES, HISTORY, AND STRATEGY

Radiologist Report. Jerald Zimmer, MD notes from a Computerized Axial Tomography (CAT SCAN) notes "a moderate central stenosis L4-L5, first-degree degenerative spondylolisthesis L4-5, moderate degenerative changes, burst fracture with moderate compression T-10 vertebral body, slight paracentral retropulsion, and osteopenia. From a *Magnetic Resonance (MRI)* of the thoracic spine, notes mild dextrorotoscoliosis, soft tissue fullness T9 and T10, left paracentral disc herniation T4-T5".

This injury resulted from a boating accident. In rough seas after being ejected from a flat launch boat (25,000 pounds) on its steep downward motion of a wave, the patient was hit in the back on the first up surging wave and the second wave up surging in the right anterior ribs and on the third up surging wave on his lower back as he was bounced around [1]. Non-surgical treatment of these conditions was recommended by Christopher Mandigo, the neurosurgeon at that time [2]. The patient had an extensive background in physical medicine, electro stimulation, rehabilitation and acupuncture, so Dr. Mandigo recommended that the patient undergoes extensive rehabilitation including myofascial pain relief procedure, physical thein which this report is based upon as well as therapist notes. Research shows inserting a steel rod fixating the spine did not do better in the long run.

The patient who had a background in physical medicine kept detailed daily records of his pain symptoms, treatment, surrounding condition such as weather, and sleep pattern.

Therapist Report: Laurence Porter, Occidental and Oriental Healer. Palpation to the patient's body created a template of understanding of symptoms and symptomatology as follows: Immobility and painful to stand, cervical stiffness and pain, lower anterior and posterior ribs not fixed on sternum and spine, injured area sensitive to touch, organs in spasm (dysfunctional, large intestine not moving), in neurological shock. Bulging cranium and pain to left temple, left jaw constriction, pain to left scapula, left inguinal hernia initiated, soft tissue injury, arrhythmia, fatigue from pain,constipation, digestive difficulty, agitation, anxiety, apprehension, and fear.

Treatment Technique: Gentle circular motions to let tissue release from tension and trauma (Fig. **3**). Practice of Nian Li (using will and intention), external Qigong and the Three Buddha healing technique (residing in the third eye and palms of both hands on the area to be healed with mind empty). Three hours a day for six months.

History and Pre-existing Conditions: Age 12, injury to thoracic left anterior rib from accidentally running into twine tied to trees at full speed in a race; age 17,18,25, three serious brain concussions from football, basketball, and head on 60 MPH car accident (hospitalized); age 20,25,29, three serious hamstring tears at full sprinting speed; age 21, stress fracture left fourth metatarsal; age 20-29, four meniscus tears to right and left knee; age 17,62, two right rib traumas; age 21, herniation of L4-5; age 27, arthritis right and left hips; age 29 right achilles tendon tear; age 23, groin muscle tear; age 50, right calcaneus bone spur; age 24-27, chronic sinus infections; age 22, migraines; age 45, neck injury car accident; age 46,48, dislocated right wrist and left wrist sesamoid bone broken; and age unknown, dextrorotoscoliosis. Leg asymmetry (right ¾ shorter than left, left foot size smaller than right). age 68, second degree Lyme infection (Borrelia burgdorferisensu stricto), antibiotic for one month; age 71, left inguinal hernia operation six months after accident. Patient had complete recovery from all accident and infections (including arthritis of hips*) from 1963 to 2013 through* yoga, meditation, stretching and strengthening (weight training and swimming).

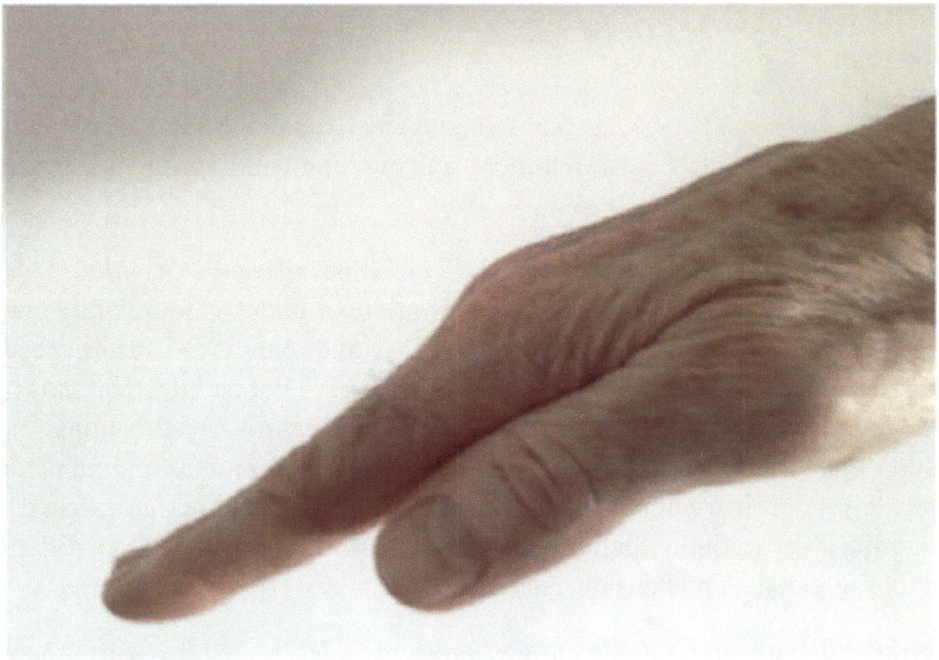

Fig. (3). This picture shows the angle of deep massage used for healing the spinal injury.

Right after the accident, the patient was stuck on the cruise liner for three days before coming back to New York. He was in shock and great pain. His only resource was breathing. Through the breath, he was able to connect to absolute energy and calm the pain down. See involuntary meditation below. Breathing through the pain, opening the rib cage and the spine slowly proved to be essential. By not avoiding the pain through heavy medication and remaining alive to the moment, the patient was able to direct energy where it was most needed. Since, the breath has guided the healing process for both the therapist and the patient. See below.

Substances for Pain Relief. This patient took Acetaminophen twice a day for the first 8 days then Oxycontin once a day for thirteen days then no manufactured drugs. After one and one half years, took Ashwagandha for one month for reactions to stress activities. To start intestine movement, after traumatic shock to the intestine nerves in the back at T11 used an ayurvedic food for three days (two liters) with success. For pain relief,1 gram per day at 8PM of cannabis, two inhalations, and two 12 ounces of Czechoslovakian or Russian beer.

Treatment Strategy. Treatment started with the injured rib cage on the right side, then the shocked digestive system, and then opening up of the hips. At first, only external Qigong was applied to the spine [3]. Shortly, it was possible to touch the fractured vertebrae without pain and move the spine. Within three months, the hips, lower and mid back released, creating a good environment for the fractured vertebrae to heal. From there on, attention was mostly needed from the mid back up to the neck and skull where tensions due to PTSD started to develop. The body continued to be treated as a whole, unifying the past, present and future to let the body take on a different form, looking at emotions and movement of the mind. Consciousness rose in the spine, allowing more flexibility, spontaneous movement.

The legs remained strong but not as predominant, more in harmony with the rest of the body. During these first months, the patient experienced a *reenactment of all old injuries listed above as if it was the day after the trauma. A past injury pain memory which had abated was recreated. Originally, the intense pain from these injuries abated in about three days, so this understanding of the acute finite characteristics of these past injuries was understood as passing.* As the months went by the old injuries subsided with treatment and the recent injuries became more painful. The movement of the painful areas moved upward in the body. Throughout the treatment the patient and the therapist experienced a wide range of emotions, accepting all that was there for the healing process to take place at all levels. The best healing sessions occurred when both patient and therapist were in complete unison. The patient, during these sessions, often went to a state of deep meditation.The therapist saw a lot of colors and in spite of the injured spine saw it as a golden or blue river several times. (Migraines, triggered from outside stress and overwork, became common).

Heart Agitation, Arrhythmia, and Relief Procedures

Over a year later, the left jaw and left neck and shoulder created a pseudo feeling of an impending heart attack with pain in heart and left shoulder. Treatment included releasing the jaw, neck shoulder, axilla and left triceps. Arrhythmia lasted two weeks, then eight days, reducing to three days, being able to correct, with early warning signs to left neck and shoulder. A year later it took just three hours to correct with the below technique. Two years later the arrhythmia was less frequent and by laying down for ten minutes it passed, usually triggered by too much time at the computer or outside agitation.

The heart treatment involved acupuncture to the posterior paravertebral muscles at the third cervical vertebrae (important cardiovascular points discovered from research for therapy) and to the Shu points on the left posterior rhomboid, superior to scapula just opposite of the fourth thoracic vertebra or known as the alarm points as seen in point 22. The patient's left shoulder, axilla and jaw went into spasm and released through easy hand stimulation (Fig. **3** above) as well as the other Shu points with acupuncture. Other symptoms included agitation, distraction, and all consuming irritability with pain in chest, tension pain across the supraorbital forehead area, a left temple pain and arrhythmia (skipped every 3-5 beats then resolved to every 18 beats then stabilized. During this period of arrhythmia a feeling of euphoria pervaded the whole organism which created the impression that this was rebellious Qi and the spine was blocking energy to the heart. Also the moment of impact, as mentioned, the patient had emotional upset which conditioned the patient to have physical and emotional pain combined, both triggering the other. In other words the pain areas brought emotional pain and emotional pain brought physical pain.

Relieve from arrhythmia by acupuncture and manual stimulation to the back of the neck near the junction of the arteries is possible (Fig. **4**).

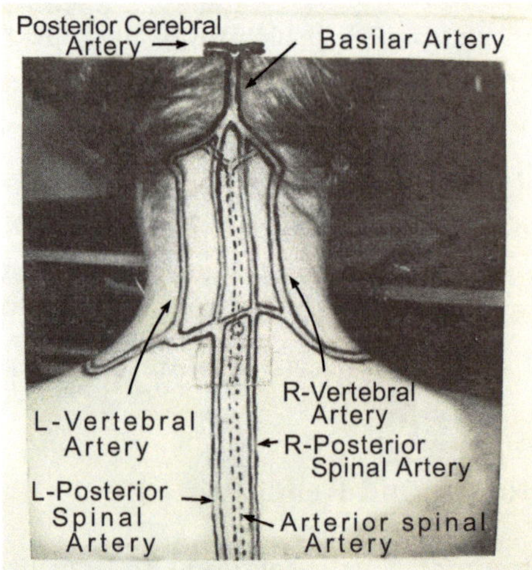

Fig. (4). Relieve from arrhythmia by acupuncture and manual stimulation to the back of the neck near the junction of the arteries is possible. (With special permission of Omura).

As one can see when cardio-vascular brain circulation is compromised with spasticity to the back of the neck, the brain's central regulation disruption stresses the heart because of lack of blood circulation (Fig. **4**). See #22 for cardiovascular treatment points (Fig. **5**). This important neck areas are cardiovascular areas discovered using heart and artery tissue on the neck, resonating with the local tissue using the O-ring Diagnostic method to map cardiovascular points on the back of the neck (Figs. **4**, **5**). These neck areas are important areas to stimulate (mechanical, external Qigong, laser, acupuncture, and massage) for heart hypertension (Fig. **6**). If the brain is under stress from lack of blood circulation the heart suffers since it is an organ under a certain central regulation. Also T4 enervates the heart and if under spasm will compromise electrical input to the heart (Voltage=Resistance x Current, V=RI, so that resistance is up current to heart goes down).

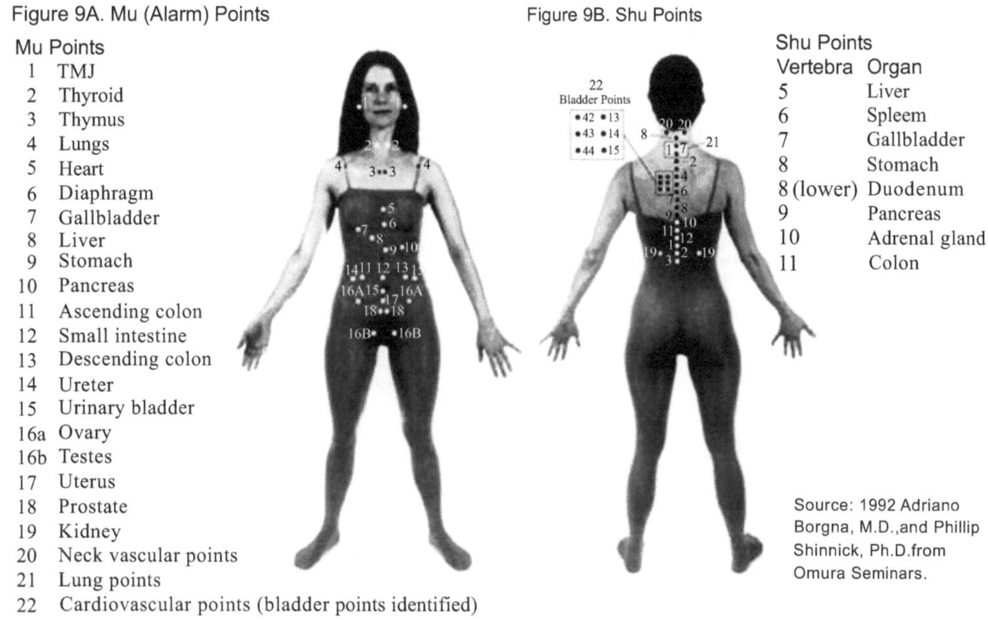

Fig. (5). This picture shows the Mu and Shu points which are the organ representation points for the organs on the back and front of a subject. See #22 for cardiovascular points. (With special permission of Shinnick).

Arrhythmia. Rebellious Qi. For the patient arrhythmia is felt with a raising energy euphoria in the chest. This energy, which is healing energy, gets stuck in the chest and will not flow through the spine because of the scoliosis, contorted from the accident; the upper thoracic and cervical spine became twisted to the right. In a Taoist seeding ceremony at the lunar moon in China ten years before by the patient, approximated this contortion (shaking) of the spine while feeling euphoric. It appears when the energy cannot move up the spine then things get stuck. Episodes of arrhythmia lasted from two weeks to recent occasions three hours (after understanding method of treatment) with long periods of calmness. Also when in a relaxed state after meditating for some time or in long therapy sessions, shaking starts throughout the body as the energy starts to move up and the spasticity let go [4].

Conditions Triggering Heart Agitation from Case Notes; Hot weather, traveling, agitation in the environment, posture, clenched jaw, spasm in the left posterior cervical, left pectorals and axilla spasms, and viscera tension.

Procedure for Relief: Sitting ZeZen, acupuncture to axilla, mandible, posterior cervical, upper posterior thoracic (T4), forehead with anterior chest massage.

Self Help Treatment

Symptoms: This patient suffers from multiple pain locations, digestion and elimination problems and mental anguish.

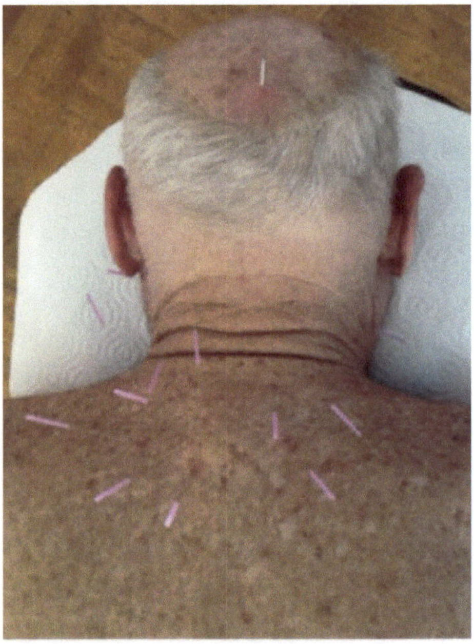

Fig. (6). Acupuncture to the cardiovascular alarm points to inhibit arrhythmia. These points differ from our Shu points due to patient differences and palpation (Fig. **6**). (With special permission of Hegda).

Patient Involuntary and Involuntary Meditation Experiences From 1963 to 1972 this patient did daily training for World and Olympic competition in jumps and sprints while self-healing numerous serious sports injuries without drugs or surgery. He trained with heavy weights, sprinting and uphill mountain running and later Yoga. In the 1980's adapted sitting Zazen meditation as a daily routine. In the 1990s learned Five Animal Forms of Kung Fu with Master Larry Tan (student of Bruce Lee) as a daily routine. In 1994 learned Qigong from He Bin Hui 2-6 hours daily. Traveled to China for a two week retreat at Lao Fu for the traditional Taoist seeding Lunar moon ceremony. From 1988 went to the Russian/Turkish baths two to three times a week to relax the body and did yoga in the heat. Learned this in Budapest in 1965 in the Turkish baths while on an international national team.

Procedure Self-Help: Involuntary and Voluntary Mediation Techniques to alleviate pain and elicit endogenous opiates, relieve pain, calm the mind, and relax the abdomen through meditation.

Involuntary Meditation:

Practices: ZaZen (Japanese), Qigong (Chinese), Yoga (India) Meditation and hot baths.

Requirement for Zazen and Qigong: In Zazen, sitting with the spine straight or erect, not moving and one pointed for long periods on the lower part of the body. In Qigong one can sit, stand, or lay down with attention to the lower abdomen.

The Physiologic Effect and Techniques: In sitting meditation the brain cools and calms down, if agitated, from energies squandered through compulsive drives, purposeless action, mental anguish and trauma. During the cold winter, hot baths and heat calm the brain and body. There is a soothing of the autonomic system creating emotional stability and not easily disturbed by outside stimulus or unresponsiveness to reactivity of the trauma. The organs are thus strengthened and inner tension decreases. Particular consciousness originates from the amount of attention (time) to different parts of the body. For the average person, the mind with it's arisal of thoughts is where attention is focused. For trauma which has mental attributes, paying too much attention to the mind results in experiencing anxiety, agitation, apprehension, and fear by re-experiencing the trauma. This emotionality and thought fishing triggers pain and suffering when too much attention is paid to feelings and thought.

In Zazen, focus is on the Hara (viscera), the stomach, digestion, and elimination. In Qigong this is the lower Dan Tian (Red Fields) or the ancestral Qi center. These meditations integrates the body, mind and spirit. In Yoga the lower body is one of the energy centers, all create the cultivation of energy in the body (not the head) by concentrating on the lower abdomen. The technique is very simple according to Qigong Master He Bin Hui, place one hand over the other with the web (men right over left, women reverse) over the umbilicus. Wherever the mind goes, energy goes, stay down in the meditation, not up, inside the body not outside. This technique was the most used in this study on an average of 3-12 hours per day for pain continuous pain relief.

The patient during the most severe pain episodes took a hot bath 3-4 times a day doing involuntary meditation while soaking. Four months later went to the Shvitz (sweat) at the Russian/Turkish baths for 2 hours of heat and did yoga after heating up successfully. Only after a year was the patient able to do hot/cold combination (220 degrees F. of radiate heat then submerging in 56 degrees F cold water) which patient had done for 20 years 2-3 times a week.

Voluntary Meditation

Symptoms Patient suffers from pain when moving. Body stiffness and limited range of motion throughout body.

Practice: To occupy the mind, by paying attention to form, avoiding reaction/action, by thoughts on positional forms for healing. These physical forms elicit endogenous opiates and increase the ability to move better. In swimming, the person needs to make peace with water, let it hold the person. Since this person had water trauma the practice was to let go in water, relax, float, then swim. In breath control, this technique uses volition to move or hold voluntary muscles, as (coordination of abdominal muscles with the breath) or asana Yoga postures. In a Yoga Asanas the best pain relief for this patient resulted from hyperextension of the spine, in balasana, "child's pose" posture, resting on the back of calves with arms out or backward, stretching the spine, holding that position resulted in pain relief (Fig. **7**).

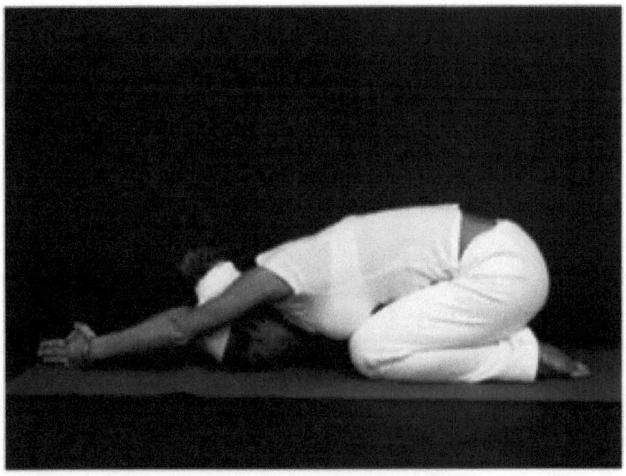

Fig. (7). Balasana, child's pose. (With special permission of Hegda).

In Yoga the patient held certain Asanas positional forms for long periods of time (Fig.**7**). Initially, held position forms for hours as pain relief. Sometimes during the early month After three months the patient could not get down from Sarvangasana without help because of pain from the fracture (Fig. **8**). After a year coming down slowly vertebrae by vertebrae pausing at each one for up to five minutes. Each vertebrae made a loud pop and readjusted going down to the sacrum. The patient did this all day.

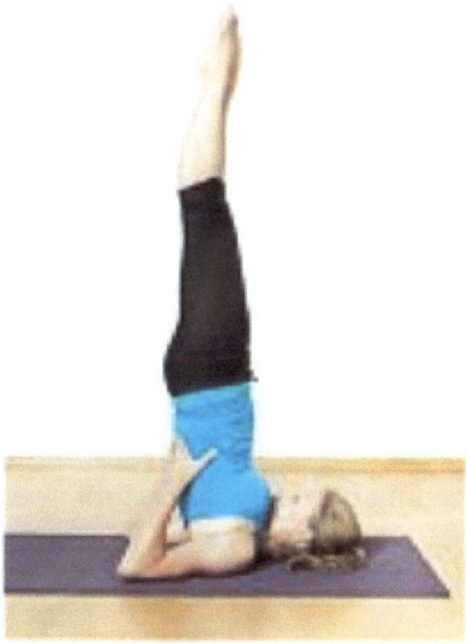

Fig. (8). Sarvangasana, shoulder stand. (With special permission of Hegda).

In Yoga tradition there is a snake curled around the spine in Kundalini yoga (Fig. **9**).

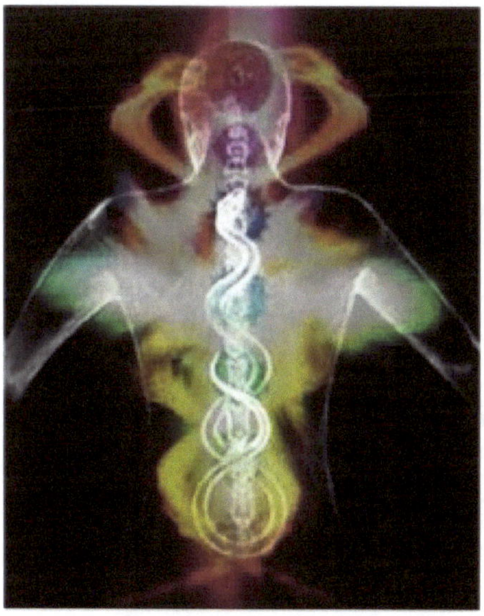

Fig. (9). In yogic tradition, a snake is curled at the base of the spine and travels up upon awakening. (With special permission of Hegda).

Breathing, Sitting and Lying -- on inhalation expanding the lower abdomen and back, exhaling relaxing the jaw, shoulders, hips. In the first three days the patient had success in ameliorating the pain by lying still and doing Qigong meditation with attention to the lower abdomen creating a vibration in the abdomen which distracted from the pain. The patient had been doing yoga and other meditations during four days before the accident, so was "charged up". Laying on his back he was aware of the accident in the back but the front was vibrating (spanda) so things were in balance with Qigong. At the end of the third day the vibration stopped and the pain came around to the front and was all consuming. In desperation the patient went one pointed into inner space and the pain intensified until he saw Anuttara a no form energy singularity of a gold ball with red and black surrounding it, still but vibrating. A deep cry for help resulted in a body contorting and a deep gasp for breath. In a flash the the patient understood that the breath was the way out. For the next four hours the breath as described above was practised with the pain receding to a quiescence and peace of body, mind and soul and never again did the patient fall into a hopeless state. Slowly the voluntary moving meditations could be practiced.

Background of Voluntary Meditation: Yoga, Kung Fu and Native Americans Animal Forms

This technique uses volition to move or hold voluntary muscles by assuming certain physical stationary and moving position in animal, Qigong or Yoga forms.

In Qigong and Shaolin Gung Fu the practitioner used a variety of animal forms while moving in and out of certain positions (Fig. **10**). To practice Native American animal forms one stays in one pointed concentration looking for an eye in the inner field with eyes closed. For this patient, a bird had appeared many years before. Later, when this eye appeared, an animal form came from no form.

We need a little background on this case before going on. The patient learned this twenty years ago from Zhang Zhang, a Rinpoche of Tibet, while visualizing the Medicine Buddha as all blue with the adornment, outside the body in front of the meditator. Chanting chi, chi, chi, continuously. Then take this form inside one's body, then become the Medicine Buddha, expanding in all directions, then raise this form up, as this happens the form, becomes no form, which is absolute energy, which fans the mind/brain/will/thought with a plasma explosion all encompassing. It does not lead to reaction, as thought, and thus this experience escapes habituation from the Law of Action/Reaction and eases its physical grip.

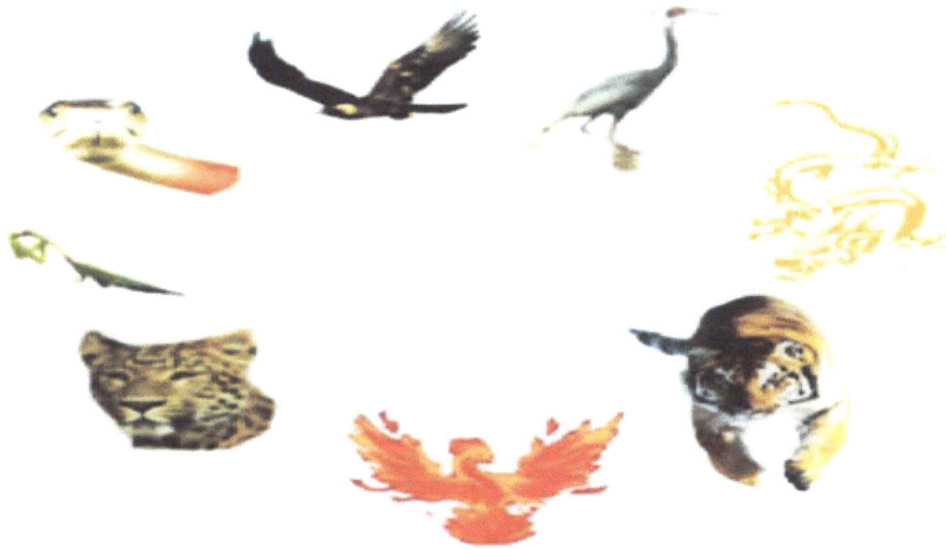

Fig. (10). Shaolin Kung Fu Animals. (With special permission of Hegda).

Animal Healing Arts

Animal spirit healing, in this case study, shows the animal form with its essence, infusing the body, uncoiling a compressed spine, creating one pointed alertness. An important instruction in practicing this art is needed. Being one pointed in inner space is a yoga technique usually through the third eye. In distant healing one becomes one pointed in inner space and tries to find the patient's eyes or face to be healed. After this happens, one knows the location and one needs just to give the proper healing necessary.

For animal healing the patient or mediator uses the plea to be released from pain in their heart while being one pointed in space. Instead of a person, one looks for just an eye, and a particular animal appears in a faint form, also, recognized by the type of animal eye. When this happens, the eyes meet and a transformation happens. The spine becomes different, expands while deep animal sounds come. In ShaoLin Kung Fu animal sounds are made when in form when attacking and striking or moving.

Another way is to goes inside the animal's eye, reversing positions, flipping to the other side, instead of looking out you are looking in, maintaining focus inside the body, thus that animal. Instead of the injury taking the energy, the body responds, as an animal, extending the spine up, opening the thoracic ribcage. The spine reacts as an animal and expands upward with essence, spirit and energy, to heal spinal injuries. It should be noted that this came after stretching the spine with the

Balasana Asana repeatedly after the accident for pain relief and years of practicing the animal forms of Gung Fu was the prelude to this. It can happen naturally, spontaneously, abruptly, since the spine has this tendency.

....

1877. *Bitterroot Mountain Range. Idaho/Montana, USA. "Grizzly Bear Youth lay in his tent suffering from the wounds received in the Big Hole fight. Here a great bird, that never alights on the earth or trees but rests only in the clouds, appeared to the sufferer in his lodge. . .it is never seen except by those wishing it for their Medicine. said, 'I see you have tears in your eyes, caused by grieving over the loss of your relatives our country, and your arm. Why do you cry? Look behind about two days' travel and you will see two creeks. These creeks are on Camas Meadow. The big chief of the Idaho soldiers, "Cut Arm" and his force are camped there, it is rather a strong force, but fear them not. The Nez Perce will kill some of the his men and get possession of his animals..." "Through the Nez Perce Eyes Trust Betrayed" by Duncan MacDonald. Macdonald lived with the Nez Perce and could write in English.*

....

Birds because of the position of their eyes can see more of the horizon and a view of the world. The first to rescue is usually the bird, others come as well to help, bear, cougar, horse, goat, snake, or wolf.

Manifestation of the Bear, Snake, Horse, Lion, Goat and Bird came naturally from extending the spine, seeing the animal in the third eye, then going behind the eye to be that animal with its noises and postures thus opening and healing the spine (Fig. **11**). In animal forms one concentrates on the lower abdomen with mind empty, which captures essence, breath and spirit of the animal body/mind/spirit for healing and opening of the spine. This appears to be a natural reaction to healing during extreme spinal pain to open up the vertebrae which are crushed. Below: The Cobra appeared all white many times to the patient and therapist with a different colored head (red, gold, blue and black). Right in Kundalini Yoga the snake coils at the bottom of the spine then raises up.

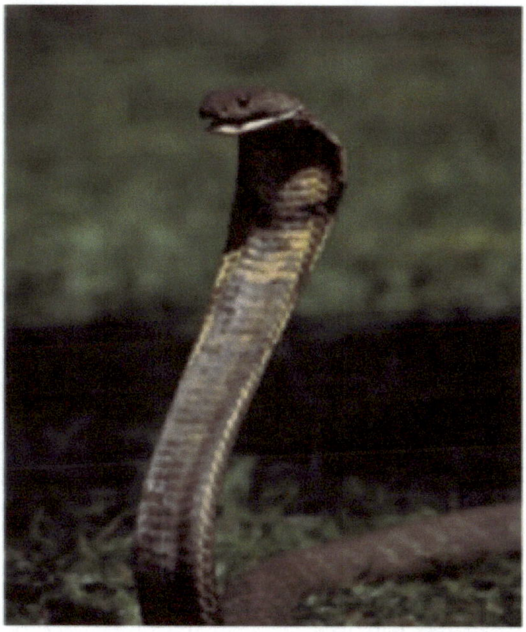

Fig. (11). The Cobra Snake in the coiled position is how the snake comes to those evoking the animal spirit thus opening up the spine, creating alertness and ease to vertebrae. The spine has an impulse to heal itself as the central spark that creates mobility Fig. **11**). (With special permission of Hegda).

Stone Carving in a Chinese cave, AD 25 -220, showing a raven/crow taking a patient's pulse and giving acupuncture (Fig.**12**). Snakes and birds have been apart of medicine in healing through the ages, in advanced stages giving teachings on healing on shown above 2,000 years ago and 150 years ago in the mountain of Idaho USA. We must assume that this has gone on for sometime. Here we see just two records, one on a stone cave, the other, in a tent, during a time of great injustice when the Nez Perce were forced off their land.

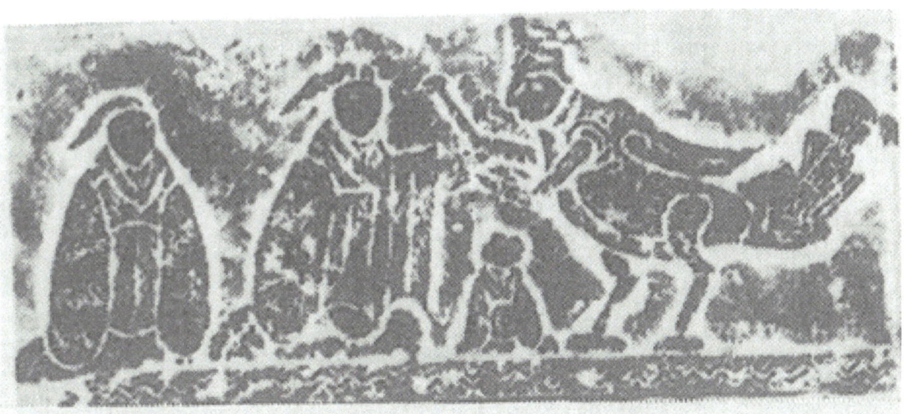

Fig. (12). The bird: ancient raven healing. (With special permission of Omura).

Perhaps in China at that time there was a great need for a new medicine which birds knew from their vast vision and understanding of space (Fig. **13**).

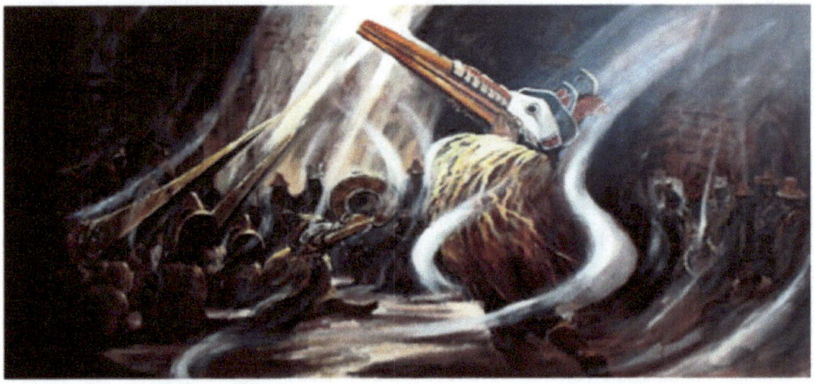

Fig. (13). Calling forth the bird spirit which is space and wind, a communal ritual in Northwest America. (With special permission of Hegda).

This patient did a traditional four day retreat into the Selkirk Mountain Range of Idaho at 12 years old, alone with his 14 year old brother in 1955 with the elk, grizzly bears, cougars, birds, deer, mountain goats and mountain fish (Fig. **14**). Also he rode cattle roundup bareback on a great white horse, four days continuous, 18 hours a day. For Native Americans doing a mountain retreat links the individual to the animal spirit. Riders of horses understand the great strength in the chest of horses and racing through space.

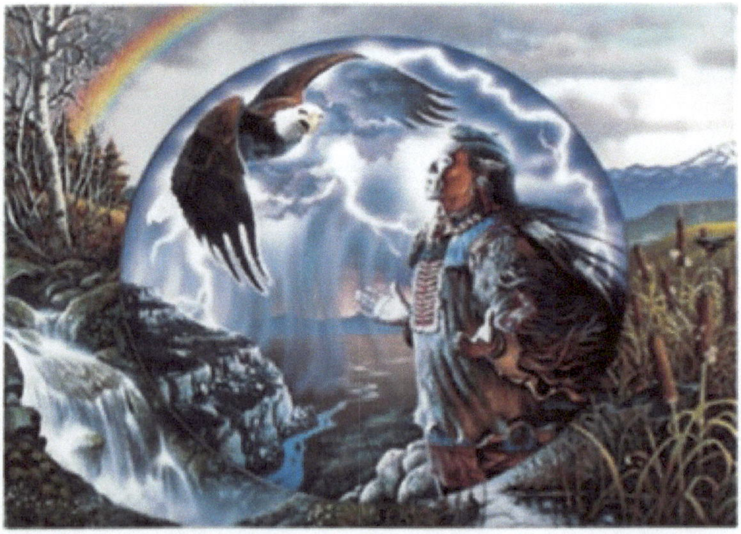

Fig. (14). Young Native Americans as a ritual go to mountains and fast to receive the animal spirit to guide them. Shamans also do this for healing (Fig. **14**). (With special permission of Hegda).

The Law of Action/Reaction in Emotional and Physical Pain

Physical and Emotional Reactivity:

Our assumption is that mind/will/thought/movement/pain/pleasure are all material. In normal action/reaction there is an experience from the senses either from outside or inside signals which translate into memory, thought and movement. In an extreme shock or traumatic injury the whole neurological system is disrupted, the bones, muscles, tendons are all impacted and the physical traumatic memory can be activated by too much movement or emotional intensification. This reactivates injury memories of pain, also, from old injuries. Emotional tension, outside and inside the person, triggers physical reactivity of pain and spasm, and, apprehension, agitation and memory loss. Each acts upon each other, from detailed daily case notes, *cause and effect, is confusing.* These reactions never seem to reproduce themselves the same way twice, so treatment is different each acute episode, as are the exact symptoms. Nevertheless each treatment detail created opportunities to change approaches to constantly changing symptoms.

Involuntary meditation goes beyond this physical response and thought which creates movement, to no form, yet in this state of synchronization there is stillness and movement but does not lead to reactivity because it is not time bound and timeless. Physical experiences create thought which moves the organism to react, in involuntary meditation of no form, one can be out of the iron claws of reactivity where vibration is felt and movement sensed and in this state there is a place to rest; this is what the patient did during the moments of great duress. This can be healing as seen in the animal spirits, which are not bound by thought and reactivity; the spine is extended, and the essence of the vertebrae expresses itself in self healing. The Shinnick painting expresses this going from no form to form to no form again. This can be natural or contrived by a deep wish to be healed. In the third day of the accident when cultivated Qi became exhausted being one focused into no form lead to an explosion of the breath from non-form (vibration and movement) to signal a direction for self healing. The breath. This is better than thought/reaction time bound from our entirely physical material existence of action/reaction.

A force of 25,000 lbs hit the spine. As a result outside lesser energies create a physiological reaction in the spine. These energy forces, based upon clinical notes, cause a reaction of the trauma when subjected to hot, cold, barometric pressure (airplanes), full moon, contentious interactions, not necessarily directed toward the patient, aggressive tone or movement toward the patient, dampness, bad posture, talking too long on the phone with arm up, lack of food, too much work, heavy lifting, emotional obsessions (triggered by past injuries,) difficult patients, financial shortcoming from lack of work, and glare from the sun or bad lighting. Recurring rough water scenes and instances of past injuries in dreams or meditations amplified the condition as well as emotional upset like paranoia, obsessive thinking, or old injustices. Disruption of nervous system create inaccurate reactions to outside and internal emotional energies.

Therapist Progress Notes

The patient's body after a year and a half has been liberated. But neck and lower back stiffness from the whiplash and first-degree degenerative spondylolisthesis L4-5. The healing energy keeps moving up. There is at times recurrence of stiffness, arthritis in the hips, pain in the mid back and arrhythmia. As mentioned before, in this healing process, the patient's old injuries from old traumas receded almost entirely, evolving into new spheres of physical consciousness. However after the original injuries subsided, as well, the upper cervical spasmed with pain with restricted motion, since the head was rotated to the left upon impact while looking backward. The spondylolisthesis, along with the occipital, activated with stiffness and pain, yet, having good flexibility because of yoga.

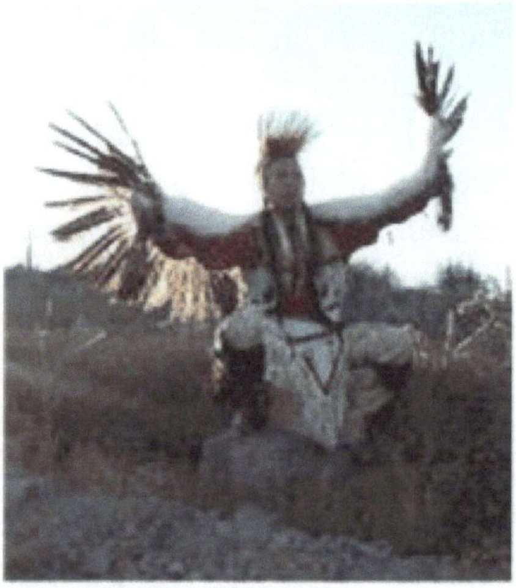

Fig. (15). In a sitting position a bird meditation is performed by a Native American. (With special permission of Hegda).

The question that we all ask when we are sick and hit hard is "why did this happened to me". In this case, the patient never felt like he was a victim and was able to deeply heal because he saw that this accident would be an important phase of evolution. With the daily notes, a lot of information became coherent and available to shed some light on a healing process away from medication, surgery and quick fixes and shows the importance to honor all the dimensions we have in ourselves. In the words of the poet Rainer Maria Rilke "Perhaps everything terrible is in it's being something that needs our love".

There are a variety of different animal meditations, wolf, hoop chanting and bear (Fig. **15 - 18**).

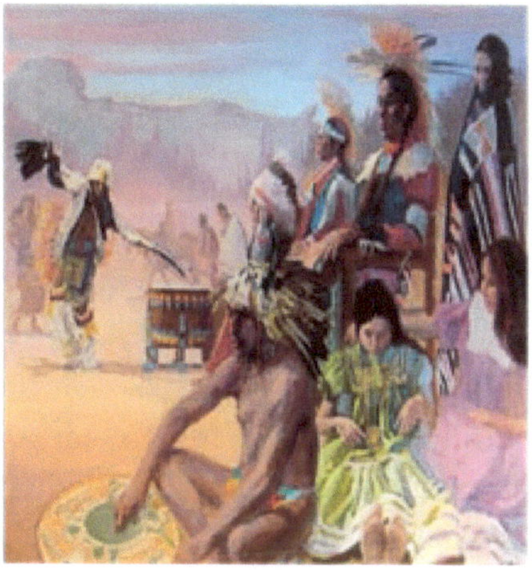

Fig. (16). Drumming, dancing, and chanting brings the bird spirit for healing from North American ceremony. (With special permission of Hegda).

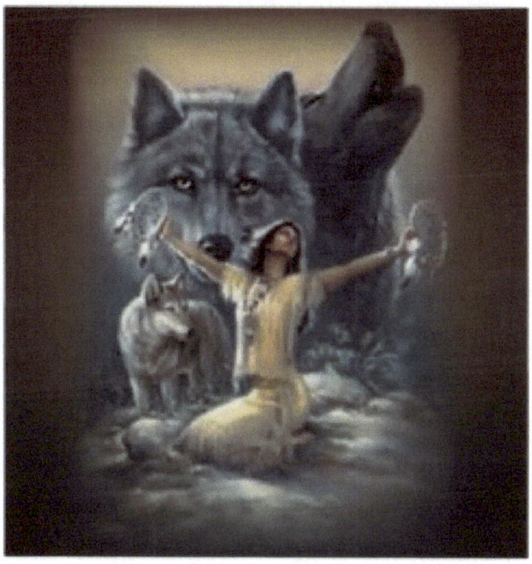

Fig. (17). Chanting and meditation for the Wolf spirit. (With special permissin of hegda).

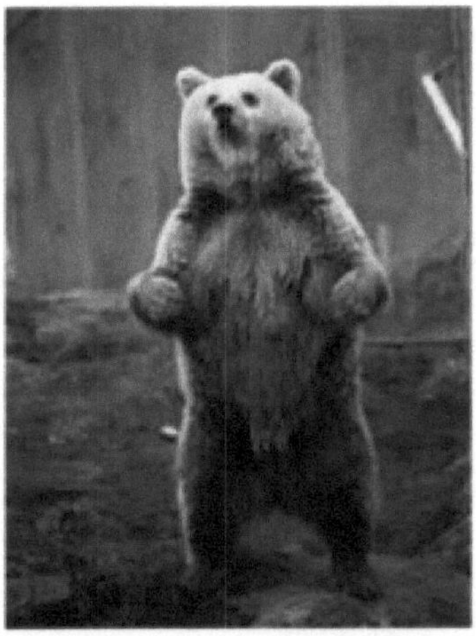

Fig. (18). For this patient bringing forth the Bear spirit caused the patient to stand up while growling. (With special permission of Hegda).

Summary

The danger in this trauma is the first several weeks, as the system shutdowns and moves in a downward spiral of pain and hopelessness. This shock can kill or paralyze. Resting in the quiescence of not moving meditation is an antidote which is not time bound by normal consciousness and therefore escapes pain and suffering by holding it at arm's length. Being one pointed in timeless space is a reprieve. Not moving, being still and being attentive to inner space suspends time and reactivity to emotional and physical pain

Healing and learning to move again requires a whole new set of meditations which recruit the voluntary muscles to distract from pain and to occupy the potential space required to move freely. Physical therapy, yoga, Tai Chi Chuan, Gung Fu, swimming, biking, golf, walking, climbing stairs, as well as heat therapy of baths and Svitz while doing stretching, lessened reactivity to movements. Cause and effect is confusing in rehabilitation of this shock injury. Since no clear relationship seems to exist between moving and reactivating pain, many approaches seemed to help. After four months it appeared as if normal activities could be assumed again, eliciting no pain, yet after three weeks of normal activities, a violent reaction occurred which took almost two months to get back to that point of no pain again. After a year and ¾ this point was never permanently reached again, but a wider range of activities and intensity became possible until almost the fourth year.

The dedication of a healer who prepares each day to heal by regeneration of compassion by mantras and other meditation techniques facilitates the patient into moving physiology to a synchronized state for healing.

Only after reviewing many times the detailed daily notes of AM, afternoon, PM and outside and inside variable of 600 pages over the year and ¾ did any relationship emerge. Physical and emotional reactivities were not so much by therapies (for example, overdoing things) but by inside and outside energy sources. For example, too much heat, too much cold, too much hot or cold wind, barometric pressure, too much time in loud noisy places, not enough food, anger in the immediate situation, too much glare, created reactivity. This was not understood until the detailed notes were examined. These outer variables also triggered emotional agitation, apprehension, fear and anxiety. Yet lack of monitoring the mind resulted in slipping into this emotional turmoil without outside variables. This internal lack of attention caused resultant physical symptoms of old injuries and tightening contortions of the spine and restricted movement.

It appears that this is permanent unless overtime this shadow lifts. However ordinary mindful awareness seems to be sufficient to manage the potential of reactivity which resides in the spine and emotions. .

An image comes from a philosophical understanding of Abhinavagupta, the Kula Ritual of Siva and Sakti (Fig. **19**).

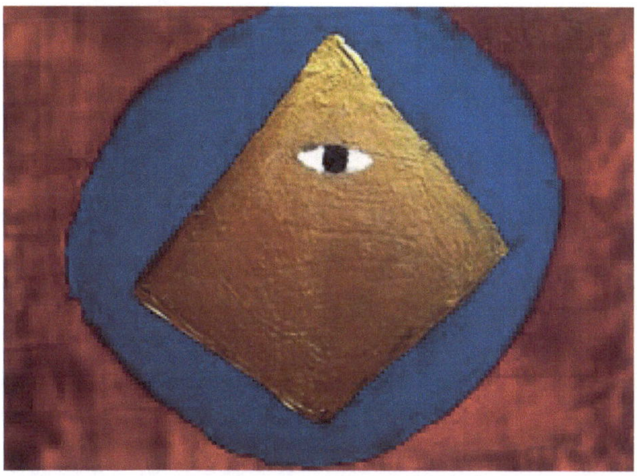

Fig. (19). Naked awareness PKS 2005. (With special permission of Shinnick).

There is no forgetting oneself with business as usual. This is not much different than a serious injury such as a hamstring tear and the constant awareness of the need to relax and stay in form in high level competition and performance at the Olympic level. When this reactivity comes, all of a sudden, sometimes it just requires sitting or lying down for ten minutes and breathing or doing Qigong and it seems to pass. This is very promising. Other times it means protecting against outside forces such as a windbreaker, extra clothing when the temperature changes suddenly, and meditating with eyes open in social situations of too much noise or anger.

Even though this process was difficult for the patient, his experiences with other sports injuries conditioned him to understand how time heals and not to take heroic therapies to escapes pain and suffering in the short run. Things pass and the patient was thankful for the opportunity to be able to see the real variables in the recovery from traumatic pain and suffering; the traditional cause of disease, hot, cold, wind, atmospheric pressure, lack of right food, physical positions, anger, expectations, and neglect of the mind/body/spirit at any time.

Mung Bean and Rice to Aid Digestion by Yogi Bhajan, Ph.D.

One cup mung beans, one cup basmati rice, 4-6 cups assorted vegetables, two chopped onions, ⅓ cup ginger root, 8-10 cloves garlic, minced, one heaping tsp. turmeric, ½ tsp. pepper one heaping tsp. garam masala, one tsp. crushed red chiles, one tbsp. sweet basil, 2 bay leaves, seeds of 5 cardamon pods, salt or soy sauce to taste. Rinse beans and rice, boil,add vegetables to cooking rice and beans, heat ½ cup oil in frying pan, add onions, garlic ginger to saute, add spices and add to beans and rice. stir.

Photonic Image

Computerized Axiomatic Thermography

Starting from the compression/fracture at T10 you can count up 6 vertebrae from the mid thoracic to see a herniation at T4. The scoliosis creates unusual configurations for the vertebrae, seen twisted further up on the cervical spine where the vertebrae seem to disappear. Down, Spondylolisthesis at L4/5 (Go 6 vertebrae down from the tenth vertebrae compression/fracture) Also one can see the spinous process, to the right of the vertebrae, are arranged differently after the accident pointing out differently. At first this seemed, by touch to the back, like kyphosis at the ninth, tenth and eleventh thoracic vertebrae yet the Thermography Scan showed the spinous process sticking straight out from the blow rather than angled downward with the vertebrae not kyphotic (Figs. **20, 21**).

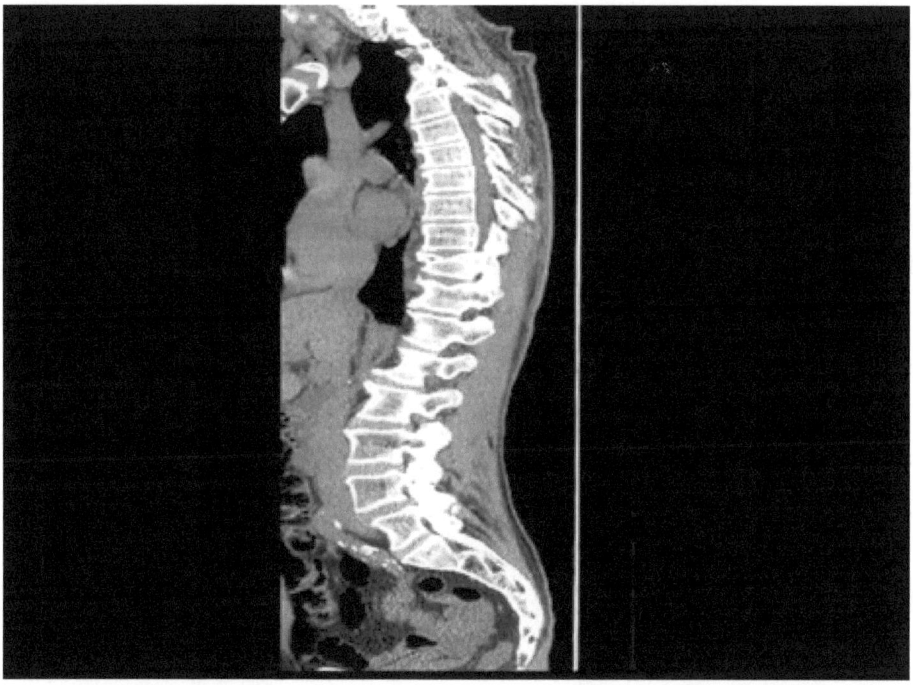

Fig. (20). The spinus process sticking out from the vertebrae are twisted in the upper back. Also you can see the crushed vertebrae in the mid back. Further up the spine the cervical vertebrae are twisted to the right.

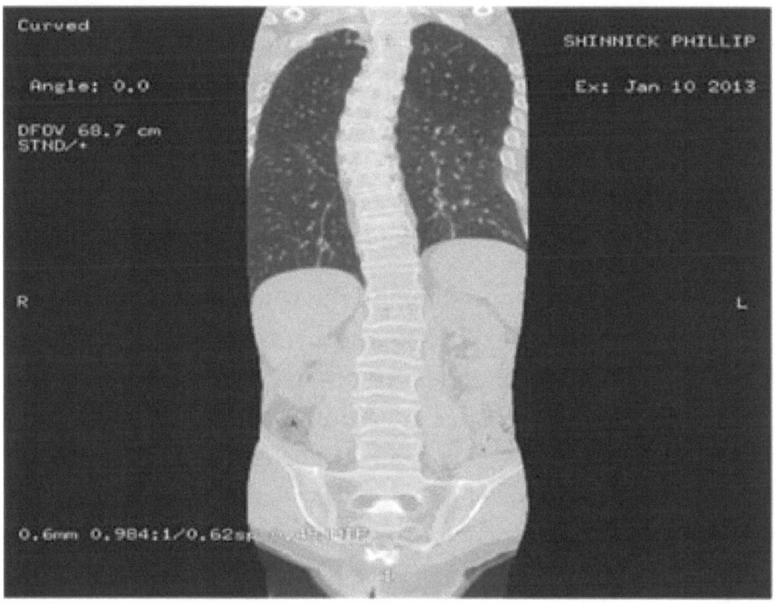

Fig. (21). Posterior view of scoliosis of the patient.

Physician Report. Christopher E. Mandigo, M.D., attending physician notes that "this injury resulted from a boating accident. In rough seas after being ejected from the boat (25,000 pounds), Dr. Shinnick was subsequently hit three times by the boat (going up and down in the 15' waves), in his mid back, then lower back, and, right anterior ribs. Non-surgical treatment of these conditions is recommended at this time. With Dr. Shinnick's extensive background in physical medicine, electro stimulation, rehabilitation and acupuncture, Dr. Mandigo recommended that the patient undergoes extensive rehabilitation including myofascial pain relief procedure, physical therapy and movement in an attempt to treat painful symptomatology PHOTONIC IMAGE below.

He requested that Dr. Shinnick sent him a daily record of his symptoms. Dr. Shinnick's prognosis is guarded and he will be prone to exacerbations in the future which may require additional treatment".

Therapist Preparation: The therapist followed Abhinavagupta's teachings of devotion and compassion to the patient, creating vibrational energy (spanda) with the aid of external Qigong to the patient by meditating on the lower Dan Tian. (Indian and Oriental practices) The therapist also did continuous chanting of the Medicine Buddha Sadhana, night and day, as a practice to create union of spirit, a oneness necessary for healing. The mantra of the Medicine Buddha Sadhana she chanted is as follows:

Om Namo Bhagavate Bhekandzyai, Guru Bendurya Prabha Randzaya, Tatha-gataya Arhate Samyaksam Buddhaya, Tayata, Om Bhenkandzyai Bhekandzyai Maha Bhenkandzyai Bhekandzyai, Randza Samungate Soha [1].

Patient Preparation. The patient gave reverence and homage for being created from no form to form then became one pointed in inner space during the therapy.

Turtle Qigong. Starting from straightening the spine and creating flexibility. The turtle should be done sitting, extending the neck up out of the shoulders then *exhaling* down with the neck extended, lower back slightly curled and shoulders back (Fig. **22**). With legs apart one goes down according to flexibility. Going back up, inhaling with chin curled on sternum and back curled going slowly up till neck is extended up. Head comes up and out from the shoulders after each round. It is Important to get as much space between the head and shoulders before going down to gravity. This is done 10 times but one can do it for half an hour or more. A good meditation.

There is a change in cranial blood circulation due to the change in the head in relationship to the heart. Sitting up, blood circulation to the cranial area is about 90 MM, parallel to heart 120 MM on the way down and when the cranial is below the heart about 150 mm depending upon distance below the heart. Calculate 7 MM for every centimeter, subtracting going up above the heart and adding going downward, below the heart. This increase in blood pressure bring fresh blood to the cranial area and creates flexibility to the spine [5].

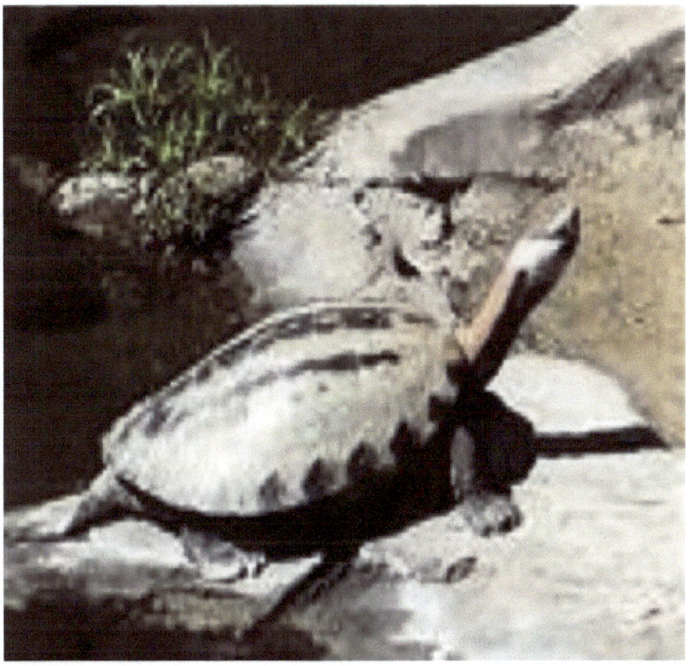

Fig. (22). Turtles extend their necks when looking about. Extending the neck out of the shoulders is a good exercise for neck pain. (With special permission of Hegda).

REFERENCES

[1] Shinnick P, Porter L. Self healing from a traumatic injury using occidental and oriental treatment for a burst fracture with compression T-10 vertebral body, L 4-5 spondylolisthesis, osteopenia, and post traumatic stress syndrome (PTSS). Proceedings Seen and Unseen Realities of the International Society for the Study of Subtle Energies and Energy Medicine. Missouri: Unity Village Lee's Summit 2014.

[2] Shinnick P, Porter L, Mandigo C. Whole person self healing: global treatments for a traumatic spinal fracture. J Sci Healing Outcomes 2014; 7: 25.

[3] Shinnick P. Qigong: where did it come from? Where does it fit in science? What are the advances? J Altern Complement Med 2006; 12(4): 351-3. [http://dx.doi.org/10.1089/acm.2006.12.351] [PMID: 16722782]

[4] Shinnick P, Freed S. A case study of the synchronization of human energy in an acute condition of chronic heart disease through complementary treatment. Subtl Ener & Ener Med 2002; 13(3): 209-32.

[5] Shinnick P, Freed S, Blumenthal C, Omura Y. Heart. New York: The Heart Disease Research Foundation 1990.

CHAPTER 10

Whole Person Considerations for Self Healing in Athletics

Abstract: Athletes can learn how to self-heal from injuries they have sustained. Therefore, we need to create an athletic culture that does not automatically use drugs and surgery as a panacea for injuries. With time, the body heals itself, and the mind can heal the body.

Keywords : Athletics, Injury, Performance enhancing drugs, Restorative drugs.

CREATING A NEW SPORTS CULTURE

Science was supposedly the big hope in athletics, but by exploiting their understanding of the biochemistry of the body, reductionists believe that pushing drugs and quickly repairing injuries is the way to great athletic performances. The rest of the world seemed to be performing on anabolic steroids, which was science's main contribution to athletes. At the time there was tremendous pressure to win against the USSR. Being the best in the world meant excelling at speed, strength and endurance, a trio that would be most difficult to beat. To achieve all three took daily practice, mental relaxation and intense focus -- remaining in the moment and not getting distracted. I kept daily journals of all my variables, which included strength, speed, endurance, flexibility, heart rate, emotional state, workout details, outside stress and performance marks. When we are consistent at making entries in a journal over long periods of time, we create a good database that will show us our variables. The greatest challenges were overcoming my fears, overcoming my injuries, and not allowing my ego to succumb to the accolades, the fame, the recognition that can come from winning (Fig. **1**).

From my organized daily journals, it was easy to explain the difficulties of injuries, recovery, mind practices and social interactions. My training has been an intensely private matter. At the urging of Dr. Rustum Roy, I agreed to discuss the impact of drugs on sports when I was on a joint International Olympic Committee and on a UNESCO committee for building a culture of peace. We wanted to

Phillip Shinnick & Laurence Porter

create a culture of sport that would be more humane and peace oriented. We looked at more natural ways for athletes to perform at the highest level in a way that is not destructive to the body, while still respecting the essence of athletics and competition [1 - 3]. Because of the need to develop an alternative to the present madness in sport, I gave a weekly lecture on drug use among athletes at Cal State College at Hayward in the early '70s under a National Institute of Mental Health grant, and I testified before and helped to organize Cong-ressional and Presidential hearings.

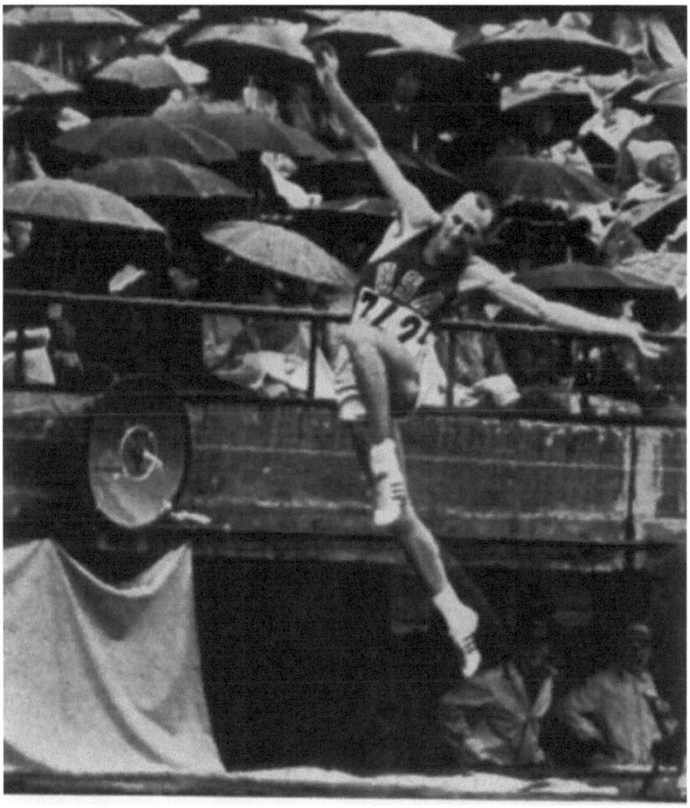

Fig. (1). 1964 Tokyo Olympic Games, US athlete Phillip Shinnick, then was called Icarus. sportspressnw.com/2154213/2013/wayback.../icarus-tokyo1964-copy

In 1999, sportspersons from all over the world gathered at the Hague to create a Culture of Peace for the years 2000-2010. The World Doping Committee increased their effort to get rid of the abuse of prescription drugs that enhance performance and those used as a restorative in sports. Drug usage has changed sports. Today, my 1963 best mark of 27 feet, 4 inches would receive a medal in World and Olympic competition (Fig. **1**). The next difficult step will be to get young, academic students to stop using performance enhancing drugs. This will come to a head when young athletes, who took such drugs to excel in their school work, are tested in higher competition. Amphetamines, which are illegal in sports, are not illegal in academics. This is where our consciousness needs to go.

A MORE NATURAL APPROACH TO ATHLETICS AND COMPETITION

My basic strategy was simple. Become the fastest, the strongest, the most flexible and the most in-shape jumper or athlete in the world. In 1971, after competing for almost 10 years at a world class level, I devised a system of training that might help me achieve such goals as hitting my mark on the runway, avoiding nagging injuries, achieving better mental alertness when competing, reaching a consistent speed where it was needed, getting adequate rest for proper recovery, overcoming my decline in strength and winning top marks in world competitions.

All great athletes know they have to be here and now in the present moment while they are performing. They cannot be distracted or emotionally upset by their thoughts of past or future problems. From my training and from my diaries, I realized it doesn't matter what state one is in before a competition. One's state only matters during the event. Prior to the 1968 Olympics, the US Olympic team competed against the German Olympic team in a pre-Olympic meet in Flagstaff, Arizona. Because the airline lost my shoes and uniform, I still didn't have them 15 minutes before the competition started. I had a headache from the altitude. The runway was lousy. The pit was lumpy. And the wind kept shifting. My jump was measured at 26 feet, 9 ½ inches. It was the third longest jump in the world that year and the fourth longest in US history. On the runway, it felt as if I was being pulled by a string attached to my solar plexus. I just needed to maintain form. The two German jumpers set new national German records, behind me, and ahead of me, Ralph Boston surpassed my world record by a fraction of an inch.

How does it happen, that we are able to be in the moment during a competition? At any given moment, if I became nervous about competition, I would stop right where I was, even on the street. I'd snuggle up against a building and I'd say, "You have 10 seconds to get ready to jump". Mentally putting myself at the end of the runway, I would start to count. Slowly I moved out onto the sidewalk and acted as if I was just about to start my jump. Then, I'd walk on. If you want the moment to be right, it might not come at the right moment. Sometimes, we wake up only when the competition is over, which meant that I needed to continually practice to prepare myself for being in the actual competitive moment.

Athletes voluntarily put themselves into training. These competitive situations can produce anxiety, stress, fear, intimidation and, inevitably, injuries. For any of these problems, voluntary or involuntary meditation can be healing. Sometimes pain advances one's conditioning in athletics. At other times, it can just wreck you. Experiencing a synchronization of mind and body that transcends what we experience in daily life is the reward for athletes. For many athletes, the only time their mind and body will work together is during the game. It empowers them to hit the ball harder, be more accurate or beat their opponent. An exceptional performance can make one a hero for a lifetime and beyond. For some, this is the motivation behind all their hard work. But in a deeper sense, using athletics to liberate oneself means integrating the whole person. This results in breaking free from habits, which are harmful to our health, and it creates greater clarity in our lives. By learning to stay in the moment, we help create a more synchronized state. Although one can perform while feeling stressed, emotionally upset or confused, it is important to realize that anyone can learn how to change states of consciousness when needed so their fears will abate.

I can tell you from experience that great performances are effortless, intensely in the present moment and happen when mind and body are synchronized. Coaches encourage their athletes to be more motivated. When athletes are engaged, they have greater access to their willpower. It is important that they can get themselves into a competitive state when it's needed but also be able to get out of it again at the right moment. Most athletes are primed to do well, but outside stress and their own internal distractions can be their demons. Desire for fame, fortune and sex are the same today as they have been for hundreds of years. Clearly, one must keep the mind engaged, remain in the process and not think of the outcome until the event is over.

Intention and direction are what make sports exciting. Direction is important in ball games. When an athlete throws the ball, he directs it through space by continuing to follow it with his mind. If you focus your concentration on it, you are less likely to drop the ball when you catch it. Much like a master projects external Qi, athletes project themselves or physical objects into space. This happens best when their physiology is not differentiated or fragmented.

If your state is differentiated, move and breathe as suggested in Chapter Seven on Chronic Heart Disease. Fear causes the abdomen to spasm and the breath to shorten. The breath control technique described in Chapter Seven is appropriate to use for training, before and during competition, and it will help with recovery afterward.

Puzzled about an episode I had while running a marathon, I called my fellow Olympic Marathon friend, Kenny Moore, for his feedback. I told him that a pallor came over me all of a sudden. I couldn't run one more step. The thought of running another 14 miles, after completing the first 11, just overwhelmed me. I couldn't breathe. I turned to tell my marathon running friend, Kevin Finneran, that I had to give up. He didn't hear me. When I tried again, my lips froze, but I managed to catch his eye. Suddenly, I felt fine. "What did you say?" he asked. "Forget it", I replied. What Kenny Moore told me was that as you gain more experience you find yourself having little bumps along the way that will disappear if you give them a few moments. He just laughed at me and said, "Hang in there. Like black clouds, they pass by, and you quickly move away from them".

Non athletes don't understand that something we're afraid of while training will haunt us until we make peace with it. Only then will it go away. At the peak of my training after age 50, I swam three mornings a week on a tri-athlete swim team. Practice started at 6:00 AM. Sometimes I woke up at 3:00 AM wondering if it was time to go to practice yet. I'd go back to sleep and wake up feeling rested, ready and raring to go only to discover it was now 3:05 AM. This could happen every five minutes till 5:15 AM finally arrived. It was pure fear. One morning this anxiety routine exhausted me so much that I skipped practice. Ten minutes after it was time to leave, I was wide awake and regretted staying home.

The best way to address this fear is by letting go once you are in the water. Let the water hold you up, synchronize your breath, do not panic for air, stay calm, stay in your form, stay longer in the water and take fewer strokes. The fewer strokes you take, the faster you go.

I can panic in the middle of a workout, especially while doing the butterfly stroke. I lose my breath. I start panting. Lactic acid builds up. The lungs get constricted by tightened muscles in the body. It gets more difficult to breathe. I feel weak. All of this causes me to push harder and breathe too fast. If I would let go, instead, I'd raise up higher in the water, not sink down. If I started to plane, it would take less effort. Then, by extending and slowing down my stroke and my breath, I would naturally go faster. This way I'd glide more, and I can rest in the glide. When I connect, I'm able to swim lifetime bests with ease and have a good laugh at the end without even feeling tired.

Stretching my spine while practicing Yoga helps diminish any anxiety I might have about an upcoming swim workout. Qigong practices are similar to what is done in training workouts. In Qigong, we also move and breathe in sync. Remain inside yourself instead of going outside. Stay down in the body instead of going up into the head and relax. In Zen meditation one just relaxes the muscles. But relaxing one's muscles when the swimming pool is 78 degrees Fahrenheit and the temperature outdoors is five degrees Fahrenheit is difficult. I had to wear a top shirt to keep warm the first year. Now I warm up after three laps. If you get it right, without tensing up in the water, the breath will warm you.

Leisure time players of sports today are learning that long-term participation in these activities can be ruinous to the joints. I experienced hip pain at an Olympic training camp in 1970. X-rays revealed advanced arthritis in my hips. Although there was no cure, I was told to take eight aspirins a day. That year I started my Yoga practice. Since then, every X-ray has shown no arthritis in my hips. By doing Yoga every day, I extended my career for years, and there were no problems from all my jumping and pounding. Now I do Yoga for one hour three times a week in temperatures up to 220 degrees Fahrenheit. The body adapts to such changes in temperature quite easily.

On a Goodwill Tour in Africa in 1968, I decided to confront the forces of Nature (or "take on the bear", as they say). I generally find it necessary to extend the limits of training about once a month. For example, I did 10 repeat runs at a 22 - 23 second pace, which is fast enough to win a high school race. Each run was 220 yards. I ran at high noon in Tanzania, on the Equator, with just enough rest time to recover from nausea. It was close to 100 degrees Fahrenheit. It took a week to recover, but I felt strong for a year. It helped that I stayed in the African heat for six weeks. If you take on the bear every once in awhile, you won't need to exert yourself as much in future practice.

Most sports injuries come from not stretching or warming up when the body is cold. Approximately one third of the training time for sports should be spent practicing Yoga, meditation and Qigong. Many people see their body as just an extension of the tennis racket they're using to pound the ball, which can be harmful to the body, to beat an opponent, who is only seen as one more number.

COACHES, MASTERS AND ATHLETIC SELF-HELP

Most sports require coordinated, synchronized movement of the body and the mind. Meditation would contribute to an athlete's improved performance and help create the optimum conditions for precision in playing, a quick response time, the overcoming of fears and difficult emotions, the easing of effort and greater clarity for the mind and the body. Aspects of one's personality, such as our fears or our anxieties, can cause one to lose control, drop the ball or stumble and fall. Inner doubts are a problem when playing sports, and they begin with physical training.

During most of my competitive career I had no coach. And what little coaching advice I got was usually wrong. By watching great athletes perform on film, I was able to actualize what I saw through my body with this vision. I also kept diaries, made observations, meditated and did Yoga. Unlike some athletes, I did not need constant guidance and coaching. Those athletes tend to fall apart if their coaches leave or if they move up to another educational level.

A study I did of football players on college teams revealed sadism in an authoritarian atmosphere, poor flow of information through the team, players being degraded for their injuries, players getting harassed to give up their scholarships, which was their only salary, and a winning-at-all-cost attitude. Professional sports are not much better. This type of training promotes a military attitude. Order, obedience, giving your body up to the cause, nationalism, racism and sexism abound. Master - student relationships in the traditional healing arts may embody similar characteristics. If athletics were unencumbered by officials, coaches and doctors, athletes would have more freedom to develop as human beings. So many athletes fall apart after quitting their sport. That shows us they didn't learn anything about the deeper significance of athletics or personal health.

This is why the healing arts must be combined with sports from an early age. Young athletes will learn how to prevent or heal their injuries, recover from hard training sessions by meditating, develop an inner voice and learn how to actualize their athletic intention. This ancient tradition of the Olympians and of the healing arts will liberate them from ignorance, fear, delusion and suffering. Sports and the healing arts fit together beautifully and represent the best the Occident and Orient have to offer. The creative spirit comes from energy, intention and consciousness.

There are gifted Masters who share their knowledge. Qigong Master, He Bin Hui, was a national caliber weight lifter. He trained cancer patients in self-help healing techniques, and he shared his wisdom with scientists. Bill Bowerman, from Oregon, could turn average athletes into Olympic champions by teaching rather than directing them.

OLYMPIC PREPARATION, COMPETITION, MEDITATION AND INJURIES

I had only one chance to qualify for my third Olympic Team in 1972. Situations like this are very important to the soul. Nine years had passed since my record leap (Fig. **2**). My head was in confusion, my back ached. Although I trained every day, I hadn't competed seriously in the long jump for several years. One week before my last opportunity to qualify for the Olympic trials, I took my written exams for a Ph.D. in social psychology and organizational theory at UC Berkeley.

Meditating on opposites can be a way of scrambling the mind in order to ferret out those comfortable patterns that seem to make us happy. After breaking the world record in 1963, I decided to confront the distractions that interfered with my heart's desire to make the Olympic team. I challenged my impulses by doing the opposite of what I wanted to do. If I was used to going to school one way, I'd walk some other way. If I went to the movies on Friday night, I stopped going. Since I liked to sleep late, I got up early. I liked to go to parties, drink beer and dance, so I stopped doing them all. This austerity was a challenge to desire. Slowly, my perceptions began to change. Light, sounds and odors started to feel different. My sleep pattern changed. I seemed awake when I slept. If someone walked by my bunk in the middle of the night, I could open my eyes and have a lucid conversation. There was no difference between night and day.

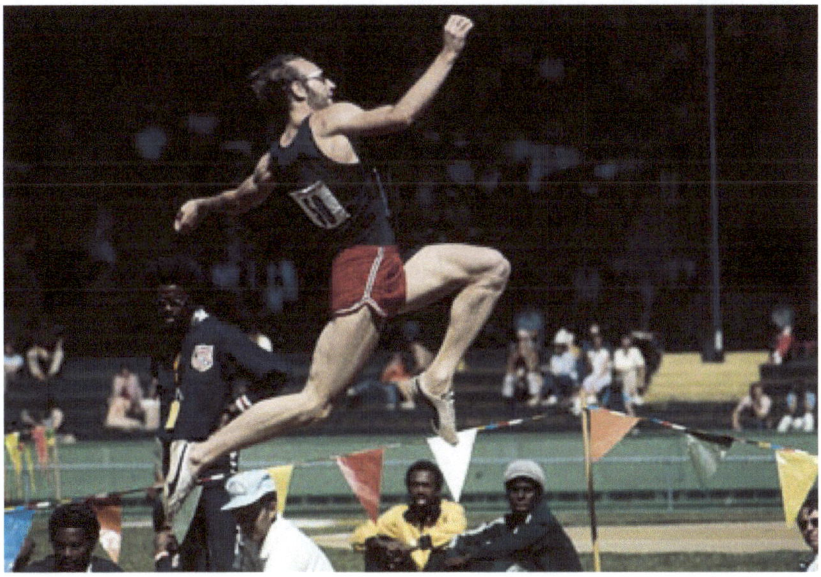

Fig. (2). 1972 U.S. Olympic Trials, Phillip Shinnick, after many injuries. gettyimages.com/photos/eugene-oregon

To prepare myself for the 1972 Olympic tryouts, I again put into practice what I have called the Meditation of Opposites (Fig. **3**). When I was not in motion, I'd think about motion. When I was in motion, I would not think at all. I went alone into a dark room, laid on my back for half an hour and slowed my breath down to about one full breath per minute. Letting go of the stress, my lactic acid went down, my oxygen consumption decreased and my brain waves harmonized. With my mind still, I practiced the Unity of Opposites (Fig. **3**). In my mind I visualized the moment when I'd start the upcoming competition, the moment before I'd start to jump. I then proceeded one step at a time. There were 20 steps in all, and I felt each one. There was the takeoff. I conceptualized the form, picturing my shoulders in their proper position. And, finally, I experienced the landing. After completing a mental runthrough, I assumed the various physical positions I'd take if I were on the runway. I maintained each posture for a while. Then, slowly, I came up to a full standing position with a clear awareness. And to complete the meditation, I walked out onto the field where I did a light, short warm-up to prepare for the upcoming competition on that hot day.

Fig. (3). Union of opposites. (With permission of Porter).

At the end of the runway, the jump I had rehearsed and practiced in the room came to me naturally. What had been in my mind became the external reality. I just actualized the form. I ran down the runway, relaxed and all out. I felt I was moving in slow motion. From this connected state, I could correct any mistake that arose the moment it happened. Four steps before the board, my left foot veered to the left. Realizing it, on the next stride I toed in my left foot. Otherwise, my jump was just like the one in my meditation, but this time I was not thinking at all. Aware of myself at each moment, I continued to self-correct as needed. After not competing seriously for two years, my jump made it to the top five jumps in the world at that time. I qualified for the Olympic trials by jumping 26 feet, 5½ inches. At that moment, I did exactly what was needed in order to perform at the highest level for those 20 minutes, but my headache and pains returned 10 minutes after I completed my jump.

Getting out of the head and into the body is no easy matter. To produce a world-class jump, speed is everything. As Charlie Green, a world-class sprinter, taught me: Focus on the solar plexus while running. Under competitive stress, sprint from a one-pointed state. Feel the vibration in the solar plexus. Let go. Stay centered. Don't interfere. Gravity and linearity will disappear. Feel the stillness. Legs and arms may be flying about as if one were escaping the jaws of a lion, but the lion is actually in the body performing an all-out attack on speed.

It is now accepted that, with repeated practice, 30 to 40 minutes of physical activity changes body and mind. The mind can also work against the body when it obsesses and makes too many demands. I used to enjoy long, hard runs in the woods to quiet my mind and feelings, but during the early Olympic years, I suffered from training too much. For years, I was a slave to my obsessions with goals, numbers and with finding ways to clear my mind of stress. This behavior crippled my body, and I was not able to function in a synchronized way.

During my Olympic training, just before attempting a new world indoor record in the long jump, I pulled my hamstrings while competing with Olympic champion, Ralph Boston. The indoor runway was made of plywood. Underneath it were support struts that acted like mini trampolines, speeding up my leg which was already going at its maximum rate. Three steps from the board, I hit a space between the struts, causing my leg to spring up too fast. The hamstrings cramped. I could not stop my leg from going forward in full flight. My hamstrings ripped apart, and I immediately knew what all inclusive pain meant.

I spent that night in a sleeping bag on the floor of a cloistered Jesuit retreat house in the Californian Mountains. I couldn't sleep. I discovered that if I continued to move around, I would find a position where I was in less pain. When I became quiet, the pain receded. I discovered a place in the mind to retreat to, away from pain, in a position of repose. That relief can last for some minutes, which is enough during a time of such extreme pain. It was necessary for me to move around until I found another position of reprieve when the pain started up again.

Injuries I've sustained while working to get in shape have caused me to feel like giving up and cursing my fate. I have lost all hope, at times, that I would ever get healthy again. As athletes grow older, they continue using sports to batter their bodies. Obsession, stemming from an emotional attachment to competition and to winning, drives them. The result is always pain and suffering. Tennis, basketball, baseball, softball, skiing, weightlifting and many other sports can cause the body to deteriorate, but the ongoing appeal is the release of psychological tension. During Olympic training, I pulled hamstrings and back muscles, sprained ankles, cracked foot bones, jammed toes, injured knees and created arthritis in my hip. I was willing to suffer all that pain to make the Olympic team. I learned, eventually, to achieve the same thing with far less emotional effort or physical damage.

Identifying the root cause of our injuries is more productive than merely allowing them to be a distraction When we are attentive, at ease and natural, it helps us to heal. If we allow time to stand still as we heal, if we are patient, let go of any preconception about where we should be, if we meditate on our healing and exercise more slowly, we will grow stronger and heal more completely. Injuries require an understanding of which parts of the body need to be stronger, more flexible and in better shape than they used to be. Certain injuries can take years to mend. If we can be patient and kind to ourselves, we'll be here for the long run. There is plenty of time in which to let things happen and to heal ourselves.

Yoga can help us when we are healing from our injuries. When we control our breath, heat rises in the body and muscles loosen, which allows our bodies to take Yoga positions more easily. If we don't learn to work with our injuries, we can end up in a situation that is worse than the injury itself. Getting medical relief, which often means surgery, can do us irreversible harm. I have escaped scalpels and drugs for many years by just being patient with my injuries.

You can feel disappointed when a re-injury occurs after your strength and energy have begun to return, and you are reminded that the shadow of the injury is still there. Injuries take time to heal. Be respectful of that. After an injury, remain within your limits if competing. Relax. Despite an injury, a good performance still might happen later on without re-injury occurring. Ignore other judgements.

I had to compete in the Olympic trials eight months after my injury, which took five years to heal completely. Slowly, I brought myself back up to full speed, but I never stayed there for long. It was not easy to overcome feeling fearful and hopeless. I worried that my body might not be ready in time for Olympic competition. How could I sprint without fear of injury? I had to condition myself to not react to situations that had caused the injury in the first place. To protect myself from further injury, I had to find a way to sprint without my body reacting. This is the conditioning for non-recognition. By running long distance, improving my flexibility and lifting weight gently, I rebuilt the torn fibers in my hamstrings so my body could absorb the internal bleeding that went from ankle to groin.

At the time when I attended college, I had no understanding of Yoga, Buddhism or Taoism. I only had my Christian upbringing. Secretly, I rose before anybody else in my fraternity. To gain spiritual strength, I went to mass, no matter the weather, to join my suffering with those in situations far worse than mine. I prayed. I never slept, afraid that if I sank into a deep sleep, I'd lose any hold I had on my "will" to make the Olympic team. Because my college gave me a scholarship that required me to compete at a lower NCAA level, further injuries resulted. I suffered from a cracked bone in my jumping foot, deep pains in my lower back, migraines, neck problems and sinus infections. I learned about pain and suffering.

While playing football, basketball, running the hurdles in track, high jumping, long jumping and sprinting, I suffered many injuries. They can happen when practice techniques are not good, with poor competing conditions, from the body lacking flexibility or by doing something out of the ordinary, from an imbalance in the posture or muscles, from any asymmetry or misalignment in the body, from feelings of anxiety, by being distracted, from lack of nourishment and as the result of an accident. Getting injured probably indicates that one's approach to flexibility and strength might need rethinking. One can be aware that injury is one possibility among many of what might be coming because accidents do happen.

I did make the Olympic team despite all my injuries by learning to relax under pressure, refraining from giving it my all, staying in control and overcoming my fear of injury. Training for the 1968 Olympics, I learned proper breathing, which transformed me. While I was training at high altitude at South Lake Tahoe, I slowed my breath to the point where I was able to count to 200 during my exhale. Then I sank into a deep relaxed state. After practicing this technique for a while, the counting drifted away. This is a good antidote for stress. My body opened up when it benefitted from practicing dance and Yoga. I went from the limitations of an iron clad mind to being at ease, feeling calm and more able to flow. By then, most competitors were using steroids, but I was still able to compete with the top three or four athletes in the world in my category by using simple meditation techniques. As I grew older, I injured myself less frequently. I solved my health problems. I adopted meditation and Yoga practices. I ate only natural foods. I pursued alternative treatment for my injuries. Not included in this way of life were performance enhancing drugs, injections of any kind, anti-inflammatory pills, muscle relaxants, antihistamines and excessive vitamin pills.

Through meditation, I began to understand gravity. It helped me control my mind and my will, and I was stronger, more steady. Obviously, I could not live on this high physical plane forever. Because of injuries and age, I stopped competing, but I continued to meditate. Meditation disciplines make sense when we are natural and at ease, which is part of the Song of Tilopa. He sings of being at ease in a natural state, of not reacting to good or bad and being alive in the moment. This is sweet to hear. When our meditation practice gets too rigid, it freezes us. To help us heal, we need to interact with outside forms of energy like stillness, motion, vibration fields and space. That will give us the hope of healing ourselves from injuries we have inflicted upon ourselves. There is no formula for this.

Meditation practice can be helped by numbers, language, mantras, repetition of words, as in prayer, primal vibratory sounds, animal sounds, movement or simply by being at ease and doing nothing. Meditation is good for quieting a confused mind or a body overburdened with strong emotions. It can help one to perform with a clearer head. After meditating, my mind was free of thoughts. I was aware of the process. I was able to adjust quickly with accuracy. I was able to move unhindered in a coordinated way.

While training, I recorded my pulse each day when I woke up. My normal rate was 40 or less. When it was higher, it meant I had overtrained. During the day, I gauged my feelings and the particulars of my workout. If I had a long warm up, workouts and competitions were not adversely affected. After a 15-minute jog, 30 minutes of Yoga and 10 minutes of easy fast running in 100-yard intervals, I would do meditative breathing exercises. After that, I was close to my top-level performance ability.

Movement creates regularity in the breath. It is as simple as watching the breath. I have done it many times when my head is filled with too much conversation and my body feels tight from so much stress. Through meditation, there are many ways to get to a place where all things come together, if only for a short while. Over time, meditation practice will create greater stability.

Many people focus on pain. When there is restricted circulation to one side of the brain, while the flow is good on the other side, the brain has to adjust. Pain results from it. Though we are one, we have two physical sides that are joined together. Look at yourself in a mirror. You will see that we each have a twin in us. The two sides of us can struggle with each other and make trouble. A great cause of problems with troubled organs, aches and pains in the body, an impairment of our mobility and digestive difficulties is asymmetry in the body.

To feel space opening and gravity receding, we must run when practicing with the same intensity as we run in competition. The basic disciplines of running fast in marathons, jumping high and far, throwing heavy weights, hurdling and spinning the disc in Olympic sports demand our undivided focus at all times, under any circumstance and in every mental or physical state. That is when heightened world-class performances happen. We condition the mind/body/spirit to handle all possible variables like hot, cold, rain, injustice, cheating and so on. I was always prepared to perform in the moment, without distractions, at the appointed date and time. I chose to do this as a gesture, to reach through time and join the ancient Olympians. I was fortunate to have been born in an ideal era to follow my heart's desire. There were perfect situations for me to jump at different locations around the world. It was the best time in history for that.

On Earth, we spin in both directions. Our orbit takes us in two directions also. Precious moments for meditation can be lost while sleeping. We believe that everything shuts down because it is dark. This is not true for the meditator. Night and day are the same.

TRAINING FOR STRENGTH, ENDURANCE, SPEED, FLEXIBILITY AND COMPETITION

My training system was simple. I worked out for three days. One day I focused on endurance, another was devoted to speed work, and the third day was for building strength. That was followed by a day of rest. Yoga I would do every single day without fail. You will compete the way you have practiced. If you get used to running at a certain speed, that will be how fast you run in competition. Which workout I would do on which of the three days could change according to my needs and abilities in each three-day cycle.

The endurance work was running uphill for four miles then racing downhill for another four miles at a fast pace. For the strength workout, I'd use the Olympic bar at 150 to 220 pounds to do clean and jerks, which is forcefully jerking the bar off the floor, lifting it to my chest and lowering it back to the floor again. I'd also step up onto a bench holding 350 pounds on my shoulders and step-up on one leg. This workout included bench presses and other exercises with heavy weights. If you lift heavy weights without concentrating fully, most likely you will injure yourself.

The speed work included one half hour of yoga and stretching, followed by 10 easy wind sprints of 100 yards each, done with easy strides. Then I did anywhere from six to 10 run throughs on the runway, where I pretended to jump with each approach. I would do several 150-yard sprints going all out but still staying relaxed. The sprint had to be at a world class sprinter's speed of about 13.5

seconds for 150 yards, which I would do two or three times.

One must get that run up the steps right in order to hit the takeoff board without going over or getting too far behind the eight-inch board. If you sprint faster in competition, your approach will be different, and you will go over the board.

How did I train at a pace similar to competition? The answer is Yoga and the flexibility it gave my body. I could train all out all the time and never be sore. One must be relaxed and mentally alert in order to achieve that. Around this time, I ran 100 yards in 9.5 seconds on a terrible track beating several athletes who had tied for the world record.

PRACTICING FOR FUTURE DISEASES

In a little study I did last year, I reviewed hundreds of my patients' cases and found that those who were successful in muting symptoms of disease in later life had previous experience in meditation or yoga and could quickly bring these skills to bear in a short time even if they had not done those practices in years.

GENERAL CONCLUSION

Information becomes valuable when we put it into practice. Otherwise it remains words on a page with no connection to our bodies or to our lives. Every day we have the choice to pay attention to how we breathe, what we eat, how we feel. We can be responsible for our energy, our movements, our thoughts, our interactions with others and be aware that they are all connected. Let's open our minds and dare to imagine a world at peace. Although we might choose to believe we are cogs in a mechanistic universe and adopt reductionist ways to live in it, wouldn't it be better to envision a reality where we all live in harmony and peace? At every moment, we have the chance to stop being mechanical. Any step is a small miracle opening the way to uncharted territories. By establishing a direct contact with the nature of life, we will live closer to a reality that requires us to take responsibility for being alive. This book is a bridge to the awareness that All Is One. We need to walk the walk, whatever the journey may be. What is the purpose for humanity if not to evolve to a higher plane of consciousness? What is the use of science, medicine and the arts if not to move things in that direction?

SHINNICK AND FREED BACKGROUND

Simon Freed, Ph.D., Co-Director of the Research Institute of Global Physiology, Behavior and Treatment, Inc., Associate Editor J. Chemical Physics. Chief Chemist Oak Ridge National Laboratory, Research Scientist, Professor of

Physiology, Mt. Sinai Medical Center, Research Scientist, Heart Disease Research Foundation.

Scientific Interests and Publications: Optical and magnetic [properties of chemical compounds: symmetry of electrical fields about ions in solution and crystals; chemistry and biochemistry at low temperature' resolution of states and reactivities in chemistry and biochemistry; radioactivity, physiological chemistry of the nervous system, cryo biochemical analysis of tissue; endogenous chemistry of animals induced through learning; comparative biology of mnemonic processes.

Phillip Shinnick, Ph.D., MPA, L.Ac. UC Berkeley Ph.D. in Social Psychology, University of Washington, M.P.A., in International Public Policy, Assistant Professor in Sociology and History Rutgers University, Assistant Clinical Professor New York Medical College (founding the physician acupuncture training program), Associate Editor, Acupuncture & Electro-Therapeutics, the International Journal, Associate Editor, The Journal of the Science of Healing Outcomes, Associate, Center for Dance and Sports Medicine in New York, a non-surgery Orthopedic practice.

Scientific Interests and Publications. Global Physiology (brain, heart pulsations, blood lactate, oxygen consumption), heart disease, Oriental and Occidental medicine, physical medicine, non-invasive diagnosis, microorganisms, organic and inorganic nature, physical and emotional trauma, drugs use in athletics, involuntary and voluntary meditation.

Athletics. Competed on the US Olympic team in track and field and yearly made national teams then became a U.S. team captain in track and field at the Pan Pacific Games in Asia. Founder of the Sports Science Program at Rutgers University. Shinnick's understanding of athletics came from recording daily heart rate, emotions, competitive performance and combined this with recording traditional techniques of training in my sport. He added a new sport, swimming (15 years ago), and Gung Fu (15 years ago), and Tai Chi Chuan (28 years ago.) The forms of meditation besides Zen which he has practiced since 1964 are Siddha (19 years ago), and Tibetan meditation (22 years ago) and a sports medicine doctor. He still serves an International Olympic Committee on peace and sports and was named a an Ambassador of UNESCO.

Laurence Porter. Laurence Porter has been Dr. Shinnick's assistant for the last 8 years. Originally a dancer, movement is essential to her. Trained in ballet, she turned to modern dance and later after she moved from France to the US to improvisation dance. She is an intuitive healer. She has a full practice, co/write with Dr. Shinnick, guides improvisation workshop and keep being engaged in the creative process however it presents itself. She also practices Yoga and QiGong in a free flowing form.

GLOSSARY

Addiction Therapy: Michael Smith, M.D. showed in the 80's that auricular therapy or acupuncture to the ear helped in withdrawal from cocaine. Kevin Chen, Ph.D., M.P.H., *et al.* showed that Qigong meditation was successful in addiction withdrawal with women having a higher rate of success in subtle energy techniques than men.

AGA Thermogram: This sensitive sensor can detect qi emission down the arm and out the fingers with a 3 degree rise in temperature.

Albumin: is responsible for much of the colloidal osmotic pressure of the blood, and thus is a very important factor in regulating the exchange of water between the plasma and the interstitial compartment (space between the cell). In heart disease instead of creating blood results in a water build up or edema and water in the lung in Chronic Heart Disease.

Alternating Current: This bi-phasic current changes polarity and is safe for electro-therapy if used for 15 minutes, since most stimulators are 60% and 40% rather than 50/50. It is expressed in bipolar waves.

Arrhythmia: This is a heart condition detected by pulse reading on the radial artery or EKG which shows a heartbeat that is irregular, that is there is a pause between beats or two beats come with little pause. In Occidental medicine there are a variety of drugs each creating changes to the biochemistry, which have to be monitored, due to unexpected other biochemical changes. They do not always make the situation better. In Oriental medicine, there are areas of the body to be stimulated, like the back of the neck and left rhomboid area and medial part of the left arm, with good success.

Asymmetrical: In humans, asymmetry results in scoliosis, or in spasticity to one side of the neck result in asymmetrical blood flow to the brain which requires compensation and requires energy for this adaptation. Asymmetry can be between the left and right side, between the front and the back or between the upper and lower body all affecting the physiology of a person.

Atrioventricular (AV) Node: The AV node follows the rhythm of the Sinoatrial (SA) node and is part of the pacemakers' cells controlling the heartbeat. During a heart attack this rhythm is disrupted. These cardiac cells potentiate a charge and are synchronized for a healthy regulation of the heart synchronized by the purkinje fiber which runs across the front of the heart. It is located in the middle part of the heart.

Auricular: Oriental medicine shows that parts of the ear reflect parts of the body and organs and can be treated, and also very effective for addiction therapy. Nogier from France showed an upside down fetus in the ear and with stimulating parts of the ear for certain disease.

Blood Lactate: In this study, blood lactate can be used as a global physiological test to show levels of stress in the body.

Compression Fracture: In one chapter, a boat hit a patient and his vertebrae compressed to one/half the size and split or fractured. This can be fatal or led to paralysis. The prognosis is guarded.

Digitalis: Common flower is Foxglove as part of Figwort and used in heart disease for water regulation.

Diaphragm: A circular dome, musculomembranous partition between abdominal and thoracic cavities, around the midsection of the body when constricted led to breath shortness and a series of respiration ailments. According to the O-Ring Test, the diaphragm has phases and is implicated in sinusitis, allergies, asthma, constricted thoracic, hypertension, and herniation of the cervical vertebrae.

Direct Current: Harmful to the body as it creates electrolysis with acid accumulating at one pole and alkaline in the other, with needles, can lead to breaking. It has continuous distribution and is not impulse, which is different than direct current.

Earth Vibration: Known as the Schuman Resonance reflected in Appendix I in Chapter 2. It is the cavity of the earth, which holds energy from lightning strikes as part of what sustains life on earth.

Electromagnetic Spectrum: This is measured by frequency f, wavelength l, and photon energy E. The longest wavelengths are radio wave but the wave can be as long as the universe and the longer the wave the less the photon energy 12.4 feV to high frequency 1.24 MeV. Sensitive instruments can pick up, for example in a stomach, wavelength from almost the whole spectrum.

Enlightenment: For Europeans this is associated with Bacon, Descartes, Locke, Spinoza, Boyles, Voltaire, Kant, Newton and summarized by Diderot. From 1650 to 1780, this lead up to the French Revolution. The key ideas were toleration, science and skepticism. However, in these ideas was reductionism which has been the downfall of Occidental medicine which does not look at the whole person. This reductionism leads to separation of the observer to what is observed. For the Ancients it was Bodhi or to awaken and understand, to have woken up and understand. This is based upon the four noble truths; life is suffering, the cause is ignorance, desire can be destroyed and the means are eightfold. The eightfold means are mental discipline, wisdom, ethical conduct or right view, intention, speech, action, livelihood, effort, mindfulness and concentration. In Bodhi, a key concept is the observer and observed are not distinct and mutually co-dependent.

Entropy: Entropy cannot be seen, it is inferred primarily from inorganic experiments of pressure, volume, and temperature in gases, as these variable change and the system changes, the system cannot be brought back to the original state without loss of energy thus entropy. This is equilibrium. This is positive entropy which modern medicine, with a reductionist legacy from the French Enlightenment, sees as the pattern of disease. “Nothing we can do”. Negative entropy are things that organic being use to maintain life, gotten from outside such as food, water in air, air, breathing, and, internally, by creating a mind that is not encumbered with obsessive thinking and agitated emotions. Also negative entropy practices such as building up one's qi or energy through bringing the mind inside the body, mutes positive entropy and creating life giving negative entropy. There is no equilibrium in organic nature and this disequilibrium is what creates the energy for adaptation.

Fragmentation: This state can be seen in EEG, EKG, and EMG as a desynchronization of brain waves, heart rhythm, and nerve speed changes.

Gaussian: A term used to describe magnetic energy.

GE Micro-pressure Detector: An instrument = which can measure the pressure of fluids and can be used to detect the pressure of qi from a Master emitting qi from various distances.

Gram: Taking electro signals from the body from the heart, brain and nerves onto a graph are the origins of the electroencephalogram (EEG), electrocardiogram (EKG) and electromyogram (EMG). The graph then shows deviations from a normal sine wave.

Habituated Condition: Human organism trauma, either emotional or physical, can cause a condition to repeat itself with an approximation of the circumstances of the original trauma. This can also be in the mind, when thoughts that are antithetical to one's life direction condition from events during upbringing, the heart seems to be a reservoir of memory for these dysfunctional conditions.

Herniated Disk: This is when the disk between the various vertebrae impinges on the spinal nerve through muscles tension caused by stress or trauma. A person can have symptoms or not and those exhibiting symptoms are in the most serious situation when the legs or arms weaken, then surgery may be required. In most of the cases, time heals when strengthening and stretching the surround muscles which hold the vertebrae in place.

Involuntary Meditation: This is when the mediator does not use volition (will) to move muscles as in sitting meditation where one does not control either the mind or body by sitting still with a straight spine and lets things settle on their own for quiescence.

Lasix: Lasix is furosemide a loop diuretic which causes salt to be expelled through the urine to overcome edema used in chronic heart disease.

Macromolecule: When helium is taken to a low temperature to almost absolute zero after a series of changes, reaches the most stable Bose-Einstein state and becomes a macromolecule which has superfluity information flow and exhibits stranger behavior.

Meridian: A term used in Oriental medicine to reflect organ's pulsation of energy on the outside and inside of the body in a distinct pattern which is codified in the twelve main meridian system having a dominate organ over sister organ *e.g.* spleen over stomach, liver over gallbladder, *etc.*

Moxibustion: Used in acupuncture in a cold syndrome by putting an herb on the end of an acupuncture inserted needle and then lighting it which heats up the surrounding tissue. Stimulation of these points is effective in organ dysfunction.

MU: The Mu points are organ representation points or alarm points on the front of the body which when stimulated change organ functioning.

Non-Equilibrium: Prigogine received the Nobel Prize to say human organisms live in a non-equilibrium world for survival on earth by using non –equilibrium to evolve to local conditions.

Non-reactivity: Many times people are conditioned to respond in a certain way to outside stimulation. For example, many times when anger comes to a person he responds with anger, a non-reactivity would be when anger comes to a person and he sees the anger as not his anger, and does not respond. Or he does not act on internal emotions, recognizing the feeling and letting it dissipate as a natural phenomenon not using reason to hold it.

One-Pointed: In meditation, keeping one's attention on an object in inner space or outer space leads to avoiding distractions. If one becomes one pointed under the sway of anger, desire, greed, infatuation, arrogance and envy the reality underlying these states alone subsists. "In reality nothing arises, and nothing subsides, only the divine Spanda-sakti which, thorough free succession, appears in different aspects as if arising and as if subsiding".

Pacemaker Cells: These cells (sinoatrial [SA] and atrioventricular [AV]) potentiate electrical charges to activate the rhythm of the heart through the left and right atrium and left and right ventricles. The purkinje fiber coordinates this.

PEMF: Pulsed Electromagnetic Fields describe the energies from coulombic, gaussian and photonic fields or electromagnetic and photonic energy. It can be used to describe pulse generators such as organs in the body, or manufactured pulse generators.

Performance Drugs: These drugs are used to increase performance such as anabolic steroids which when taken promote protein uptake in the muscles to build strength, athletes take these to perform at a level beyond their capability. Uppers or amphetamines are taken to raise awareness during competition or to increase endurance. Blood doping means that blood is taken out of the system then put back later to increase blood oxygen levels.

Photonic: This is primarily electro-magnetic wave form energy.

Post Traumatic Stress Disorder (PTSD): A reaction to a past trauma creates a rerun of the trauma triggered by outside agitation, pain, hot or cold, dehydration, lack of food, and other variables when the original trauma is activated. It can also be activated by recurrent thoughts of the incident.

Purkinje Fiber: The purkinje Fiber runs across the front of the heart and sequences the Atrioventricular (AV) nodes and Sinoatrial (SA) nodes to create a synchronization of the electrical rhythm of the heart implicated in traumatic injury reactivation.

Qigong: Qigong is a term used to define human energy that can be cultivated for health, or emitted to heal others, through a series of moving and non-moving meditations.

Restorative Drugs: These drugs are taken for injuries which can include anabolic steroids, anti-inflammatory, muscle relaxers, or opiates for pain relief.

Samadhi: Samadhi is the last stage of Buddhism through practice of ahyana reaches a non dualistic state with concentration on the divine and complete absorption.

Sinoatrial Nodes: The sinoatrial node (SA) is located on the right atrium and has pacemaker cells which set the rhythm of the atrioventricular (AV) node of the heart.

Shu: Shu points are organ representation points on the spine which correspond generally to the enervation of the organs. These can be stimulated to release tension in the abdomen and particular organs.

Spondylolisthesis: This is a condition of a vertebra when one vertebra is forward placed usually the 5th lumbar and out of alignment.

Stable State: This stable state is the most efficient defined as lowering of blood lactate, oxygen consumption and synchronization of the heart and brain which requires the least amount of energy in either organic or inorganic nature.

Superfluid Helium: When taking this gas to the lowest temperature near absolute zero, the gas turns to superfluity as a macro-molecule which has super fast information, responds accurately to stimulation and acquires strange behavior. Inorganic nature is the most stable at lower temperatures.

Subject/Object: In the last stages of Buddhism or Samadhi, the observer and observed dissolve and become mutually co-dependent. In physics, when an experiment is conducted the nature of reality changes upon examination. From the influence of the French Enlightenment, scientists see themselves apart from nature with a belief that reductionism, or reducing things to the most particular advances medicine. They are commanders of nature through biochemical changes rather than understanding negative entropy practices for pain and suffering.

Synchronization: When the human organism is synchronized, the brain, heart, and other systems work together and this can be detected through EEG, EKG, EMG and is optimal for health and overcoming disease.

Trauma: In this book, we deal with physical trauma but one can see aspects of emotional trauma from a physical accident and this trauma can be conditioned to reactivate upon approximation of the circumstance of the original trauma.

Vibration: In yoga, this is the Spandakarika which can be found under one-pointed concentration. Pulse generators such as stars, the earth, trees, worms, inorganic and organic nature emit vibration waves.

Voluntary Meditation: This meditation is when a person uses their volition or will to move their voluntary muscles as in movement of yoga, Qigong, running, biking, or a physical activity which causes the mind to use forms such as Tai Chi, traditional dance or sport.

Yoga: Yoga has a whole system of physical and mental practices but primarily the US yoga is done through asana or yoga postures. This is much easier for women than men and can be painful and over the long run loosen the body and mind to synchronize. The more advanced practices such as chanting, sitting meditation, and so forth, are not as popular.

Zazen: This is an involuntary meditation, where you sit, with spine straight and focus the mind, or not, to synchronize the whole person over time. However, an abrupt awakening can happen in the unforeseen future anytime. Practitioners may experience calmness and descend to the great vacuity, an expansive space with stillness but underlying movement.

REFERENCES

[1] Shinnick P. Statement of Phil Shinnick, director of athletics, livingston college, rutgers, new brunswick, nj: Proper and improper use of drugs by athletes: hearing before the subcommittee to investigate juvenile delinquency of the committee of the judiciary united states senate ninety-third Congress 1st Session,. 18 June 12, 13 July 1973.

[2] Shinnick P. Testimony. Proceedings of the White house commission on complementary and alternative medicine policy. June 4, 2003

[3] Shinnick P. Testimony of ambassador shinnick on drug use among athletes. Proceedings of the International Year for the Culture of Peace. 1999; 2000.

SUBJECT INDEX

A

Absolute measurement 16, 17
Absorbing attention, given long 39, 41
Acetylcholine 25, 139
Acupuncture 15, 24, 26, 30, 162, 165, 166, 170
  area 166, 170
  circular 162, 165
  effectiveness of 26, 30
  electro 15, 24
  traditional heart 166
Acupuncture needle 21, 192
Acupuncture point recedes 146
Acupuncture points 7, 26, 28, 122, 141, 146, 147, 148, 160
  traditional 28
Acupuncture point ST 148
Acupuncture stimulation 22, 146
Addiction therapy 3, 95, 117, 234, 235
AGA thermogram 95, 99, 234
Amino acids 140
Animal spirit 8, 192, 207, 208
Antibiotics 75, 120, 138, 140, 177, 186, 195
  right 138
Antidote 83, 84, 120, 212
Appetite 156
Arm strength 121
Arrhythmia 136, 192, 195, 197, 198, 199, 200, 210, 234
Arteries, posterior cerebral 135
Arthritis 14, 133, 195, 210, 223, 228
Artists 9, 10, 53
Asclepius 193, 194
Asthma 103, 120, 128, 129, 235
Athletes, world class 52, 53
Atomic time, reversible 24
Atomic time spin-vector 33
Auricular therapy 12, 28, 234

B

Balance, torsion 16
Balasana 202
Biological materials 6, 101, 103
Bladder prostate 133
Blood circulation 15, 75, 116, 135, 138, 198, 216
Blood lactate 5, 31, 41, 69, 156, 159, 160, 163, 233, 235, 239
Body erect 110
Body movements 87, 105, 112, 192
Body postures 104, 105
Body temperature 101, 157, 162, 167
Bose-Einstein stable state 3
Brain blood-flow 52
Brain circulation 22, 134, 135, 192
Brain fields 44, 159, 160
  homogeneous 44
Breast implants 27, 120, 124
Breath, uncoordinated 163, 169
Breath control 162, 164, 202
Breath count 156
Breathing 11, 25, 52, 57, 58, 114, 115, 170, 189
  abdominal 114, 115, 156, 162, 163
  conscious 11, 57, 58
  deep 170, 189
  fetal 25, 52, 59, 60
  nostril 52, 60
  rapid 156, 162, 163
Breathing experience, first 62
Breathing techniques 7, 52, 59, 162
Breath-listening 114

C

Cancer cells 30, 98, 103
Cancer growth, effect of EQ on 102
Capillary electrometer 18
Cardiovascular points 80, 186, 198, 199
Cell phones 23, 24, 31, 32, 143
Cervical vertebras 113, 161
Chemical reaction 95, 146
Chinese energy exercises, traditional 95, 97
Chronic heart disease and treatment strategies 167
Circulation disturbance 138, 139
Cold weather 192

Collateral damage 175
Compression fracture 192, 235
Concentration, deep mind meditation 96
Conditioned stimuli 39, 41, 46, 47
Connections, natural 85, 176
Cortical thickness 77
Cultures, lung cancer cell 101
Curiosity, emotional 45, 46

D

Degrees Fahrenheit 222, 223
Denmark B-K corp's infrasonic sound detector 100
Desynchronization 20, 31, 44, 236
Detectors, physical signal 98
Devices, electrical 18, 19
Dextrorotoscoliosis 194, 195
Diffuse boundaries 142, 143
Digestive system 82, 185, 189
Directions to the body 175
Discoveries, scientific 149
Disk, herniated 81, 192, 237
DNA Synthesis 95, 98, 101
Downwards, facing 106, 107
Drugs 3, 4, 6, 76, 77, 218, 219, 239
  enhancing 3, 218, 219, 229
  prescription 76, 77, 219
  restorative 3, 4, 6, 218, 239
Duality, time-bound 49
Dynamic time 33

E

Earth's electromagnetic cavity 33, 34
Earth vibration 52, 235
Edema 167, 169, 234, 237
Elbows outwards 107
Electrical stimulation, painful 20
Electric force 15, 16
Electrocardiogram 12, 18, 236
Electroencephalogram 12, 19, 41, 43, 236
Electrolysis 21, 23, 24, 235
Electromagnetic energies 13, 26
Electromagnetic therapy 12
Electromagnetism 14, 95
Electromyography 12, 18, 19
Electrotherapy 3, 21, 169
Emotional state 77, 86, 159, 163, 218
Emotions, strong 86, 87, 230
Energy 5, 13, 47, 57, 78, 79, 184, 188, 196, 204, 235
  absolute 196, 204
  healthy 57
  lowest 5, 47
  natures 13
  photon 235
  transmit 78, 79, 184, 188
  zero-point 47
Energy force, life-giving 189
Energy pulse signatures 26
Energy techniques 234
Enlightenment, awakening of 40, 45, 47
Entropy, positive 4, 5, 33, 236
EQ, effect of 101, 102
Existential energy 39, 41
Expanded awareness 52, 63

F

Five elements palm 111, 112
Fluid in lungs 161, 168, 171
Fluid retention 156
Fragmented global physiology 3
French enlightenment 236, 239
Fungus 74, 138

G

GE micro-pressure detector 95, 99, 236
Global physiology 11, 32, 159, 232, 233
Governor vessels 113, 114, 115
Grip force 121, 140
Groups 100, 103
  aldehyde 100
  treated 103

H

Healing energy 70, 190, 199, 210
Healing pain 14
Healing process 81, 157, 196, 197, 210, 211
Heal ourselves 82, 83, 93, 190, 228
Health care 4, 120, 121

Healthcare system 3
Health Preserving Qigong 111
Heart attack 25, 136, 197, 235
Heart disease, symptoms of chronic 156, 160
Heart disease research foundation 7, 233
Heart hypertension 120, 136, 198
Heart representation areas 135
Heart rhythms 157, 236
Heart treatment 197
Hegda, special permission of 14, 17, 19, 27, 104, 202, 203, 205, 207, 208, 210, 211, 212, 217
helicobacter pylori 137
Hip pain, experienced 223
Hippocrates 175, 176, 190
Hot weather 192, 199
Hui hypothesis 142, 143
Hydrogen peroxide 100
Hypertension 129, 130, 135, 235
Hypnosis 78, 79
Hypotension 60
Hysteria 52, 78, 79

I

Imitated Qigong healer's movement 102
Immune response 52, 74
Immune system 74, 75, 139, 183
Impulse 25, 34, 54, 56
  electrical 25, 34
  natural 54, 56
Infrasonic sound detectors 95
Injuries, fear of 228, 229
Inner space suspends time 212
Inorganic energies 3
Inorganic sciences 14, 40
Internal bleeding 175, 228
Internal Qigong 6, 97, 143, 162, 164
Ionosphere 34
Ions 24, 69, 78
  negative 24, 69, 78
  positive 78
Iron clad mind 229

J

Jaw relaxation 52

K

Keeping the mind on 114
Kneeling, straight 110
Kundalini Yoga, spine in 8, 203

L

Laparoscopic surgery 175
Lattice, hexagonal 148
Left calf, medial 132
Left nostril 60
Left sinus 60
Levels of reality 178, 180, 182
Life 12, 90, 185
  healthy 185
  healthy spiritual 90
  organic 12
Life direction condition 237
Life energy 39, 41, 50, 58
Life-simulating Qigong type 111
Light 73, 100, 101
  strong 100, 101
  white 73
Limbs 20, 116
  artificial 20
  lower 116
Liquid, quantum 39, 41, 47
Liquid helium 48
Listening, withdrawing the sight and reversing 113
Liver cancer 95, 101
Liver cancer cells 101
Long term meditators 77, 78, 81
Lung pathway 26, 120, 124, 125
Lying posture 105, 109

M

Machine mechanization 175
Macromolecule 39, 40, 237
Magnetic field 15, 16, 23
Magnetic force 16
Magnetic Resonance (MRIs) 122, 137, 194
Magnetic resonance instrument 192
Maneuver 105, 112, 113
  external 105, 112

internal 105, 112, 113
Mass, gravitating 33
Matter 5, 32, 33, 56, 61, 71, 78
grey 61
inorganic 5, 32, 33, 56
white 71, 78
Measurements, global 159, 160
Medial prefrontal cortex 77
Medicine, physical 194, 195, 216, 233
Medicine buddha 72, 175, 176, 204
Meditation 6, 57, 67, 163, 164, 196, 201, 209, 221, 237, 240
first experienced breathing 57
involuntary 6, 67, 163, 164, 196, 201, 209, 221, 237, 240
voluntary 192, 202, 204, 233, 240
Meditational state 39, 40, 47
Meditation experience 65, 80
Meditation group 117
Meditation practice 56, 61, 69, 81, 230
Meditation techniques 3, 52, 156, 212
Meditative breathing exercises 230
Meditative state 62, 73, 77, 86, 93, 157, 163
Mental anguish 200, 201
Metals, heavy 139, 140
Metastasis 102
Meters, microwave radiation 95, 99
Methods, acupuncture treatment 162
Metronome 30
Microcirculation 138
Micro reductionist 52, 56
Microscopic slides 123, 134, 149
Microwave ovens 23, 31, 140
Mind 64, 85, 230
active 164
confused 230
quiet 85
Mind-body sciences-psychology 97
Mind-boggling forces 71
Mind exercises 90
Mindfulness 42, 47, 49, 117, 236
attained all-important 49
total 42
Mindfulness-of-breathing 42
Mind involvement 97
Mind practices 218
Mind quiets 62
Mind's activity 65
Mind work 62
Modern medicine 12, 75, 76, 96, 236
Modern science 6
Modern scientists 19
Molecular identification 120
Movement 57, 59, 61, 70, 71, 73, 80, 83, 85, 87, 89, 93, 97, 104, 107, 110, 111, 112, 113, 116, 122, 142, 143, 145, 146, 164, 166, 180, 182, 183, 197, 209, 210, 212, 216, 230, 232, 233, 240
external 112, 113
flexible 111, 116
linear 142, 146
spontaneous 110, 112, 197
Moxibustion 156, 162, 168, 170, 237
Muscles, voluntary 162, 164, 202, 204, 212, 240
Myofascial pain relief procedure 194, 216

N

Natural energy 68
Natural foods 91, 229
Natural powers 72, 188, 190
Natural process 64, 87, 97
Nature 5, 9, 15, 40, 41, 48, 50, 54, 63, 64, 66, 67, 68, 69, 70, 71, 82, 85, 91, 175, 178, 180, 182, 186, 188, 190, 223, 232, 233, 236, 239
inorganic 233, 239
organic 5, 236
Nature of reality 9, 10, 239
Negative entropy 3, 4, 5, 13, 24, 32, 33, 175, 236
Negative phases time 22
Nerve fibers 19, 21
Nerves, sensory 20
Non-drug treatment 192
Non-Qigong subject 98
Non-surgical treatment 192, 194, 216

O

Occidental medicine 14, 233, 234, 236
Olympians, fellow 66
Olympic team 52, 54, 57, 225, 228, 229
Olympic training 227, 228

Olympic Trials 68, 224, 225, 226, 228
Omura, special permission of 135, 136, 141, 142, 198, 200, 207
Oneness, state of 47, 70, 72, 86, 89
Oneness of being 77
Opposites, dualities of 39, 41
Organ energies bifurcate 70
Organic energy 4
Organic sciences 14
Organism 4, 5, 10, 23, 32, 53, 75, 101, 102, 103, 143, 159, 175, 186, 190, 198, 209, 237, 239
  human 4, 237, 239
  living 10, 75, 101, 102, 103, 186, 190
Organ meridians 120
Organ PEMF 120, 122
Organ representation points 122, 125, 126, 127, 199, 237, 239
  subject's 122
Organs 24, 25, 26, 28, 29, 30, 32, 67, 69, 72, 75, 78, 82, 122, 123, 124, 127, 131, 133, 134, 136, 140, 141, 143, 145, 148, 149, 165, 195, 199, 201, 235, 237, 238, 239
  internal 123, 131, 133
Organ stress 12, 59
Organ tissues 7, 123, 127
Oriental medicine 13, 120, 123, 125, 131, 134, 234, 235, 237
O-Ring test 120, 122, 142, 235
Oscilloscope 22
Outward splayfoot 116
Overactive mind 74
Oxygen consumption 31, 42, 59, 69, 156, 157, 159, 160, 163, 225, 233, 239

P

Pacemaker cells 13, 24, 238, 239
Pain 22, 77, 89, 129, 138, 198, 201, 209, 212, 214
  chest 129
  emotional 89, 198
  escapes 212, 214
  person's 77
  physical 198, 209, 212
  relieve 22, 138, 201
  traumatic 214
Pain areas 148, 149, 198
Pain conditions 120, 131
Pain state 159
Pain symptoms 192, 195
  lumbar spine 192
Palpation 3, 4, 8, 12, 175, 184, 195, 200
Parallelism 32, 39, 40
Paravertebral muscles 166, 170
Past injuries 197, 210
Pathological phases 120
Pathways 54, 69, 70, 120, 122, 123, 124, 126, 128, 129, 130, 131, 134, 140, 141, 148
  energetic 70
  multiple 126
  normal 131, 134
  toxins.The heart 130
Perfusates 25
Permission, special 13, 20, 30, 31, 32, 40, 42, 43, 44, 45, 53, 92, 96, 123, 124, 125, 126, 127, 128, 129, 130, 131, 132, 133, 142, 144, 145, 146, 147, 149, 150, 151, 158, 177, 179, 181, 182, 184, 187, 189, 193, 199, 213
Person, non-Qigong 101
Personal experiences 56
Photonic energy 27, 238
Photonic fields 3, 12, 13, 14, 23, 238
Physiological state 39, 40
Physiologic state 39, 40, 41
  stable 39, 41
Physiologic state of enlightenment 41
Physiology curvature 115
Position 109, 110
  lateral recumbent 109, 110
  supine 109
Post traumatic shock disorder (PTSD) 192, 197, 238
Posture maneuver 105
Practicing holding-ball type 106, 107
Practicing yoga 62, 222, 223
Practitioners, non-Qigong 99, 100
Pressure, infrasonic sound 100
Prigogine, Ilya 33
Probes, conducting 137, 149, 150, 151
Problems, mechanical 53, 129, 131
Psoas insufficiency 133
Psychosomatic responses 12, 165, 166

Pulsed electromagnetic fields 3, 4, 12, 13, 39, 120, 238
Pulse generators 23, 24, 26, 143, 238, 240
Purkinje fibers 13, 25, 235, 238

Q

Qi emission 99, 101, 234
Qigong 79, 97, 111, 112, 113, 146, 157, 164, 195, 196, 198, 216
  dynamic 111, 112, 113
  external 79, 97, 146, 157, 164, 195, 196, 198, 216
  static 105, 107, 113
Qigong and breathing techniques 7
Qigong definition 95, 97
Qigong effect 97, 102
Qigong energy 157
Qigong healer 99, 100, 101, 102, 103
  well-trained 103
Qigong master 90, 201, 224
Qigong meditation 6, 117, 157, 203, 234
Qigong movement 111
Qigong practice 103, 104, 105, 107, 111, 112, 113, 114, 115, 116, 162, 192, 222
  dynamic 112
  static 107, 113
Qigong practitioners 98, 99, 101
Qigong research 5, 97
Qigong science 98
Qigong state 98, 104, 106, 157
Qigong studies 102, 157
Qigong techniques 96, 103
Qigong theory 96, 100
Quantum physics 56, 175, 176, 178
Quantum superfluid of helium 50
Quaternion equations 16
Quiet in total body-mind 49

R

Reactivity 25, 39, 192, 201, 209, 212, 213, 233
Regulation of breath and relaxation of muscles 70
Reversing listening 113, 114
Rhythm 19, 24, 43, 44, 45, 80, 112, 136, 159, 167, 235, 238, 239
  alpha 43, 44, 45, 159

S

Science and human transformation 31
Science of healing outcomes 233
Science prigogine 143
Scientific community 138
Scientific delineation, clear 12
Scientific disparities, extreme 39, 41
Scientific experiments, given modern 13
Scientific Interests 233
Scientific studies 95
Scientific work 56
Scientists, creative 11
Shinnick, right 125
Shinnick borgna book 126
Shinnick glides 10
Shinnick painting 209
Shinnick's assistant 233
Shinnick's prognosis 216
Shinnick's treatment 181, 182
Shinnick's understanding 233
Shock, electrical 30
Sinoatrial Nodes 239
Societal injustice 175
Solar plexus 79, 166, 220, 227
Space, vibration of 67, 180
Space time 146, 147
  normal 146, 147
  reciprocal 146, 147
Spark of life and electromagnetic energy 13
Spasms, abdominal 156, 161, 162, 163
Spectrum, electromagnetic 12, 26, 235
Spinal column 115, 116
Spinal cord 21, 127
Spin vector 33
Splayfoot, inward 116
Spondylolisthesis 8, 192, 194, 210, 214, 239
Spontaneous dynamic Qigong 112
Spontaneous Qigong movements 112
Spontaneous synchronization 39
Sports injuries 54, 200, 214, 223
Sports science program 233
Sputum production 156, 161

Stable stationary states 39
Standing posture 105, 106, 116
Standing style 114
State 7, 9, 33, 58, 65, 70, 75, 89, 93, 95, 98, 143, 159, 176, 178, 186, 230
  dangerous 176, 186
  differentiated 75, 159
  diseased 7, 95, 98
  natural 9, 33, 89, 93, 143, 178, 230
  pointed 58, 70
  timeless 65
Stationary quantum state, stable 39, 41
Steroids, anabolic 6, 218, 238, 239
Stillness and movement 89, 183, 209
Stress, emotional 84, 120, 129, 131, 136
Superfluid component 47
Superfluid helium 39, 40, 239
Superfluid of Helium 47, 48
Swim lifetime bests 222
Symptomatology photonic image, painful 216
Synchronize space-time 72

T

Techniques 96, 97, 157, 221
  breath control 221
  internal Qigong 157
  modern 96, 97
Techniques of qigong practice 103
Tendon changing classics 111
Terminal illnessr 156, 157
Tested acupoints 100
Thermodynamics 3, 24, 33
Thermography 27
Thighs, opposite 108
Thought/reaction time 209
Thromboxane B2 139, 140
Thromboxane-B2 138
Time constraints 4
Time oxygen consumption 159
Time players 223
Traditional Chinese medicine (TCM) 3, 14, 122, 134, 141, 143, 156, 159, 162
Traditional Chinese medicine and Qigong 97
Transcends duality 39
Transitions, abrupt 47, 49, 50
Transplantation 102
Trauma 25, 60, 86, 87, 136, 143, 158, 195, 197, 201, 209, 212, 237, 238, 240
Treatment, electro-acupuncture 23
Treatment outcomes 117
Treatment strategies 167, 168, 196
Tree leaf sensors 101

V

Vanquishing devil 108
Ventricle, right 18, 238
Vertebrae, fractured 192, 197
Visceral dysfunction 192
Visions, global scientific 4

W

Waves, organic nature emit vibration 240
Weight lifting 52
Western science 134
Whiplash 192, 210

Z

Zen masters 45, 46, 49
Zen meditation 163, 164, 172, 222

www.ingramcontent.com/pod-product-compliance
Lightning Source LLC
LaVergne TN
LVHW070935210926
848482LV00003B/242